Adult and Pediatric Neuromodulation

Jason P. Gilleran · Seth A. Alpert
Editors

Adult and Pediatric Neuromodulation

Springer

Editors
Jason P. Gilleran
Department of Urology
Oakland University William
Beaumont School of Medicine
Royal Oak, MI, USA

Seth A. Alpert
Section of Urology
Nationwide Children's Hospital and
The Ohio State Wexner Medical Center
Columbus, OH, USA

ISBN 978-3-319-73265-7 ISBN 978-3-319-73266-4 (eBook)
https://doi.org/10.1007/978-3-319-73266-4

Library of Congress Control Number: 2018932539

Printed on acid-free paper

This Springer imprint is published by the registered company Springer International Publishing AG part of Springer Nature.
The registered company address is: Gewerbestrasse 11, 6330 Cham, Switzerland

Dedication/Acknowledgments

In no particular order, I would like to acknowledge the multitude of clinicians who have supported me through my early career and continue to do so today, starting with Drs. Philippe Zimmern and Gary Lemack at the University of Texas Southwestern, Dr. Tony Buffington at The Ohio State University, and to all of the knowledgeable professionals at Medtronic, including Ailyn Chapman.

To my colleagues at William Beaumont Hospital, most notably Dr. Kenneth Peters, who has and continues to "push the envelope" in the field of neuromodulation for pelvic floor disorders, and also Dr. Larry Sirls; Dr. Jamie Bartley; Nicole Stanczak, NP; Katherine Turner, NP; and the entire OR staff at Beaumont.

To all the authors who tirelessly contributed to this textbook, bringing together some of the brightest young minds in the field of neuromodulation, and to everyone at Springer, who made this textbook possible.

I would be remiss if I did not acknowledge my wife, Robyn, and my boys, Spencer and Elliott, who have always been there for me during the many hours involved with the writing of this textbook and the countless more hours of my profession. Thank you.

Jason P. Gilleran

To my colleagues on the urology team at Nationwide Children's Hospital: Thank you for all your help and support not only with this project but also on a daily basis, as we seek to improve the health and well-being of the children entrusted to our care.

To my patients and families: Thank you for allowing me the honor of caring for and performing surgery on your children. The trust you place in me cannot be underestimated, and I strive to care for your children as if they were my own.

To my current and former residents, fellows, and medical students: I hope that you have learned as much from me as I have from you. You constantly challenge me to think of why I am doing what I do and make me reevaluate that I am doing the right things for the right reasons.

To Julie, Justin, Scott, and Roxie: Thank you for your love, patience, and support of my career, now and always. This textbook is dedicated to you for all of your understanding of the times I must be somewhere else, caring for other people's children. You are my world and my everything.

Seth A. Alpert

Preface

Throughout medical history, surgical treatments of various conditions involve removal of abnormal tissues and reconstruction of normal (or nearly normal) anatomy in order to improve a patient's functional status. Such invasive procedures are highly morbid and may not accomplish the goal of correcting organ dysfunction. With the advent of neuromodulation, clinicians are now armed with minimally invasive techniques to identify and modify abnormal nerve conduction impulses to organ systems, which in turn provide either symptom relief or improvement.

The technology of neuromodulation continues to advance, and its applications are ever expanding. While this modality is currently indicated to treat a limited number of diseases and/or organ dysfunction, we hope this textbook demonstrates the depth and breadth of conditions that can respond to neuromodulation. We also look forward to the future of neuromodulation and its interface with modern digital technology, which can lead to noninvasive approaches that can be used at home and empower patients of all ages to manage these difficult conditions.

Royal Oak, MI, USA — Jason P. Gilleran
Columbus, OH, USA — Seth A. Alpert

Contents

Contributors

Dadrie Baptiste Department of Colorectal Surgery, Beaumont Health, Royal Oak, MI, USA

Kevin Benson Female Pelvic Medicine and Reconstructive Surgery, Sanford Health, Sioux Falls, SD, USA

Christopher J. Chermansky Department of Urology, University of Pittsburgh Medical Center Magee Women's Hospital, Pittsburgh, PA, USA

Chirag Dave Department of Urology, Beaumont Hospital/Oakland University William Beaumont School of Medicine, Royal Oak, MI, USA

Mirret M. El-Hagrassy Spaulding Neuromodulation Center, Department of Physical Medicine & Rehabilitation, Spaulding Rehabilitation Hospital and Massachusetts General Hospital, Charlestown, MA, USA

Kassem Faraj Department of Urology, Beaumont Hospital/Oakland University William Beaumont School of Medicine, Royal Oak, MI, USA

Kevin M. Feber Department of Urology, Beaumont Hospital/Oakland University William Beaumont School of Medicine, Royal Oak, MI, USA

Felipe Fregni Spaulding Neuromodulation Center, Department of Physical Medicine & Rehabilitation, Spaulding Rehabilitation Hospital and Massachusetts General Hospital, Charlestown, MA, USA

Joel T. Funk Division of Urology, Department of Surgery, University of Arizona College of Medicine, Tucson, AZ, USA

Natalie Gaines Urology San Antonio, San Antonio, TX, USA

Jason P. Gilleran Department of Urology, Oakland University William Beaumont School of Medicine, Royal Oak, MI, USA

Paul J. Guidos Department of Urology, University of Iowa Hospitals and Clinics, Iowa City, IA, USA

Adonis Hijaz Center of Female Pelvic Medicine and Surgery, University Hospitals Cleveland Medical Center, Urology Institute, Cleveland, OH, USA

Spencer C. Hiller Department of Urology, William Beaumont Hospital, Royal Oak, MI, USA

Felipe Jones Spaulding Neuromodulation Center, Department of Physical Medicine & Rehabilitation, Spaulding Rehabilitation Hospital and Massachusetts General Hospital, Charlestown, MA, USA

Sunchin Kim Division of Urology, Department of Surgery, University of Arizona College of Medicine, Tucson, AZ, USA

Ryan M. Krlin Department of Urology, Lousiana State University Health Sciences Center, New Orleans, LA, USA

Jessica C. Lloyd Glickman Urological Institute, Cleveland Clinic, Cleveland, OH, USA

Peter L. Lu Division of Gastroenterology, Hepatology and Nutrition, Department of Pediatrics, Nationwide Children's Hospital, Columbus, OH, USA

John R. Michalak Division of Urology, Department of Surgery, University of Arizona College of Medicine, Tucson, AZ, USA

Jonathan P. Miller Department of Neurological Surgery, University Hospitals Cleveland Medical Center/Case Western Reserve University, Cleveland, OH, USA

Courtenay K. Moore Glickman Urological Institute, Cleveland Clinic, Cleveland, OH, USA

Laura N. Nguyen Department of Urology, Beaumont Health, Royal Oak, MI, USA

Karen Noblett Department of Obstetrics and Gynecology, Division Female Pelvic Medicine and Reconstructive Surgery, University of California, Irvine, Orange, CA, USA

Kenneth M. Peters Department of Urology, Beaumont Health, Royal Oak, MI, USA

C.R. Powell Department of Urology, Indiana University School of Medicine, Indianapolis, IN, USA

Gleysson Rosa Spaulding Neuromodulation Center, Department of Physical Medicine & Rehabilitation, Spaulding Rehabilitation Hospital and Massachusetts General Hospital, Charlestown, MA, USA

Ragheed M. Saoud Division of Urology, Department of Surgery, American University of Beirut Medical Center, Beirut, Lebanon

Megan S. Schober Division of Pediatric Urology, William Beaumont Hospital, Royal Oak, MI, USA

Jason Shellnut Colon and Rectal Surgery, William Beaumont Hospital, Royal Oak, MI, USA

Larry T. Sirls Department of Urology, Beaumont Health, Royal Oak, MI, USA

Michael D. Staudt Department of Neurological Surgery, University Hospitals Cleveland Medical Center/Case Western Reserve University, Cleveland, OH, USA

Douglas W. Storm Department of Urology, University of Iowa Hospitals and Clinics, Iowa City, IA, USA

Neha Talreja Sudol Department of Obstetrics and Gynecology, Division Female Pelvic Medicine and Reconstructive Surgery, University of California, Irvine, Orange, CA, USA

Lauren Tennyson Department of Urology, University of Pittsburgh Medical Center, Pittsburgh, PA, USA

Christian O. Twiss Division of Urology, Department of Surgery, University of Arizona College of Medicine, Tucson, AZ, USA

Gillian Frances Wolff Division of Urology, Albany Medical Center, Albany, NY, USA

Desale Yacob Division of Gastroenterology, Hepatology and Nutrition, Department of Pediatrics, Nationwide Children's Hospital, Columbus, OH, USA

Part I

Adults

Basic Neuroanatomy and Neurophysiology of the Lower Urinary Tract

1

Lauren Tennyson and Christopher J. Chermansky

Key Points

- Review normal sympathetic and parasympathetic neural connections within the lower urinary tract.
- Review pathophysiology of urologic dysfunction that results from common neurologic disorders, such as cerebrovascular accident, Parkinson's disease, multiple sclerosis, and spinal cord injury.
- Review landmark basic science studies and relevant animal studies on neuromodulation from the last 10 years.

Overview of the Lower Urinary Tract Neural Activity During Bladder Storage and Voiding

The lower urinary tract (LUT) serves to store and periodically eliminate urine through complex mechanisms coordinated by local, spinal, and brain circuits. These neural circuits coordinate the activities of the bladder and urethra, alternating between two primary modes of operation: urine storage and urine elimination [1]. The bladder remains in storage mode for the majority of the time, where it accommodates increasing volumes of urine at low pressures. Continence is maintained through neural reflexes that inhibit detrusor contractions and promote external urethral sphincter (EUS) activation. To initiate voiding, the neural reflex switches to allow EUS relaxation and bladder contraction, resulting in the flow of urine. This switch is triggered by the sensation of bladder fullness, and it is mediated by a long loop spinalbulbospinal reflex pathway [1]. Three sets of peripheral nerves are responsible for the coordination of events involved in urine storage and expulsion: pelvic parasympathetic nerves, lumbar sympathetic nerves, and pudendal somatic nerves. These nerves contain afferent (sensory) fibers, which monitor bladder volume and the amplitude of bladder contractions.

Discrete neurologic lesions typically result in predictable patterns of LUT dysfunction. The nature of the dysfunction depends on the nervous system area affected, the function of that area, and whether the neurologic lesion is destructive, inflammatory, or irritative [2]. The pathophysiology of the neurologic disorders commonly affecting LUT function will be described later in this chapter.

L. Tennyson
Department of Urology, University of Pittsburgh Medical Center, Pittsburgh, PA, USA
e-mail: ginsburgle@upmc.edu

C. J. Chermansky (✉)
Department of Urology, UPMC Magee Womens Hospital, Pittsburgh, PA, USA
e-mail: chermanskycj2@upmc.edu

J. P. Gilleran, S. A. Alpert (eds.), *Adult and Pediatric Neuromodulation*,
https://doi.org/10.1007/978-3-319-73266-4_1

Neural Connections to the Lower Urinary Tract

Efferent Innervation to the LUT

Efferent pathways of the LUT include the pelvic, hypogastric, and pudendal nerves (Fig. 1.1). The motor innervation to the bladder is through pelvic parasympathetic nerves, which originate in the intermediolateral gray matter of the sacral spinal cord (S2–S4) and promote bladder emptying and urethral relaxation [3]. Both pre- and postganglionic parasympathetic nerves release acetylcholine (ACh), an excitatory neurotransmitter that acts on muscarinic receptors (M2 and M3) within the detrusor to result in bladder contraction. Detrusor contraction and resultant urinary flow is mediated primarily by M3 receptors.

Bladder sympathetic nerves arise from the thoracic and lumbar spinal cord between T11-L2 [3]. During bladder filling, these noradrenergic nerves provide inhibitory input to the bladder body and excitatory input to the urethra and bladder base, resulting in bladder relaxation and urethral contraction. Peripheral sympathetic nerves travel a complex route through the sympathetic

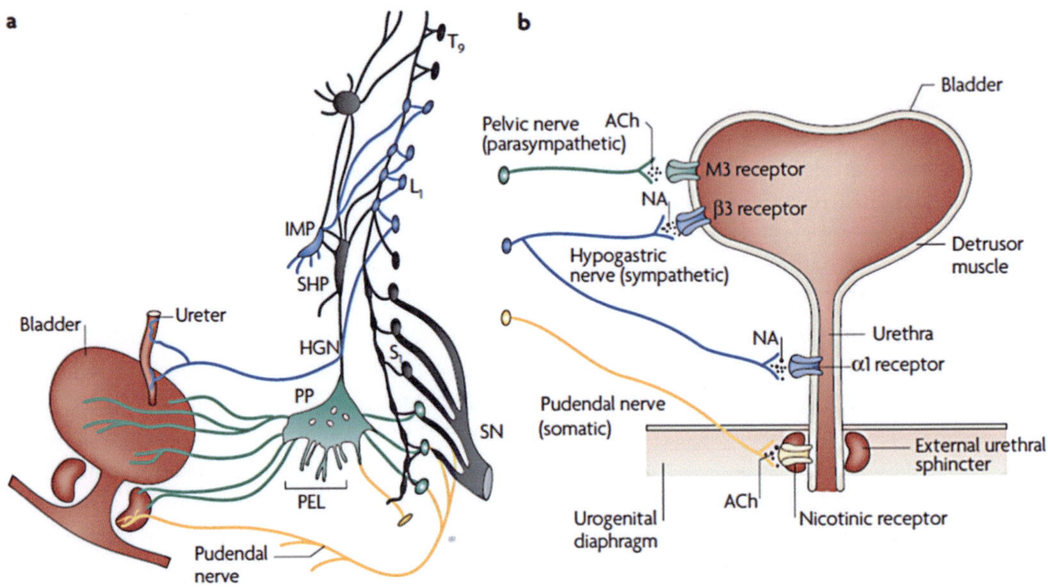

Fig. 1.1 Efferent pathways of the LUT. (**a**) Innervation of the female lower urinary tract. Sympathetic fibers (shown in blue) originate in the T11-L2 segments in the spinal cord and run through the inferior mesenteric ganglia (inferior mesenteric plexus, IMP) and hypogastric nerve (HGN) or through the paravertebral chain to enter the pelvic nerves at the base of the bladder and the urethra. Parasympathetic preganglionic fibers (shown in green) arise from the S2–S4 spinal segments and travel in sacral roots and pelvic nerves (PEL) to ganglia in the pelvic plexus (PP) and in the bladder wall. This is where the postganglionic nerves that supply parasympathetic innervation to the bladder arise. Somatic motor nerves (shown in yellow) that supply the striated muscles of the external urethral sphincter arise from the S2–S4 motor neurons and pass through the pudendal nerves. (**b**) Efferent pathways and neurotransmitter mechanisms that regulate the lower urinary tract. Parasympathetic postganglionic axons in the pelvic nerve release acetylcholine (ACh), which produces a bladder contraction by stimulating M_3 muscarinic receptors in the bladder smooth muscle. Sympathetic postganglionic neurons release noradrenaline (NA), which activates β_3 adrenergic receptors to relax bladder smooth muscle and activates α_2 adrenergic receptors to contract urethral smooth muscle. Somatic axons in the pudendal nerve also release ACh, which produces a contraction of the external sphincter striated muscle by activating nicotinic cholinergic receptors. Parasympathetic postganglionic nerves also release ATP, which excites bladder smooth muscle (not shown). L_1 first lumbar root, S_1 first sacral root, *SHP* superior hypogastric plexus, *SN* sciatic nerve, T_9 ninth thoracic root. From: de Groat WM. Neuroanatomy and neurophysiology: innervation of the lower urinary tract. In: Female Urology (Third Edition). Raz S, Rodríguez LV, eds. W.B. Saunders, Philadelphia;2008:26–46. Reprinted with permission from Elsevier

chain ganglia to the inferior mesenteric ganglia and then through the hypogastric nerves to the pelvic ganglia [4]. Sympathetic input to the LUT is not essential for micturition to occur; however, sympathetic stimulation allows the bladder to accommodate larger volumes during filling/storage [5]. Under normal conditions, the guarding reflex inhibits parasympathetic innervation of the detrusor during filling until bladder capacity is reached, at which point micturition begins. Surgical injury or pharmacologic blockade of bladder sympathetic nerves reduces outflow resistance, decreases bladder capacity, and increases the frequency and amplitude of bladder non-voiding contractions [6].

The motor nerves of the EUS originate in Onuf's nucleus within S2–S4 and travel through the pudendal nerve to innervate the striated muscles of the EUS and pelvic floor [7]. The pudendal nerve terminals release ACh, which acts on nicotinic cholinergic receptors to induce muscle contraction during storage/filling [8]. The activity of the sphincter EMG increases with bladder filling, reflecting an increase in efferent firing from the pudendal nerve which in turn increases bladder outlet resistance and contributes to urinary continence [9]. During voiding, relaxation of urethral smooth muscle occurs by activation of a parasympathetic pathway, which triggers the release of nitric oxide, and by removal of adrenergic and somatic cholinergic excitatory inputs.

Afferent Innervation to the LUT

The pelvic, hypogastric, and pudendal nerves carry afferent information from the LUT to the lumbosacral spinal cord. The majority of the afferent input from the bladder and urethra travel in the pelvic nerve, with a smaller component from the hypogastric nerve [10]. Signals from the striated muscles of the sphincter and pelvic floor travel through the pudendal nerve. Afferent nerves consist of small myelinated (Aδ) and unmyelinated (C) fibers. The Aδ-fibers in the bladder are located in the detrusor smooth muscle and respond to detrusor stretching during bladder filling to convey a sense of fullness [11]. Unmyelinated C-fibers are located in both the detrusor muscle and lamina propria, and these C fibers lie directly adjacent to urothelial cells [12]. In humans, the somata of the pelvic and pudendal afferent nerves are located within the S2–S4 dorsal root ganglion (DRG), and the somata of the hypogastric nerve are within the T11-L2 DRG. Afferent fibers enter the spinal cord through the dorsal horn where they diverge and project either locally to interneurons or to second order neurons which ascend to supraspinal centers involved in the control of micturition [13]. Interneurons make excitatory or inhibitory connections that either facilitate segmental spinal reflexes or send longer projections to supraspinal centers.

The periaqueductal gray (PAG) and pontine micturition center (PMC) are two important supraspinal centers that control the micturition reflex (Fig. 1.2). The neural pathways between the PAG and PMC integrate afferent signals and descending commands from higher brain centers to transition from bladder storage to micturition [14, 15]. Chemical or electrical stimulation of the PMC in a feline model produces voiding that is similar to the micturition reflex, supporting the critical role the PMC in the micturition reflex pathway [16]. Experiments by Takasaki et al. sought to better define the role of the PAG in reflex micturition. They interrupted connections between the PAG and PMC in various places within the feline midbrain, and reflex bladder contractions were found to persist [17]. The authors concluded that the PAG does not have a critical role in reflex micturition, but rather the PAG transmits sensory information about bladder filling to higher brain centers. Stone et al. questioned these findings after they showed in a male rat model that the PAG was essential for micturition [18]. Thus, the role of the PAG in the micturition pathway remains unclear and may differ between species.

Electrophysiological studies in cats and rats have shown that the normal micturition reflex is triggered by myelinated Aδ-fibers that respond to both passive distension and active bladder contraction [19–22]. These nerves are silent when the bladder is empty, and during slow bladder filling

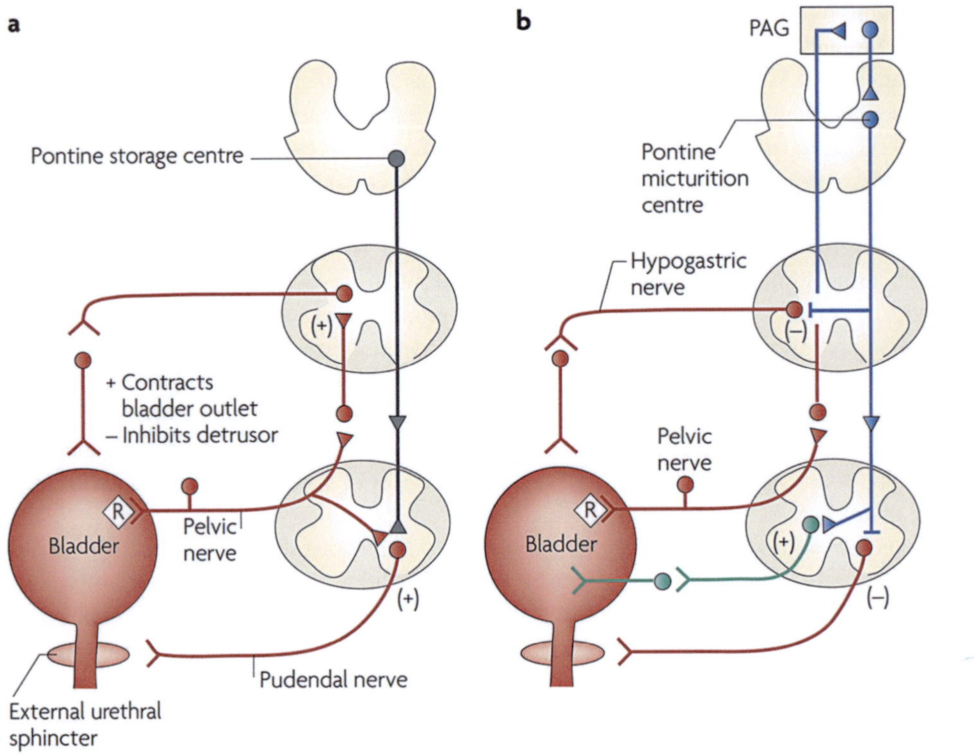

Fig. 1.2 Neural circuits that control continence and micturition. (**a**) Urine storage reflexes. During the storage of urine, distention of the bladder produces low-level vesical afferent firing. This in turn stimulates the sympathetic outflow in the hypogastric nerve to the bladder outlet (the bladder base and the urethra) and the pudendal outflow to the external urethral sphincter. These responses occur by spinal reflex pathways and represent guarding reflexes, which promote continence. Sympathetic firing also inhibits contraction of the detrusor muscle and modulates neurotransmission in bladder ganglia. A region in the rostral pons (the pontine storage center) might increase striated urethral sphincter activity. (**b**) Voiding reflexes. During the elimination of urine, intense bladder-afferent firing in the pelvic nerve activates spinobulbospinal reflex pathways (shown in blue) that pass through the pontine micturition center. This stimulates the parasympathetic outflow to the bladder and to the urethral smooth muscle (shown in green) and inhibits the sympathetic and pudendal outflow to the urethral outlet (shown in red). Ascending afferent input from the spinal cord might pass through relay neurons in the periaqueductal gray (PAG) before reaching the pontine micturition center. Note that these diagrams do not address the generation of conscious bladder sensations, nor the mechanisms that underlie the switch from storage to voiding, both of which presumably involve cerebral circuits above the PAG. R represents receptors on afferent nerve terminals. From Fowler CJ, Griffiths D, de Groat WC. The neural control of micturition. Nat Rev Neurosci 2008;9:453–66 (Nature Publishing Group)

they gradually increase in discharge frequency at intravesical pressures below 25 mmHg [23, 24]. Multiunit recordings have shown a successive recruitment of mechanoreceptors with different thresholds during bladder filling, and these thresholds correlate with the intravesical pressures at which humans report the first sensation of bladder filling [1]. In cats, C-fibers are generally mechanoinsensitive and have been termed "silent C-fibers" [20]. They are nociceptive and respond to cold, chemical, or other noxious stimuli such as high potassium, low pH, and high osmolality [25, 26]. Evidence exists that C-fibers become sensitized and drive reflex bladder contractions after spinal cord injury (SCI) [27–29]. Animal models of SCI have provided convincing evidence that the spinal reflex that develops is clearly different from animals with intact spinal cords. In SCI cats, the spinal reflex occurs after a short delay of approximately 5 milliseconds (ms), and it is triggered by C-fibers. This is in contrast to the micturition reflex in normal animals that occurs after a longer central delay of 60–70 ms, and this reflex is triggered by Aδ-fibers [30]. The sensitization of "silent" C-fibers is mediated by alterations in central neural connections and the properties of peripheral afferent receptors [31].

Neurogenic Dysfunction of the Lower Urinary Tract

Neurologic lesions generally affect LUT function in a predictable manner, depending on location of injury within the nervous system. Lesions above the brainstem that affect micturition typically result in involuntary bladder contractions, referred to as neurogenic detrusor overactivity (NDO). Coordinated sphincter function is maintained with these lesions. Following a cerebrovascular accident (CVA), the most common type of LUT dysfunction is NDO, experienced by patients as urinary urgency and frequency with possible urgency urinary incontinence (UUI) [32, 33]. Detrusor areflexia may occur initially after CVA. Patients with aphasia, diabetes mellitus, and a lower functional status have higher rates of urinary retention [34]. Additionally, although urinary retention related to detrusor areflexia is very common in the acute phase following CVA, over 95% of these patients will see resolution of their urinary retention within 2 months [35].

The relatively high rate of UUI after CVA has prompted investigators to look more closely at sphincter function. Khan et al. correlated urodynamic findings with stroke location on computed tomography, and they found that only patients with lesions in the basal ganglia and thalamus had normal sphincter function [32]. Patients who had strokes involving the cerebral cortex, internal capsule, or both were unable to generate adequate sphincter contraction in this setting, and these patients leaked. Another study evaluating geriatric patients with UUI found that half had reduced sensation of bladder filling. Thus, another possible mechanism for UUI after CVA is decreased bladder fullness and early urgency [36].

Parkinson's disease (PD) is a movement disorder that is associated with the degradation of dopaminergic neurons in the substantia nigra of the basal ganglia. Researchers believe dopamine normally exerts an inhibitory effect on the micturition reflex, and therefore decreased dopamine leads to an exaggeration of voiding reflexes, manifested as LUTS. Studies on PD patients report that bladder storage symptoms are present in 57–83% of patients and voiding symptoms are seen in 17–27% [37]. The most common symptom in PD patients is nocturia in >60%, followed by urgency in 33–54%, and frequency in 16–36% [38–40]. Urodynamic evaluation revealed neurogenic detrusor overactivity (NDO) in 67% of patients and detrusor hyporeflexia in 16%. Detrusor-external sphincter dyssynergia (DESD) and NDO with impaired contractile function were observed in 9% and 3%, respectively, and only at advanced stages. Normal detrusor function was seen in 6% [41].

Multiple sclerosis (MS), the most common neuroinflammatory disorder of the central nervous system (CNS), is characterized by neural demyelination within the brain and spinal cord. Plaques are seen scattered throughout the white matter of the CNS, and they cause impaired axonal conduction. Autopsy studies of MS patients have demonstrated evidence of cervical spinal cord demyelination, but lumbar and sacral cord involvement occurs in approximately 40% and 18%, respectively [42]. Litwiller and colleagues published a comprehensive literature review of the genitourinary effects of MS on the LUT, and they reported urinary frequency and urgency in 31–85% of patients, UUI in 37–72%, and urinary retention in 2–52% [43]. Recent urodynamic studies suggest that 62% of MS patients have NDO, 25% have NDO with DESD, 20% have detrusor underactivity, and 10% have no abnormal urodynamic findings. Bladder filling sensations remain intact. Finally, it is important to distinguish pseudodyssynergia caused by straining to void from true DESD [44].

Spinal cord injury (SCI) interrupts normal bladder function by impairing both the transmission of afferent information from the LUT to the higher brain centers and the efferent information that drives LUT function. Initially, SCI above the lumbosacral cord eliminates voluntary and supraspinal control of voiding, and this leads to a period of bladder areflexia during spinal shock [30, 31]. Urinary retention can last from hours to years depending whether the suprasacral spinal cord lesion is complete or incomplete, and incomplete lesions generally result in shorter periods of retention [45]. After spinal shock recovery, there is synaptic reorganization between the sacral cord and the bladder. The urodynamic findings of SCI patients with lesions between T6-S2 include absent bladder filling sensations, NDO, and DESD; there is no detrusor internal sphincter dyssynergia (DISD).

Patients with injuries above T6 typically have NDO, DESD, and DISD. Furthermore, they can develop autonomic hyperreflexia, during which sympathetic nervous system reflexes become exaggerated in response to stimuli below the T6 lesion. The symptoms from autonomic hyperreflexia include hypertension, bradycardia, headache, and flushing/sweating above the lesion. The UI seen in these patients results from NDO and urinary retention (caused by DESD) with overflow. Sacral SCI below S2 results in detrusor areflexia with either normal or decreased compliance, which develops from neurologic decentralization and bladder wall fibrosis [46].

Because SCI results in damaged circuitry that regulates bladder and urethral sphincter function, there has been interest in artificially modulating the nervous system to both contract the detrusor and relax the external urethral sphincter [47]. An implantable device was created in the late 1970s by Brindley to stimulate the anterior sacral nerve roots S2–S4. Electrical stimulation at low frequencies (10–30 Hz) was noted to induce detrusor contraction with concurrent external sphincteric contraction [48]. Furthermore, with intermittent stimulation, there was both sphincteric relaxation and detrusor contraction, thereby allowing bladder emptying at low detrusor pressures. Several stimulation/relaxation cycles were typically necessary to achieve adequate emptying [49]. While this device has shown promise, it has not been widely adopted as a treatment for detrusor underactivity (DU) in SCI patients. More recently, Sievert et al. investigated the benefit of early implantation of sacral nerve modulators during the acute phase of DU following thoracic SCI [50]. They found that early implantation of these devices helped to mitigate the development of NDO and improved urinary continence rates. Unfortunately, there has been limited success in advancing the application of neuromodulation to the treatment of SCI patients because of the complexity of neurogenic LUT dysfunction, associated comorbidities, and the invasiveness and risks with current neuromodulation techniques [51, 52].

Experimental Studies of Neuromodulation

Neuromodulation, either sacral or tibial, is a US Food and Drug Administration (FDA)-approved treatment for pelvic organ disorders, including OAB (both approved) and fecal incontinence (only sacral approved). Pelvic neuromodulation stimulates somatic afferent fibers, thereby influencing continence and voiding reflex pathways within the spinal cord.

Sacral neuromodulation (SNM) and percutaneous tibial nerve stimulation (PTNS) are the two FDA-approved therapies currently on the market. It should be noted that SNM and PTNS are approved only for the treatment of LUT dysfunction that is nonneurogenic in nature. Experimental neurmodulation techniques that remain under investigation include pudendal nerve stimulation, transcutaneous tibial nerve stimulation, direct electrical stimulation of the bladder and urethra, and dorsal genital nerve stimulation [53].

The mechanisms underlying the effects of neuromodulation on LUT function have not been fully understood, but it is thought that stimulation of somatic afferent nerves entering the spinal cord modulate abnormal visceral sensations and/or involuntary motor responses [53]. Multiple studies have contributed to an increased understanding of the mechanisms involved in the inhibition of reflex bladder activity [54–58]. Differences exist based on the experimental model (nociceptive versus non-nociceptive, intact versus transected spinal cord versus decerebrate), stimulation parameters, site of action, and response to drugs [53]. In cats, tibial nerve stimulation (TNS) and pudendal nerve stimulation (PNS) have been shown to inhibit the spinobulbospinal micturition reflex passing through the pontine micturition center (PMC); however, evidence suggests that they target different areas of the CNS through different neurotransmitters [59–61]. Initial studies suggested that PNS inhibited the bladder via activation of sympathetic efferents within the hypogastric nerve [62]. The notion has since been challenged by studies demonstrating that bilateral hypogastric nerve transection weakens and not abolishes PNS inhibition on the bladder [63]. Tai et al. demonstrated that the inhibitory neurotransmitter $GABA_A$ within the lumbosacral spinal cord is required for PNS bladder inhibition, and they suggested that glycineric, adrenergic, and opioidergic mechanisms may not be necessary [64]. In addition, Tai et al. showed that opioid receptors play an important role in tibial neuromodulation but not pudendal neuromodulation [59, 65]. In the cat model, Rogers et al. showed that PNS inhibition remains effective in spinal cord transected and TNS inhibition does not [61]. This study provides evidence that tibial nerve afferents cannot directly inhibit the nociceptive C-fiber-mediated bladder reflexes within the lumbosacral spinal cord. Thus, TNS requires intact supraspinal pathways. Additional investigations are necessary to further elucidate sites and mechanisms of action.

PNS is frequency dependent, and it has an inhibitory effect at low frequencies (3–10 Hz) and an excitatory effect at higher frequencies (20–30 Hz). PNS is only effective during the period of stimulation, and the effects cease within minutes of stimulus termination. This lack of a post-stimulatory effect limits the clinical translatability of PNS [54, 62]. TNS has an inhibitory effect across a broad range of frequencies (5–30 Hz) [52]. Tai et al. recently showed that the inhibitory effects of TNS persist for more than 2 h after termination of stimulus [60]. These basic science results were consistent with clinical reports demonstrating prolonged inhibitory effects following PTNS in OAB patients.

Zhang et al. recently established a feline animal model to compare the effects of sacral neuromodulation on reflex bladder activity to other types of neuromodulation [54]. They found that S1–S3 dorsal root stimulation, and not S1–S3 ventral root stimulation, inhibited reflex bladder activity. They also discovered that similar to TNS, there was a poststimulation inhibitory effect that maintained an increase in bladder capacity. They concluded that SNM inhibition of reflex bladder activity occurs in the CNS via inhibition of ascending or descending pathways of the spinobulbospinal micturition reflex.

Evidence that neuromodulation is at least in part acting on the afferent pathway of the micturition reflex is offered by experiments that showed increased bladder capacity without changes in the amplitudes of reflex bladder contractions [5]. This is because afferent signaling delays the gating of the all-or-nothing PAG-PMC switch in the reflex circuit without affecting efferent pathways. These results are consistent with the clinical findings that neuromodulation reduces urinary urgency and urinary frequency without impacting voiding efficiency [53]. Although not FDA approved, pudendal neuromodulation has been shown in preliminary studies to rival sacral neuromodulation for patients with OAB and non-obstructive urinary retention [66].

Conclusion

The information presented in this chapter reveals the complexity of the neural control of micturition, incorporating nicely the role of neuromodulation in correcting LUT dysfunction. Future research will hopefully answer these remaining questions: (1) Does neuromodulation result in permanent changes in neural control (neuroplasticity)? (2) Does neuromodulation treat symptoms alone, or can it also correct pathophysiologic processes? Uncovering and confirming pelvic neuromodulatory mechanisms of action in animal models and validating them in humans will expand potential treatment options for LUT dysfunction.

References

1. de Groat WC, Griffiths D, Yoshimura N. Neural control of the lower urinary tract. Compr Physiol. 2015;5(1):327–96.
2. Wein AJ, Dmochowski RR. Neuromuscular dysfunction of the lower urinary tract. In: Wein AJ, editor. Campbell-Walsh urology. Philadelphia: Elsevier; 2016. p. 1761–95.
3. Fowler CJ, Griffiths D, de Groat WC. The neural control of micturition. Nat Rev Neurosci. 2008;9(6):453–66.
4. Chai TC, Birder LA. Physiology and pharmacology of the bladder and urethra. In: Wein AJ, editor. Campbell-Walsh urology. Philadelphia: Elsevier; 2016. p. 1631–84.
5. de Groat WC, Wickens C. Organization of the neural switching circuitry underlying reflex micturition. Acta Physiol. 2013;207(1):66–84.
6. de Groat WC, Booth AM. Synaptic transmission in pelvic ganglia. In: Maggi CA, editor. The autonomic nervous system. London: Harwood Academic; 1993. p. 291–347.
7. Thor KB, Morgan C, Nadelhaft I, Houston M, De Groat WC. Organization of afferent and efferent pathways in the pudendal nerve of the female cat. J Comp Neurol. 1989;288(2):263–79.
8. Yoshimura N, Chancellor MB. Neurophysiology of lower urinary tract function and dysfunction. Rev Urol. 2003;5(8):S3–S10.
9. Thor KB, de Groat WC. Neural control of the female urethral and anal rhabdosphincters and pelvic floor muscles. Am J Physiol Regul Integr Comp Physiol. 2010;299:R416–38.
10. de Groat WC, Yoshimura N. Afferent nerve regulation of bladder function in health and disease. Handb Exp Pharmacol. 2009;194:91–138.
11. Sengupta JN, Gebhart GF. Mechanosensitive properties of pelvic nerve afferent fibers innervating the urinary bladder of the rat. J Neurophysiol. 1994;72:2420–30.
12. Wakabayashi Y, Tomoyoshi T, Fujimiya M, et al. Substance P-containing axon terminals in the mucosa of the human urinary bladder: pre-embedding immunohistochemistry using cryostat sections for electron microscopy. Histochemistry. 1993;100:401.
13. Steers WD, Ciambotti J, Etzel B, Erdman S, de Groat WC. Alterations in afferent pathways from the urinary bladder of the rat in response to partial urethral obstruction. J Comp Neurol. 1991;310:401–10.
14. Griffiths DJ. Cerebral control of bladder function. Curr Urol Rep. 2004;5:348–35.
15. Griffiths DJ, Fowler CJ. The micturition switch and its forebrain influences. Acta Physiol. 2013;207(1):93–109.
16. Sugaya K, Matsuyama K, Takakusaki K, Mori S. Electrical and chemical stimulations of the pontine micturition center. Neurosci Lett. 1987;80(2):197–201.
17. Takasaki A, Hui M, Sasaki M. Is the periaqueductal gray an essential relay center for the micturition reflex pathway in the cat? Brain Res. 2011;1317:108–15.
18. Stone E, Coote JH, Allard J, Lovick TA. GABAergic control of micturition within the periaqueductal grey matter of the male rat. J Physiol. 2011;589:2065–78.
19. de Groat WC, Nadelhaft I, Milne RJ, Booth AM, Morgan C, Thor K. Organization of the sacral parasympathetic reflex pathways to the urinary bladder and large intestine. J Auton Nerv Syst. 1981;3:135–60.
20. de Groat WC, Ryall RW. Reflexes to sacral parasympathetic neurons concerned with micturition in the cat. J Physiol. 1969;200:87–108.
21. Häbler HJ, Jänig W, Koltzenburg M. Activation of unmyelinated afferent fibres by mechanical stimuli and inflammation of the urinary bladder in the cat. J Physiol. 1990;425:545–62.
22. Mallory B, Steers WD, de Groat WC. Electrophysiological study of micturition reflexes in rats. Am J Phys. 1989;257:R410–21.
23. Bruns TM, Gaunt RA, Weber DJ. Multielectrode array recordings of bladder and perineal primary afferent activity from the sacral dorsal root ganglia. J Neural Eng. 2011;8:056010.
24. Jänig W, Morrison JFB. Functional properties of spinal visceral afferents supplying abdominal and pelvic organs, with special emphasis on visceral nociception. Prog Brain Res. 1986;67:87–114.
25. McMahon SB, Abel C. A model for the study of visceral pain states: chronic inflammation of the chronic decerebrate rat urinary bladder by irritant chemicals. Pain. 1987;28:109–27.
26. Fall M, Lindström S, Mazieres L. A bladder-to-bladder cooling reflex in the cat. J Physiol. 1990;427:281–300.
27. de Groat WC, Booth AM, Yoshimura N. Neurophysiology of micturition and its modification in animal models of human disease. In: Maggi CA, editor. The autonomic nervous system, nervous control of the urogenital system, vol. 3. London: Harwood Academic; 1993. p. 227–89.
28. de Groat WC. Mechanism underlying the recovery of lower urinary tract function following spinal cord injury. Paraplegia. 1995;33:493–505.
29. de Groat WC, Kawatani M, Hisamitsu T, et al. Mechanisms underlying the recovery of urinary bladder function following spinal cord injury. J Auton Nerv Syst. 1990;30(Suppl):s71–7.
30. de Groat WC, Yoshimura N. Plasticity in reflex pathways to the lower urinary tract following spinal cord injury. Exp Neurol. 2012;225:123–32.
31. de Groat WC, Yoshimura N. Mechanisms underlying the recovery of lower urinary tract function following spinal cord injury. Prog Brain Res. 2006;152:59–84.
32. Khan Z, Starer P, Yang WC, et al. Analysis of voiding disorders in patients with cerebrovascular accidents. Urology. 1990;35:265–70.

33. Fowler CJ. Neurological disorders of micturition and their treatment. Brain. 1999;122:1213–31.
34. Kim TG, Chun MH, Chang MC, et al. Outcomes of drug-resistant urinary retention in patients in the early stage of stroke. Ann Rehabil Med. 2015;39:262–7.
35. Kong KH, Young S. Incidence and outcome of post-stroke urinary retention: a prospective study. Arch Phys Med Rehabil. 2000;81:1464–7.
36. Griffiths D. Clinical studies of cerebral and urinary tract function in elderly people with urinary incontinence. Behav Brain Res. 1998;92:151–5.
37. Yeo L, Singh R, Gundeti M, et al. Urinary tract dysfunction in Parkinson's disease: a review. Int Urol Nephrol. 2012;44(2):415–24.
38. Araki I, Kuno S. Assessment of voiding dysfunction in Parkinson's disease by the international prostate symptom score. J Neurol Neurosurg Psychiatry. 2000;68(4):429–33.
39. Lemack GE, Dewey RB, Roehrborn CG, et al. Questionnaire-based assessment of bladder dysfunction in patients with mild to moderate Parkinson's disease. Urology. 2000;56:250–4.
40. Campos-Sousa RN, Quagliato E, da Silva BB, et al. Urinary symptoms in Parkinson's disease: prevalence and associated factors. Arq Neuropsiquiatr. 2003;61(2B):359–63.
41. Sakakibara R, Fowler CJ, Hattori T. Voiding and MRI analysis of the brain. Int Urogynecol J Pelvic Floor Dysfunct. 1999;10:192–9.
42. Blaivas JG, Kaplan SA. Urologic dysfunction in patients with multiple sclerosis. Semin Neurol. 1988;8:159–65.
43. Litwiller SE, Frohman EM, Zimmern PE. Multiple sclerosis and the urologist. J Urol. 1999;161:743–57.
44. Ukkonen M, Elovaara I, Dastidar P, et al. Urodynamic findings in primary progressive multiple sclerosis are associated with increased volumes of plaques and atrophy in the central nervous system. Acta Neurol Scand. 2004;109:100–5.
45. Thomas DG, O'Flynn KJ. Spinal cord injury. In: Mundy AR, Stephenson T, Wein AJ, editors. Urodynamics: principles, practice and application. London: Churchill Livingstone; 1994. p. 345–58.
46. Fam B, Yalla SV. Vesicourethral dysfunction in spinal cord injury and its management. Semin Neurol. 1988;8:150–5.
47. Ren J, Chew DJ, Biers S, et al. Electrical nerve stimulation to promote micturition in spinal cord injury patients: a review of current attempts. Neurourol Urodyn. 2016;35(3):365–70.
48. Brindley GS. An implant to empty the bladder or close the urethra. J Neurol Neurosurg Psychiatry. 1977;40:358–69.
49. Brindley GS, Polkey CE, Rushton DN. Sacral anterior root stimulators for bladder control in paraplegia. Paraplegia. 1982;20:365–81.
50. Sievert KD, Amend B, Gakis G, et al. Early sacral neuromodulation prevents urinary incontinence after complete spinal cord injury. Ann Neurol. 2010;67:74–84.
51. Yoshimura N, Smith CP, Chancellor MD, et al. Pharmacologic and potential biologic interventions to restore bladder function after spinal cord injury. Curr Opin Neurol. 2000;13:677–81.
52. Kutzenberger J, Domurath B, Sauerwein D. Spastic bladder and spinal cord injury: seventeen years of experience with sacral deafferentation and implantation of an anterior root stiumlator. Artif Organs. 2005;29:239–41.
53. de Groat WC, Tai C. Impact of bioelectronic medicine on the neural regulation of pelvic visceral function. Bioelectron Med. 2015;22:25–36.
54. Zhang F, Zhao S, Shen B, et al. Neural pathways involved in sacral neuromodulation of reflex bladder activity in cats. Am J Physiol Renal Physiol. 2013;304:F710–7.
55. Larson JA, Ogagan PD, Chen G, et al. Involvement of metabotropic glutamate receptor 5 in pudendal inhibition of nociceptive bladder activity in cats. J Physiol. 2011;589:5833–43.
56. Tai C, Chen M, Shen B, et al. Irritation induced bladder overactivity is suppressed by tibial nerve stimulation in cats. J Urol. 2011;186:326–30.
57. Tai C, Shen B, Mally AD, et al. Inhibition of micturition reflex by activation of somatic afferents in posterior femoral cutaneous nerve. J Physiol. 2012;590:4945–55.
58. Tai C, Shen B, Chen M, et al. Suppression of bladder overactivity by activation of somatic afferent nerves in the foot. BJU Int. 2011;107:303–9.
59. Tai C, Larson JA, Ogagan PD, et al. Differential role of opioid receptors in tibial nerve inhibition of nociceptive and nonnociceptive bladder reflexes in cats. Am J Physiol Renal Physiol. 2012;302:F1090–7.
60. Tai C, Shen B, Chen M, et al. Prolonged poststimulation inhibition of bladder activity induced by tibial nerve stimulation in cats. Am J Physiol Renal Physiol. 2011;300:F385–92.
61. Rogers MJ, Xiao Z, Shen B, et al. Propranolol, but not naloxone, enhances spinal reflex bladder activity and reduces pudendal inhibition in cats. Am J Physiol Regul Integr Comp Physiol. 2015;308:R42–9.
62. Tai C, Smerin SE, de Groat WC, et al. Pudendal-to-bladder reflex in chronic spinal-cord-injured cats. Exp Neuro. 2006;197:225–34.
63. Woock JP, Yoo PB, Grill WM. Mechanisms of reflex bladder activation by pudendal afferents. Am J Physiol Regul Integr Comp Physiol. 2011;300:R398–407.
64. Xiao Z, Reese J, Schwen Z, et al. Role of spinal GABAA receptors in pudendal inhibition of nociceptive and nonnociceptive bladder reflexes in cats. Am J Physiol Renal Physiol. 2014;306(7):F781–9.
65. Mally AD, Matsuta Y, Zhang F, et al. Role of opioid and metabotropic glutamate 5 receptors in pudendal inhibition of bladder overactivity in cats. J Urol. 2013;189:1574–9.
66. Peters KM, Killinger KA, Boguslawski BM, et al. Chronic pudendal neuromodulation: expanding available treatment options for refractory urologic symptoms. Neurourol Urodyn. 2010;29:1267–71.

Neuromodulation for Non-urologic Chronic Pain

2

Michael D. Staudt and Jonathan P. Miller

Neuromodulation for Pain

Chronic pain is a disabling condition that has a variety of clinical presentations and confers an enormous personal, social, and economic burden. Despite medical and technical advancements, the treatment of chronic pain syndromes continues to be challenging and often frustrating for both the patient and healthcare provider. In response to these challenges, the field of neuromodulation has emerged as a critical component of a multidisciplinary approach to pain management. Neuromodulation refers to the modification or alteration of normal nervous system activity via the precise delivery of electrical stimulation or pharmacological agent to the brain, spinal cord, or peripheral nerves.

The introduction of the "gate control" theory of pain in 1965 was instrumental in the formulation of modern understandings of pain mechanisms [1] and laid the foundation for the development of unique neurosurgical treatments and the use of neuromodulation. According to this theory, stimulation of large-diameter afferent fibers that carry light touch and proprioception sensory information to the dorsal horn of the spinal cord has an inhibitory effect on small-diameter fibers that relay noxious pain-related signals and have a higher threshold of activation. Thus, pain pathways were hypothesized to be dynamic and potentially modifiable. Prior to this revelation, the surgical treatment of pain primarily involved ablative and irreversible procedures [2], but the discovery that pain pathways are modifiable allowed a shift in focus from destructive ablation of pain pathways to reversible neuromodulation procedures.

The gate control theory directly led to two pivotal studies in the development of neuromodulation as a pain management paradigm: peripheral nerve stimulation (PNS) by Wall and Sweet [3], and dorsal column stimulation by Shealy et al. [4], both published in 1967. The theory behind dorsal column stimulation, now referred to as spinal cord stimulation (SCS), is that retrograde transmission of a stimulation impulse to the dorsal root entry zone of the affected spinal level "closes the gate" and inhibits pain neurotransmission. In effect, stimulation can be adjusted to provide a non-painful instead of painful sensation. The successes of these initial experiments were realized by the development of implantable stimulator devices [5, 6] and the foundation of modern neuromodulation procedures.

M. D. Staudt · J. P. Miller (✉)
Department of Neurological Surgery, University Hospitals Cleveland Medical Center/Case Western Reserve University, Cleveland, OH, USA
e-mail: michael.staudt@londonhospitals.ca; jonathan.miller@uhhospitals.org

J. P. Gilleran, S. A. Alpert (eds.), *Adult and Pediatric Neuromodulation*,
https://doi.org/10.1007/978-3-319-73266-4_2

Subsequently, additional modalities of neurostimulation have been utilized in the neurosurgical treatment of pain, including deep brain stimulation (DBS) and motor cortex stimulation (MCS). Although the primary use of DBS is in the treatment of movement disorders, its role in pain management has its foundations in the early observations by Heath and Mickle that septal stimulation was able to alleviate intractable pain related to cancer or rheumatoid arthritis [7]. Stimulation of additional components of the mesolimbic pathway, including the medial forebrain bundle, has also been demonstrated to alleviate cancer-related pain [8]. However, the modern use of DBS in the treatment of intractable pain owes much to the discovery of the sensory thalamus [9, 10] and periventricular areas [11, 12] as targets for chronic stimulation. Stimulation of the motor cortex was then developed in response to the inadequacy of treating central deafferentation pain with DBS [13], although its clinical efficacy continues to be debated.

Another facet of neuromodulation is chemical modulation via precise drug delivery. This was first described in 1979 when lasting anesthesia was found following the intrathecal (IT) or epidural administration of morphine [14, 15]. The use of IT therapy and implantable intrathecal drug delivery systems in the treatment of spasticity and pain syndromes has since rapidly expanded to utilize a variety of opioid and non-opioid agents.

Since development of the first implantable neuromodulation devices, the technology has continued to improve and, despite increasing sophistication and complexity, implantable devices have become smaller and more user-friendly. In addition, the indications for the use of neuromodulation in the treatment of chronic pain have expanded and become more diverse. The aim of this chapter is to review the indications for and evidence underlying commonly employed neuromodulation procedures in the treatment of chronic non-urologic pain.

Spinal Cord Stimulation

The initial case reported by Shealy et al. involved the placement of an epidural electrode at the T3 thoracic level for the alleviation of chest and abdominal pain related to metastatic bronchogenic carcinoma [4]. Subsequently, SCS has been studied in the treatment of many presentations of chronic pain, and in its current form, SCS has shown to be most efficacious in the treatment of neuropathic extremity pain. The effect of SCS on neuropathic axial pain is more controversial and is generally thought to be ineffective for nociceptive pain; pain related to ischemia in an exception, but these effects are likely to be due to induced changes in blood flow rather than direct modification of pain pathways. The use of SCS in the treatment of chronic pain is FDA approved and is most commonly utilized in the context of failed back surgery syndrome (FBSS) and complex regional pain syndrome (CRPS) [16].

FBSS refers to the development of chronic pain in a patient who has previously undergone back surgery and is also known as post-laminectomy syndrome. When considering treatment of FBSS, it is important to recognize that SCS is effective for primarily appendicular pain, with axial pain being less responsive. In appropriately selected patients, SCS has been demonstrated to provide superior pain relief and improved quality-of-life outcomes when compared to standard therapy alone [17–19]. The long-term cost-effectiveness of SCS has also been demonstrated, despite high initial costs of the hardware [20]. In addition to FBSS, SCS is highly effective in the initial treatment of patients with CRPS, with randomized control trials demonstrating improved pain control and quality of life [21, 22]. Long-term observations have described diminishing effectiveness over time although with a high rate of patient satisfaction [23]. Although the majority of studies examining the effectiveness for SCS in the treatment of neuropathic pain syndromes are observational or retrospective in nature, it appears that at least

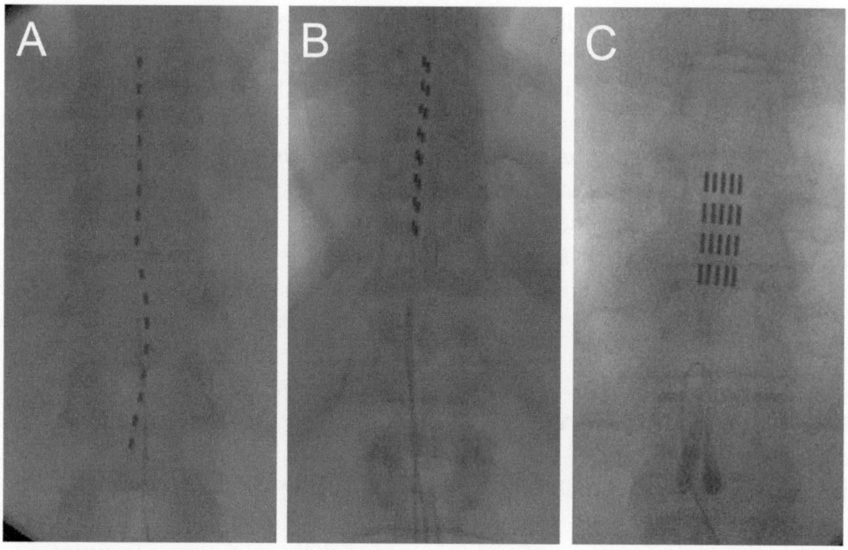

Fig. 2.1 Intraoperative fluoroscopy demonstrating percutaneous placement of thoracic epidural spinal cord stimulator electrodes in a vertical (**a**) and side-by-side (**b**) orientation. Placement of epidural paddle lead via thoracic laminotomy (**c**)

50% of patients are satisfied with the quality of pain relief [24–26].

Interestingly, SCS has also been demonstrated to provide significant benefit in those patients with nociceptive ischemic pain conditions, particularly peripheral vascular disease and angina pectoris. One of the first clinical reports on the treatment of peripheral vascular disease with SCS was published in 1976 [27] although its use would not gain prominence until the 1980s and 1990s [28, 29]. In addition to the effects of SCS on pain alleviation associated with ischemic disease, much clinical interest has also been related to the potential for improved limb salvage and wound healing, which has been demonstrated in a number of randomized and prospective studies [30, 31]. The efficacy of SCS on ischemic pain is actually greater than that for neuropathic pain; in fact, up to 90% of patients will describe significant relief from pain related to angina, as well as fewer angina attacks and emergency room visits [29, 32]. These anti-anginal and anti-ischemic effects have a physiological correlate, such as reducing myocardial oxygen consumption [33]. These patients also have better exercise tolerance and reduced nitrate consumption [34] and have an improved New York Heart Association functional class [35].

Stimulation is delivered via epidural leads placed either percutaneously or as a surgically placed paddle lead (Fig. 2.1). Conventional stimulation parameters involve the tonic delivery of current, usually within 40–80 Hz. Newer neurostimulator technology has recently been developed that is capable of delivering paresthesia-free stimulation. One technology involves the delivery of high pulses rates up to 10,000 Hz [36, 37], whereas the other delivers non-tonic "bursts" of stimulation [38, 39]. Early clinical observations demonstrate a greater ability to target axial neuropathic pain, in addition to salvaging patients who have failed or are non-responders to conventional SCS. Furthermore, there is interest in additional SCS targets, including the dorsal root ganglion (DRG). Preliminary studies indicate that DRG stimulation may be able to provide highly targeted pain control to treat focal neuropathic or nociceptive pain [40, 41].

Despite decades of clinical experience, our understanding of the mechanisms underlying SCS remain elusive. This is complicated by the fact that preclinical models are not truly translational due to the reliance on animal analogs of pain, described as "pain-like behaviors" and including measures such as withdrawal reflexes [42, 43]. In addition to the gate control theory, numerous other mechanisms have been hypothesized, including modulation of neurotransmitters, supraspinal centers, and sympathetic outputs [40]. Despite the lack of a clear mechanism, there is ample clinical and observational evidence for the effectiveness of SCS.

Peripheral Nerve Stimulation

In the same year that Shealy et al. published their landmark study on dorsal column stimulation, Wall and Sweet stimulated their own infraorbital nerves to test the gate control theory of pain [3]. Subsequently, they implanted subcutaneous or surface electrodes in patients with chronic cutaneous pain, resulting in suppression of pain signals during stimulation [3]. Encouraged by these early results, a permanent PNS device was implanted into a patient with a previous median nerve injury [44], establishing PNS as a viable treatment modality in management of chronic pain. For the next few decades, PNS devices were implanted via open surgery until the introduction of percutaneous lead placement in 1999 [45, 46]. Due to the diversity of neuropathic pain syndromes attributable to peripheral nerve etiology, there have been numerous attempts at defining a variety of indications for PNS. However, the use of PNS is not as widespread as other neuromodulation modalities, and thus the literature lacks robust, long-term data. Currently, the vast majority of PNS devices are not FDA approved and are used off-label.

The most common indication for PNS is percutaneous occipital nerve stimulation (ONS) for occipital neuralgia, which is a pain syndrome characterized predominantly by sharp and electrical pain in the distribution of the occipital nerves. Weiner and Reed described the first use of percutaneous ONS in the treatment of occipital neuralgia as an alternative to traditional open techniques [45]. This was followed by numerous prospective and retrospective case series [47–50], defining ONS as a viable treatment option in the treatment of medically intractable occipital neuralgia [51]. However, there are few robust prospective studies, and most contain small patient populations without a control or comparison group [51]. Despite these limitations, significant pain alleviation has often been described, with sustained resolution up to 1 year.

Additional indications for the use of PNS include broadly defined headaches and facial pain. ONS has been used in the treatment of chronic migraines, as stimulation of the occipital nerves can modulate areas innervated by the cervical and trigeminal nerves [46, 52]. Previous studies have demonstrated the feasibility of this treatment modality in chronic migraines [53], although the long-term effectiveness is debatable and warrants further study [54]. Sphenopalatine ganglion stimulation has been investigated for the treatment of cluster headaches, with promising early results [55]. Facial pain syndromes which are considered indications for PNS include pain secondary to peripheral nerve injury, trigeminal neuralgia, post-stroke central pain, and post-herpetic neuralgia [40]; with the exception of this latter indication of post-herpetic neuralgia [56], the effectiveness of PNS has consistently been demonstrated. Typical targets include branches of the trigeminal nerve [57] or the trigeminal ganglion itself [56].

A distinction must be made between PNS and peripheral nerve field stimulation; the former directly targets the nerve itself whereas the latter targets a non-dermatomal area or "field" of pain, typically via a subcutaneously inserted electrode [40]. There are a wide variety of indications for this type of stimulation, including joint, low back, chest wall, and abdominal wall pain [46]. The use of peripheral nerve field stimulation has also been described as an adjunct to SCS, potentially offering superior back pain control when SCS as monotherapy is ineffective [58, 59].

The percutaneous surgical technique of PNS device implantation is relatively simple, with few contraindications and a low risk of injuring neurovascular structures. As such, there is continued interest in this field to develop new stimulation devices and define appropriate clinical indications. As this field lacks robust and standardized data, this will necessitate the development of adequately powered studies in the future.

Deep Brain Stimulation

The discovery of DBS as a potential pain treatment modality predates SCS [7], but studies to identify appropriate stimulation targets were not performed until the 1970s. Common targets for intracranial stimulation with DBS include the sensory thalamus [9, 60] and periventricular-periaqueductal gray (PVG-PAG), which are generally targeted for neuropathic and nociceptive pain, respectively (Fig. 2.2). Additional targets have been described but are not commonly used, including internal capsule [61] and centromedian nucleus [62]. Currently, DBS is not FDA approved for pain [63] and is considered off-label.

Stimulation of the sensory thalamus is one of the primary indications for the use of DBS in the treatment of neuropathic pain. The thalamus has a well-studied role in pain signaling, and certain stimulation parameters are known to induce painful sensations [64]. Some of the earliest studies by Hosobuchi et al. [9] and Mazars et al. [65] targeted the sensory thalamus in the treatment of facial anesthesia dolorosa, phantom limb pain, and post-stroke central pain. Although these early studies reported alleviation of pain in the early post-operative period, the effects of stimulation were observed eventually to wane and pain almost invariably recurred. It has been suggested that much of the early therapeutic effect may have been related to electrode insertion as opposed to ongoing stimulation [66].

Early preclinical studies in rats identified that PVG-PAG stimulation can provide an anti-nociceptive role without the need for additional chemical anesthetic agents [67] although stimulation has also been observed to be effective in certain neuropathic pain syndromes as well [68]. This therapeutic effect on anti-nociception has been hypothesized to be mediated by endorphin release [12]; however, the role of endogenous opioids has been debated, as the therapeutic effect of stimulation has been demonstrated to be reversed by both naloxone [69] and placebo [70]. Thus, the analgesic effects of PVG-PAG stimula-

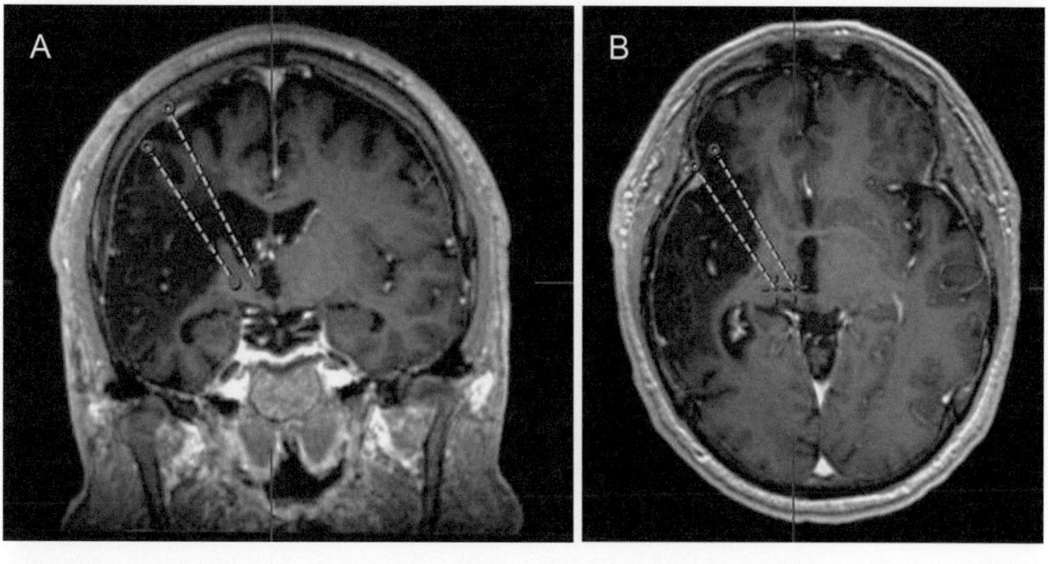

Fig. 2.2 Preoperative planning for deep brain stimulator electrode insertion in a patient with previous left middle cerebral artery infarction and post-stroke central pain. Coronal (**a**) and axial (**b**) T1-weighted MRI demonstrates trajectory for electrodes targeting the left ventrocaudal nucleus of the thalamus (lateral) and periventricular gray matter (medial)

tion are believed to be multifactorial, encompassing both opioid and non-opioid mechanisms. Functional imaging has also demonstrated activation of the anterior cingulate cortex, suggesting a potential modulatory role of the emotional response to pain [71]. Interestingly, a potential side effect of PVG-PAG stimulation in humans is characterized by a fearful response, or an "impending sense of dread" [66].

Despite initial enthusiasm and generally high reported rates of success, the clinical efficacy of DBS as a pain treatment modality has not held up to scrutiny [63] although the efficacy may be dependent on patient selection and clinical indication [72]. As a result, clinical efficacy has been reported in the range of 20–80% of treated patients [68, 73, 74]. In general, nociceptive pain appears to respond better than neuropathic or deafferentation pain [72]. Unfortunately, PVG-PAG stimulation is particularly susceptible to tolerance, with the need for higher stimulation parameters over time to achieve the same therapeutic effect [61]. Currently, DBS continues to be used clinically in the treatment of pain, and electrodes are often inserted to target both the sensory thalamus and PVG-PAG simultaneously.

The field of DBS continues to evolve as potential new targets and clinical indications are identified. The anterior limb of the internal capsule and ventral capsule and ventral striatal area have been identified as potential therapeutic targets for obsessive-compulsive disorder [75] and treatment-refractory depression [76, 77], respectively, although the clinical effectiveness has not been realized in larger clinical studies. It has been hypothesized that targeting the affective component of pain may be as important as the sensory-discriminative components, suggesting a potential avenue for future study [78].

Motor Cortex Stimulation

Motor cortex stimulation (MCS) was developed in response to the inadequacy of DBS in treating central deafferentation pain syndromes, including atypical trigeminal neuropathic pain and post-stroke central pain. These are less common forms of neuropathic pain which manifest as a result of spinothalamic tract injury and sensory conduction interruption, causing sensitization and hyperactivity of normal sensory neurons; these syndromes tend to be refractory to conservative and interventional management [79]. The use of MCS has been expanded to a number of other neuropathic pain syndromes, including pain related to peripheral nerve injury, spinal cord injury and phantom limb pain, although robust, long-term data are lacking [80]. As with DBS, the use of MCS in the treatment of pain is not FDA approved and is thus considered off-label.

The initial preclinical studies of MCS in the treatment of central deafferentation pain utilized ablation of the anterior spinothalamic tract in a cat model, resulting in hypersensitivity of the thalamic sensory nucleus [81]. With MCS, a decrease in mean spike density was observed, suggesting that thalamic hyperactivity had been reduced. These preclinical results were then translated into human studies, primarily in patients with pain secondary to hemorrhagic or ischemic stroke [13, 82]. These results were again promising, with some patients having partial or complete alleviation of pain. An early attempt to reproduce these results in three patients unfortunately did not result in clinical pain relief, but interestingly had a significant effect on atypical trigeminal neuropathic pain [83]. However, numerous case reports and case series evaluating the use of MCS to treat post-stroke central pain have since followed these initial clinical trials, with variable improvement in pain scores [84–86].

The other primary indication for the use of MCS is the treatment of trigeminal neuropathic pain, which is constant facial pain secondary to injury of the trigeminal nerve or ganglion. This type of pain may be caused by failed treatment for trigeminal neuralgia, dental or sinus surgery, or trauma. Unlike trigeminal neuralgia, there are few effective treatment paradigms for trigeminal neuropathic pain. In an early study by Meyerson et al., five patients with trigeminal neuropathic pain reported significant and lasting pain relief with MCS [83]. Subsequent studies have supported these initial findings by demonstrating lasting pain relief and safety in this patient population [87–89].

It is generally reported that 50–75% of patients with trigeminal neuropathic pain or post-stroke central pain will achieve significant pain relief from MCS [90, 91]. However, the duration of benefit is highly variable, and intensive reprogramming is often required to restore beneficial stimulation parameters [92]. Reports of long-term pain relief continue to be inconsistent, usually due to small patient populations and the potential for publication bias [93]. An important potential complication of stimulation is the development of seizures during programming and is related to both stimulation amplitude and frequency [92]. It has been suggested that final stimulation parameters should be slightly less than the motor threshold, which is the lowest voltage that produces motor contractions [94].

Despite evidence of clinical efficacy with MCS, the therapeutic mechanisms involved in pain relief remain poorly understood [95]. Positron emission tomography studies have demonstrated increased cerebral blood flow in the cingulate cortex, orbitofrontal cortex, thalamus, brainstem, and periaqueductal gray matter [96, 97]. As these are diverse regions with numerous cortico-thalamic or cortico-cortical connections, it has been suggested that MCS may act via both emotional modulation and descending inhibition toward the spinal cord [97].

Intrathecal Drug Delivery

The use of IT drug therapy has revolutionized the medical treatment of patients with spasticity, with increasing enthusiasm for the treatment of chronic pain. Currently, there are only three IT agents approved by the FDA: morphine (an opioid) and ziconitide (a non-opioid calcium channel antagonist) are approved in the treatment of pain, and baclofen (a $GABA_B$ receptor agonist) is approved for the treatment of spasticity. Numerous other IT therapies are utilized off-label by pain practitioners as alternative monotherapies, or combination therapy to synergistically target multiple pain receptors. These agents include opioids (hydromorphone, fentanyl), local anesthetics (bupivacaine, ropivacaine), adrenergic agonists (clonidine), and GABA agonists (baclofen), among others.

The use of IT morphine was first described in the treatment of cancer-related pain [14], but has since been applied to patients with chronic refractory neuropathic or nociceptive pain. Conventional treatment with oral opioids may fail due to inadequate pain relief, the use of high dosages and development of tolerance, or the development of serious side effects. The IT administration of morphine is recognized as first-line therapy in chronic neuropathic or nociceptive pain, and extensive preclinical and clinical evidence has demonstrated excellent pain relief with fewer side effects than systemic opioid therapy and potentially longer overall survival, possibly due to less toxicity from systemic treatment [98]. However, IT morphine therapy will be inadequate in a subset of patients, necessitating the use of alternative agents or combination therapy with multiple agents.

In response to the complexity of treating this patient population, a comprehensive IT treatment algorithm based on clinical evidence and expert experience has been developed [98]. Typically, IT morphine is first trialed and additional agents are added in a stepwise fashion if pain control is not adequate. It is estimated that only 20–25% of patients' pain is adequately controlled with morphine or ziconitide; thus many patients are treated off-label and with combination therapy [99]. It is important to carefully consider the dosing of multiple agents, as each compound has its own therapeutic window and complication profile.

As monotherapy, ziconotide provides significant pain relief in patients refractory to opioid therapy [100]. Combination therapy with IT morphine has been demonstrated to safely and effectively treat cancer and non-cancer-related pain [101]. Combination IT therapy with other agents has also been reported, including baclofen to treat concurrent neuropathic pain and spasticity [102]. A primary concern in combination therapy is drug stability, as opioids can induce ziconotide degradation and necessitate more frequent pump refills [101]. Optimal stability can be achieved with lower opioid dosages, necessitating careful titration and individualized patient regimens.

The use of local anesthetics, particularly bupivacaine, has been widely adopted as an adjunct in chronic pain treatment. Combination therapy with IT opioids and bupivacaine has been demonstrated to provide superior pain relief when compared to IT opioids alone, in addition to decreased healthcare-associated costs such as clinic and emergency room visits, and decreased oral opioid use [103]. In patients tolerant to systemic opioid therapy, combination IT morphine and levobupivacaine provides significant pain relief with lower side effects than systemic therapy [104]. Another promising agent is clonidine, an alpha-2 adrenergic agonist that modulates neurotransmission at the dorsal horn. IT clonidine has been extensively studied as an anesthetic adjunct, and also as monotherapy in chronic pain patients [105]. However, its efficacy as monotherapy has been debated [106], and is thus recommended as third-line monotherapy for neuropathic pain or second line when used in combination with opioids [98]. Combination therapy with IT morphine has been reported to provide superior pain relief compared to either agent alone in the treatment of neuropathic pain [106, 107].

The use of IT therapy with both on- and off-label agents is widely used and supported by clinical experience. It is important to carefully consider the dosing of multiple agents, as each compound has its own therapeutic window and complications. However, most challenges are technical in nature, including accelerated motor stalling and device failures in commercial pumps using off-label agents [108], as well as the inability to adjust drug concentrations without completely emptying and refilling the chamber [99]. Additional clinical experience with a variety of IT agents is necessary to expand the efficacy of monotherapy and combination therapy, as well as the indications for patient selection.

Summary

There is good evidence to support the use of neuromodulation in the treatment of chronic pain syndromes with sustained long-term success in carefully selected patients and clinical indications. SCS is currently the most commonly used neuromodulation modality and is supported by decades of research and clinical interest. However, certain pain syndromes may not adequately be treated by a single modality, and it is possible that a combination of neuromodulation techniques may be beneficial. Although PNS, DBS, and MCS do not have the same robust literature base as SCS, there is good evidence to support their use in appropriate clinical scenarios. As neuromodulation technology improves, device implantation will become more straightforward, and this is likely to lead to the development of high-quality evidence with even more diverse clinical indications.

References

1. Melzack R, Wall PD. Pain mechanisms: a new theory. Science. 1965;150(3699):971–9; Epub 1965/11/19.
2. Raslan AM, Cetas JS, McCartney S, Burchiel KJ. Destructive procedures for control of cancer pain: the case for cordotomy. J Neurosurg. 2011;114(1):155–70; Epub 2010/08/10.
3. Wall PD, Sweet WH. Temporary abolition of pain in man. Science. 1967;155(3758):108–9; Epub 1967/01/06.
4. Shealy CN, Mortimer JT, Reswick JB. Electrical inhibition of pain by stimulation of the dorsal columns: preliminary clinical report. Anesth Analg. 1967;46(4):489–91; Epub 1967/07/01.
5. Sweet WH, Wepsic JG. Treatment of chronic pain by stimulation of fibers of primary afferent neuron. Trans Am Neurol Assoc. 1968;93:103–7; Epub 1968/01/01.
6. Gildenberg PL. History of electrical neuromodulation for chronic pain. Pain Med. 2006;7(S1):S7–13.
7. Heath RG, Mickle WA. Evaluation of seven years' experience with depth electrode studies in human patients. In: Ramey ER, O'Doherty D, editors. Electrical studies on the unanesthetized brain. New York: Harper & Brothers; 1960. p. 214–47.

8. Ervin FR, Mark VH, Stevens J. Behavioral and affective responses to brain stimulation in man. Proc Annu Meet Am Psychopathol Assoc. 1969;58:54–65; Epub 1969/01/01.
9. Hosobuchi Y, Adams JE, Rutkin B. Chronic thalamic stimulation for the control of facial anesthesia dolorosa. Arch Neurol. 1973;29(3):158–61; Epub 1973/09/01.
10. Mazars GJ. Intermittent stimulation of nucleus ventralis posterolateralis for intractable pain. Surg Neurol. 1975;4(1):93–5; Epub 1975/07/01.
11. Richardson DE, Akil H. Pain reduction by electrical brain stimulation in man. Part 1: acute administration in periaqueductal and periventricular sites. J Neurosurg. 1977;47(2):178–83; Epub 1977/08/01.
12. Richardson DE, Akil H. Long term results of periventricular gray self-stimulation. Neurosurgery. 1977;1(2):199–202; Epub 1977/09/01.
13. Tsubokawa T, Katayama Y, Yamamoto T, Hirayama T, Koyama S. Chronic motor cortex stimulation for the treatment of central pain. Acta Neurochir Suppl. 1991;52:137–9; Epub 1991/01/01.
14. Wang JK, Nauss LA, Thomas JE. Pain relief by intrathecally applied morphine in man. Anesthesiology. 1979;50(2):149–51; Epub 1979/02/01.
15. Behar M, Magora F, Olshwang D, Davidson JT. Epidural morphine in treatment of pain. Lancet. 1979;1(8115):527–9; Epub 1979/03/10.
16. Krames E. Spinal cord stimulation: indications, mechanism of action, and efficacy. Curr Rev Pain. 1999;3(6):419–26; Epub 2000/09/22.
17. Kumar K, Taylor RS, Jacques L, Eldabe S, Meglio M, Molet J, et al. Spinal cord stimulation versus conventional medical management for neuropathic pain: a multicentre randomised controlled trial in patients with failed back surgery syndrome. Pain. 2007;132(1–2):179–88; Epub 2007/09/12.
18. Burchiel KJ, Anderson VC, Brown FD, Fessler RG, Friedman WA, Pelofsky S, et al. Prospective, multicenter study of spinal cord stimulation for relief of chronic back and extremity pain. Spine. 1996;21(23):2786–94; Epub 1996/12/01.
19. Kumar K, Taylor RS, Jacques L, Eldabe S, Meglio M, Molet J, et al. The effects of spinal cord stimulation in neuropathic pain are sustained: a 24-month follow-up of the prospective randomized controlled multicenter trial of the effectiveness of spinal cord stimulation. Neurosurgery. 2008;63(4):762–70; discussion 70; Epub 2008/11/05.
20. Kumar K, Malik S, Demeria D. Treatment of chronic pain with spinal cord stimulation versus alternative therapies: cost-effectiveness analysis. Neurosurgery. 2002;51(1):106–15; discussion 15–6; Epub 2002/08/17.
21. Kemler MA, Barendse GA, van Kleef M, de Vet HC, Rijks CP, Furnee CA, et al. Spinal cord stimulation in patients with chronic reflex sympathetic dystrophy. N Engl J Med. 2000;343(9):618–24; Epub 2000/08/31.
22. Kemler MA, De Vet HC, Barendse GA, Van Den Wildenberg FA, Van Kleef M. The effect of spinal cord stimulation in patients with chronic reflex sympathetic dystrophy: two years' follow-up of the randomized controlled trial. Ann Neurol. 2004;55(1):13–8; Epub 2004/01/06.
23. Kemler MA, de Vet HC, Barendse GA, van den Wildenberg FA, van Kleef M. Effect of spinal cord stimulation for chronic complex regional pain syndrome type I: five-year final follow-up of patients in a randomized controlled trial. J Neurosurg. 2008;108(2):292–8; Epub 2008/02/05.
24. Grabow TS, Tella PK, Raja SN. Spinal cord stimulation for complex regional pain syndrome: an evidence-based medicine review of the literature. Clin J Pain. 2003;19(6):371–83; Epub 2003/11/06.
25. Kumar K, Hunter G, Demeria D. Spinal cord stimulation in treatment of chronic benign pain: challenges in treatment planning and present status, a 22-year experience. Neurosurgery. 2006;58(3):481–96; discussion 481–96; Epub 2006/03/11.
26. North RB, Kidd DH, Zahurak M, James CS, Long DM. Spinal cord stimulation for chronic, intractable pain: experience over two decades. Neurosurgery. 1993;32(3):384–94; discussion 94–5; Epub 1993/03/01.
27. Cook AW, Oygar A, Baggenstos P, Pacheco S, Kleriga E. Vascular disease of extremities. Electric stimulation of spinal cord and posterior roots. N Y State J Med. 1976;76(3):366–8; Epub 1976/03/01.
28. Murphy DF, Giles KE. Dorsal column stimulation for pain relief from intractable angina pectoris. Pain. 1987;28(3):365–8; Epub 1987/03/01.
29. Eliasson T, Augustinsson LE, Mannheimer C. Spinal cord stimulation in severe angina pectoris—presentation of current studies, indications and clinical experience. Pain. 1996;65(2–3):169–79; Epub 1996/05/01.
30. Jivegard LE, Augustinsson LE, Holm J, Risberg B, Ortenwall P. Effects of spinal cord stimulation (SCS) in patients with inoperable severe lower limb ischaemia: a prospective randomised controlled study. Eur J Vasc Endovasc Surg. 1995;9(4):421–5; Epub 1995/05/01.
31. Claeys LG, Horsch S. Transcutaneous oxygen pressure as predictive parameter for ulcer healing in endstage vascular patients treated with spinal cord stimulation. Int Angiol. 1996;15(4):344–9; Epub 1996/12/01.
32. Jessurun GA, DeJongste MJ, Blanksma PK. Current views on neurostimulation in the treatment of cardiac ischemic syndromes. Pain. 1996;66(2–3):109–16; Epub 1996/08/01.
33. Mannheimer C, Eliasson T, Andersson B, Bergh CH, Augustinsson LE, Emanuelsson H, et al. Effects of spinal cord stimulation in angina pectoris induced by pacing and possible mechanisms of action. BMJ. 1993;307(6902):477–80; Epub 1993/08/21.

34. Hautvast RW, Brouwer J, DeJongste MJ, Lie KI. Effect of spinal cord stimulation on heart rate variability and myocardial ischemia in patients with chronic intractable angina pectoris—a prospective ambulatory electrocardiographic study. Clin Cardiol. 1998;21(1):33–8; Epub 1998/02/25.
35. TenVaarwerk IA, Jessurun GA, DeJongste MJ, Andersen C, Mannheimer C, Eliasson T, et al. Clinical outcome of patients treated with spinal cord stimulation for therapeutically refractory angina pectoris. Heart. 1999;82(1):82–8; Epub 1999/06/23.
36. Van Buyten JP, Al-Kaisy A, Smet I, Palmisani S, Smith T. High-frequency spinal cord stimulation for the treatment of chronic back pain patients: results of a prospective multicenter European Clinical Study. Neuromodulation. 2013;16(1):59–65; discussion 65–6; Epub 2012/12/04.
37. Tiede J, Brown L, Gekht G, Vallejo R, Yearwood T, Morgan D. Novel spinal cord stimulation parameters in patients with predominant back pain. Neuromodulation. 2013;16(4):370–5; Epub 2013/02/26.
38. de Vos CC, Bom MJ, Vanneste S, Lenders MW, de Ridder D. Burst spinal cord stimulation evaluated in patients with failed back surgery syndrome and painful diabetic neuropathy. Neuromodulation. 2014;17(2):152–9; Epub 2014/03/25.
39. De Ridder D, Vanneste S, Plazier M, van der Loo E, Menovsky T. Burst spinal cord stimulation: toward paresthesia-free pain suppression. Neurosurgery. 2010;66(5):986–90; Epub 2010/04/21.
40. Deer TR, Krames E, Mekhail N, Pope J, Leong M, Stanton-Hicks M, et al. The appropriate use of neurostimulation: new and evolving neurostimulation therapies and applicable treatment for chronic pain and selected disease states. Neuromodulation Appropriateness Consensus Committee. Neuromodulation. 2014;17(6):599–615; Epub 2012/12/04.
41. Liem L, Russo M, Huygen FJ, Van Buyten JP, Smet I, Verrills P, et al. One-year outcomes of spinal cord stimulation of the dorsal root ganglion in the treatment of chronic neuropathic pain. Neuromodulation. 2015;18(1):41–8; discussion 8–9; Epub 2014/08/26.
42. Hansson P. Difficulties in stratifying neuropathic pain by mechanisms. Eur J Pain. 2003;7(4):353–7; Epub 2003/06/25.
43. Mao J. Translational pain research: bridging the gap between basic and clinical research. Pain. 2002;97(3):183–7; Epub 2002/06/05.
44. White JC, Sweet WH. Pain and the neurosurgeon: a 40-year experience. Springfield, IL: Charles C. Thomas; 1969. 1000p.
45. Weiner RL, Reed KL. Peripheral neurostimulation for control of intractable occipital neuralgia. Neuromodulation. 1999;2(3):217–21; Epub 1999/07/01.
46. Goroszeniuk T, Pang D. Peripheral neuromodulation: a review. Curr Pain Headache Rep. 2014;18(5):412; Epub 2014/03/29.
47. Slavin KV, Nersesyan H, Wess C. Peripheral neurostimulation for treatment of intractable occipital neuralgia. Neurosurgery. 2006;58(1):112–9; discussion 112–9; Epub 2005/12/31.
48. Magown P, Garcia R, Beauprie I, Mendez IM. Occipital nerve stimulation for intractable occipital neuralgia: an open surgical technique. Clin Neurosurg. 2009;56:119–24; Epub 2009/01/01.
49. Oh MY, Ortega J, Bellotte JB, Whiting DM, Alo K. Peripheral nerve stimulation for the treatment of occipital neuralgia and transformed migraine using a c1-2-3 subcutaneous paddle style electrode: a technical report. Neuromodulation. 2004;7(2):103–12; Epub 2004/04/01.
50. Melvin EA Jr, Jordan FR, Weiner RL, Primm D. Using peripheral stimulation to reduce the pain of C2-mediated occipital headaches: a preliminary report. Pain Physician. 2007;10(3):453–60; Epub 2007/05/26.
51. Sweet JA, Mitchell LS, Narouze S, Sharan AD, Falowski SM, Schwalb JM, et al. Occipital nerve stimulation for the treatment of patients with medically refractory occipital neuralgia: congress of neurological surgeons systematic review and evidence-based guideline. Neurosurgery. 2015;77(3):332–41; Epub 2015/07/01.
52. Mueller O, Hagel V, Wrede K, Schlamann M, Hohn HP, Sure U, et al. Stimulation of the greater occipital nerve: anatomical considerations and clinical implications. Pain Physician. 2013;16(3):E181–9; Epub 2013/05/25.
53. Saper JR, Dodick DW, Silberstein SD, McCarville S, Sun M, Goadsby PJ. Occipital nerve stimulation for the treatment of intractable chronic migraine headache: ONSTIM feasibility study. Cephalalgia. 2011;31(3):271–85; Epub 2010/09/24.
54. Silberstein SD, Dodick DW, Saper J, Huh B, Slavin KV, Sharan A, et al. Safety and efficacy of peripheral nerve stimulation of the occipital nerves for the management of chronic migraine: results from a randomized, multicenter, double-blinded, controlled study. Cephalalgia. 2012;32(16):1165–79; Epub 2012/10/05.
55. Schoenen J, Jensen RH, Lanteri-Minet M, Lainez MJ, Gaul C, Goodman AM, et al. Stimulation of the sphenopalatine ganglion (SPG) for cluster headache treatment. Pathway CH-1: a randomized, sham-controlled study. Cephalalgia. 2013;33(10):816–30; Epub 2013/01/15.
56. Taub E, Munz M, Tasker RR. Chronic electrical stimulation of the gasserian ganglion for the relief of pain in a series of 34 patients. J Neurosurg. 1997;86(2):197–202; Epub 1997/02/01.
57. Slavin KV, Colpan ME, Munawar N, Wess C, Nersesyan H. Trigeminal and occipital peripheral nerve stimulation for craniofacial pain: a single-institution experience and review of the literature. Neurosurg Focus. 2006;21(6):E5; Epub 2007/03/08.
58. Navarro RM, Vercimak DC. Triangular stimulation method utilizing combination spinal cord

stimulation with peripheral subcutaneous field stimulation for chronic pain patients: a retrospective study. Neuromodulation. 2012;15(2):124–31; Epub 2012/02/15.
59. Hamm-Faber TE, Aukes H, van Gorp EJ, Gultuna I. Subcutaneous stimulation as an additional therapy to spinal cord stimulation for the treatment of low back pain and leg pain in failed back surgery syndrome: four-year follow-up. Neuromodulation. 2015;18(7):618–22; discussion 22; Epub 2015/05/07.
60. Hosobuchi Y, Adams JE, Rutkin B. Chronic thalamic and internal capsule stimulation for the control of central pain. Surg Neurol. 1975;4(1):91–2; Epub 1975/07/01.
61. Kumar K, Wyant GM, Nath R. Deep brain stimulation for control of intractable pain in humans, present and future: a ten-year follow-up. Neurosurgery. 1990;26(5):774–81; discussion 81–2; Epub 1990/05/01.
62. Andy OJ. Parafascicular-center median nuclei stimulation for intractable pain and dyskinesia (painful-dyskinesia). Appl Neurophysiol. 1980;43(3–5):133–44; Epub 1980/01/01.
63. Coffey RJ. Deep brain stimulation for chronic pain: results of two multicenter trials and a structured review. Pain Med. 2001;2(3):183–92; Epub 2004/04/23.
64. Lenz FA, Seike M, Richardson RT, Lin YC, Baker FH, Khoja I, et al. Thermal and pain sensations evoked by microstimulation in the area of human ventrocaudal nucleus. J Neurophysiol. 1993;70(1):200–12; Epub 1993/07/01.
65. Mazars G, Merienne L, Cioloca C. Treatment of certain types of pain with implantable thalamic stimulators. Neuro-Chirurgie. 1974;20(2):117–24; Epub 1974/03/01. Traitement de certains types de douleurs par des stimulateurs thalamiques implantables.
66. Hamani C, Schwalb JM, Rezai AR, Dostrovsky JO, Davis KD, Lozano AM. Deep brain stimulation for chronic neuropathic pain: long-term outcome and the incidence of insertional effect. Pain. 2006;125(1–2):188–96; Epub 2006/06/27.
67. Reynolds DV. Surgery in the rat during electrical analgesia induced by focal brain stimulation. Science. 1969;164(3878):444–5; Epub 1969/04/25.
68. Owen SL, Green AL, Nandi DD, Bittar RG, Wang S, Aziz TZ. Deep brain stimulation for neuropathic pain. Acta Neurochir Suppl. 2007;97(Pt 2):111–6; Epub 2007/08/19.
69. Adams JE. Naloxone reversal of analgesia produced by brain stimulation in the human. Pain. 1976;2(2):161–6; Epub 1976/06/01.
70. Young RF, Chambi VI. Pain relief by electrical stimulation of the periaqueductal and periventricular gray matter. Evidence for a non-opioid mechanism. J Neurosurg. 1987;66(3):364–71; Epub 1987/03/01.
71. Rezai AR, Lozano AM, Crawley AP, Joy ML, Davis KD, Kwan CL, et al. Thalamic stimulation and functional magnetic resonance imaging: localization of cortical and subcortical activation with implanted electrodes. Technical note. J Neurosurg. 1999;90(3):583–90; Epub 1999/03/06.
72. Bittar RG, Kar-Purkayastha I, Owen SL, Bear RE, Green A, Wang S, et al. Deep brain stimulation for pain relief: a meta-analysis. J Clin Neurosci. 2005;12(5):515–9; Epub 2005/07/05.
73. Nandi D, Aziz TZ. Deep brain stimulation in the management of neuropathic pain and multiple sclerosis tremor. J Clin Neurophysiol. 2004;21(1):31–9; Epub 2004/04/21.
74. Kumar K, Toth C, Nath RK. Deep brain stimulation for intractable pain: a 15-year experience. Neurosurgery. 1997;40(4):736–46; discussion 46–7; Epub 1997/04/01.
75. Nuttin B, Cosyns P, Demeulemeester H, Gybels J, Meyerson B. Electrical stimulation in anterior limbs of internal capsules in patients with obsessive-compulsive disorder. Lancet. 1999;354(9189):1526; Epub 1999/11/07.
76. Malone DA Jr, Dougherty DD, Rezai AR, Carpenter LL, Friehs GM, Eskandar EN, et al. Deep brain stimulation of the ventral capsule/ventral striatum for treatment-resistant depression. Biol Psychiatry. 2009;65(4):267–75; Epub 2008/10/10.
77. Dougherty DD, Rezai AR, Carpenter LL, Howland RH, Bhati MT, O'Reardon JP, et al. A randomized sham-controlled trial of deep brain stimulation of the ventral capsule/ventral striatum for chronic treatment-resistant depression. Biol Psychiatry. 2015;78(4):240–8; Epub 2015/03/03.
78. Machado AG, Baker KB, Plow E, Malone DA. Cerebral stimulation for the affective component of neuropathic pain. Neuromodulation. 2013;16(6):514–8; Epub 2012/10/26.
79. Andersen G, Vestergaard K, Ingeman-Nielsen M, Jensen TS. Incidence of central post-stroke pain. Pain. 1995;61(2):187–93; Epub 1995/05/01.
80. Brown JA, Barbaro NM. Motor cortex stimulation for central and neuropathic pain: current status. Pain. 2003;104(3):431–5; Epub 2003/08/21.
81. Hirayama T, Tsubokawa T, Katayama Y, Yamamoto Y, Koyama S. Chronic changes in activity of the thalamic relay neurons following spinothalamic tractotomy in cats. Effects of motor cortex stimulation. Pain. 1990;5(Suppl):273.
82. Tsubokawa T, Katayama Y, Yamamoto T, Hirayama T, Koyama S. Treatment of thalamic pain by chronic motor cortex stimulation. Pacing Clin Electrophysiol. 1991;14(1):131–4; Epub 1991/01/01.
83. Meyerson BA, Lindblom U, Linderoth B, Lind G, Herregodts P. Motor cortex stimulation as treatment of trigeminal neuropathic pain. Acta Neurochir Suppl. 1993;58:150–3; Epub 1993/01/01.
84. Nguyen JP, Lefaucher JP, Le Guerinel C, Eizenbaum JF, Nakano N, Carpentier A, et al. Motor cortex stimulation in the treatment of central and neuropathic pain. Arch Med Res. 2000;31(3):263–5; Epub 2000/10/19.
85. Nguyen JP, Lefaucheur JP, Decq P, Uchiyama T, Carpentier A, Fontaine D, et al. Chronic motor

cortex stimulation in the treatment of central and neuropathic pain. Correlations between clinical, electrophysiological and anatomical data. Pain. 1999;82(3):245–51; Epub 1999/09/17.
86. Mertens P, Nuti C, Sindou M, Guenot M, Peyron R, Garcia-Larrea L, et al. Precentral cortex stimulation for the treatment of central neuropathic pain: results of a prospective study in a 20-patient series. Stereotact Funct Neurosurg. 1999;73(1–4):122–5; Epub 2000/06/15.
87. Rainov NG, Fels C, Heidecke V, Burkert W. Epidural electrical stimulation of the motor cortex in patients with facial neuralgia. Clin Neurol Neurosurg. 1997;99(3):205–9; Epub 1997/08/01.
88. Rainov NG, Heidecke V. Motor cortex stimulation for neuropathic facial pain. Neurol Res. 2003;25(2):157–61; Epub 2003/03/15.
89. Henderson JM, Lad SP. Motor cortex stimulation and neuropathic facial pain. Neurosurg Focus. 2006;21(6):E6; Epub 2007/03/08.
90. Henderson JM, Lad SP, Chao K. Motor cortex stimulation. In: Winn HR, editor. Youmans neurological surgery. 6th ed: Saunders; 2011. p. 1831–4.
91. Monsalve GA. Motor cortex stimulation for facial chronic neuropathic pain: a review of the literature. Surg Neurol Int. 2012;3(Suppl 4):S290–311; Epub 2012/12/12.
92. Henderson JM, Boongird A, Rosenow JM, LaPresto E, Rezai AR. Recovery of pain control by intensive reprogramming after loss of benefit from motor cortex stimulation for neuropathic pain. Stereotact Funct Neurosurg. 2004;82(5–6):207–13; Epub 2004/12/08.
93. Sachs AJ, Babu H, Su YF, Miller KJ, Henderson JM. Lack of efficacy of motor cortex stimulation for the treatment of neuropathic pain in 14 patients. Neuromodulation. 2014;17(4):303–10; discussion 10–1; Epub 2014/04/30.
94. Chang S, Ranjan M, Slotty PJ, Honey CR. The influence of positioning and muscle activity on motor threshold during motor cortex stimulation programming. Stereotact Funct Neurosurg. 2015;93(2):122–6; Epub 2015/02/28.
95. Meyerson B. Motor cortex stimulation—effective for neuropathic pain but the mode of action remains illusive. Pain. 2005;118(1–2):6–7; Epub 2005/10/06.
96. Peyron R, Faillenot I, Mertens P, Laurent B, Garcia-Larrea L. Motor cortex stimulation in neuropathic pain. Correlations between analgesic effect and hemodynamic changes in the brain. A PET study. NeuroImage. 2007;34(1):310–21; Epub 2006/10/24.
97. Garcia-Larrea L, Peyron R. Motor cortex stimulation for neuropathic pain: from phenomenology to mechanisms. NeuroImage. 2007;37(Suppl 1): S71–9; Epub 2007/07/24.
98. Deer TR, Prager J, Levy R, Rathmell J, Buchser E, Burton A, et al. Polyanalgesic consensus conference 2012: recommendations for the management of pain by intrathecal (intraspinal) drug delivery: report of an interdisciplinary expert panel. Neuromodulation. 2012;15(5):436–64; discussion 64–6; Epub 2012/07/04.
99. Lamer TJ, Deer TR, Hayek SM. Advanced innovations for pain. Mayo Clin Proc. 2016;91(2):246–58; Epub 2016/02/06.
100. Staats PS, Yearwood T, Charapata SG, Presley RW, Wallace MS, Byas-Smith M, et al. Intrathecal ziconotide in the treatment of refractory pain in patients with cancer or AIDS: a randomized controlled trial. JAMA. 2004;291(1):63–70; Epub 2004/01/08.
101. Alicino I, Giglio M, Manca F, Bruno F, Puntillo F. Intrathecal combination of ziconotide and morphine for refractory cancer pain: a rapidly acting and effective choice. Pain. 2012;153(1):245–9; Epub 2011/11/16.
102. Saulino M, Burton AW, Danyo DA, Frost S, Glanzer J, Solanki DR. Intrathecal ziconotide and baclofen provide pain relief in seven patients with neuropathic pain and spasticity: case reports. Eur J Phys Rehabil Med. 2009;45(1):61–7; Epub 2009/01/22.
103. Deer TR, Caraway DL, Kim CK, Dempsey CD, Stewart CD, McNeil KF. Clinical experience with intrathecal bupivacaine in combination with opioid for the treatment of chronic pain related to failed back surgery syndrome and metastatic cancer pain of the spine. Spine J. 2002;2(4):274–8; Epub 2003/11/01.
104. Mercadante S, Intravaia G, Villari P, Ferrera P, Riina S, David F, et al. Intrathecal treatment in cancer patients unresponsive to multiple trials of systemic opioids. Clin J Pain. 2007;23(9):793–8; Epub 2007/12/14.
105. Hassenbusch SJ, Gunes S, Wachsman S, Willis KD. Intrathecal clonidine in the treatment of intractable pain: a phase I/II study. Pain Med. 2002;3(2):85–91; Epub 2004/04/23.
106. Ackerman LL, Follett KA, Rosenquist RW. Long-term outcomes during treatment of chronic pain with intrathecal clonidine or clonidine/opioid combinations. J Pain Symptom Manag. 2003;26(1):668–77; Epub 2003/07/10.
107. Siddall PJ, Molloy AR, Walker S, Mather LE, Rutkowski SB, Cousins MJ. The efficacy of intrathecal morphine and clonidine in the treatment of pain after spinal cord injury. Anesth Analg. 2000;91(6):1493–8; Epub 2000/11/30.
108. Galica R, Hayek SM, Veizi IE, Lawrence MM, Khalil AA, McEwan MT. Sudden intrathecal drug delivery device motor stalls: a case series. Reg Anesth Pain Med. 2016;41(2):135–9; Epub 2016/02/13.

3 Sacral Neuromodulation for Overactive Bladder

John R. Michalak, Sunchin Kim, Joel T. Funk, and Christian O. Twiss

Abbreviations

AUA	American Urologic Association
BoNT-A	Botulinum Toxin A
CIC	Clean intermittent catheterization
EAU	European Urologic Association
FDA	Food and drug administration
LUTD	Lower urinary tract dysfunction
LUTS	Lower urinary tract symptoms
MRI	Magnetic resonance imaging
MS	Multiple sclerosis
OAB	Overactive bladder
OMT	Optimal medical therapy
PTNS	Percutaneous tibial nerve stimulation
QAYL	Quality adjusted life years
QoL	Quality of life
SNM	Sacral neuromodulation

Introduction

Overactive bladder (OAB) is a common urologic condition that affects both men and women, with a prevalence of 16.5–23.3% in the United States [1, 2]. This represents a significant public health burden which carries an associated $65.9 billion annual expenditure on the management of OAB [3]. The social burden of OAB is also notable. The symptoms of OAB are detrimental to a patient's work, relationships, social events, exercise, and sleep, and they ultimately lead to reduced quality of life and productivity [4]. While lifestyle changes and oral medication have been successful in the management of OAB, sacral neuromodulation (SNM) was developed for patients refractory to these interventions. This chapter will focus on the use of SNM in patients with overactive bladder syndrome.

J. R. Michalak · S. Kim · J. T. Funk · C. O. Twiss (✉)
Division of Urology, Department of Surgery, University of Arizona College of Medicine, Tucson, AZ, USA
e-mail: johnmichalak@email.arizona.edu; sunchinkim@email.arizona.edu; jfunk@surgery.arizona.edu; ctwiss@surgery.arizona.edu

Summary of OAB

Definitions and Terminology

OAB has been defined by the International Continence Society (ICS) Standardization Committee as urinary urgency, with or without incontinence, usually with increased daytime frequency and nocturia in the absence of infection or other obvious pathology [5]. Other terms that have been used interchangeably with OAB include urge syndrome or urgency-frequency syndrome. It should be noted that OAB is a symptomatic diagnosis, distinct from detrusor overactivity, which is a urodynamic observation characterized by involuntary detrusor contractions during the filling phase of the cystometrogram [5].

J. P. Gilleran, S. A. Alpert (eds.), *Adult and Pediatric Neuromodulation*, https://doi.org/10.1007/978-3-319-73266-4_3

Urgency is the hallmark symptom of OAB, causing patients the most bother and carrying the greatest influence on quality of life, anxiety, and depression [6, 7]. Urgency is a sudden compelling desire to pass urine that is difficult to defer [5]. This is often accompanied by a fear of leakage. Involuntary leakage of urine which accompanies or immediately precedes the sensation of urgency is termed urge urinary incontinence (UUI) [5].

Epidemiology

The National Overactive Bladder Evaluation (NOBLE) study was a nationwide, randomized, case-controlled study demonstrating that the prevalence of OAB in the United States is 16.5%. Further breakdown revealed that 10.4% had OAB without UUI ("dry OAB"), and that 6.1% had OAB with UUI ("wet OAB"). The overall prevalence of OAB was similar in men (16%) and women (16.9%). Men were found to have a higher rate of dry OAB (13.4% in men vs. 7.6% in women), while women were more likely to experience wet OAB (2.6% in men vs. 9.3% in women) [2].

Data from other epidemiologic studies, including EpiLUTS and OAB-POLL, have shown higher prevalence rates in the United States, the UK, and Sweden, with rates increasing as the population ages [4, 7]. These studies also focused on factors contributing to OAB, including age and race. African-Americans had a higher prevalence of OAB compared to Caucasian, Hispanic, or Asian participants.

Pathophysiology

The origin of OAB is multifactorial, with neurogenic, myogenic, or idiopathic components likely contributing to its etiology. Disturbances of the nervous system, urothelium, or any component of the urinary bladder can contribute to the development of OAB.

The sensation of urgency is thought to originate in the urothelium and suburothelium, where the firing of afferent nerves is mediated by the release of inflammatory cytokines and growth factors [8–10]. These afferent nerve fibers include fast-conduction A delta fibers, which convey a sensation of distention and contraction, and slow-conduction unmyelinated C fibers, which respond primarily to chemical irritation or thermal stimuli of the bladder mucosa [11–13]. In the physiologic state, C fibers are significantly less active than A delta fibers. During certain pathophysiologic states, C fibers are recruited or overexpressed, leading to an increase in their contribution to afferent sensory information [14]. It is theorized that this inappropriately high level of sensory activity manifests as the symptoms of OAB.

Additional hypotheses have been proposed regarding the pathophysiology of OAB. The neurogenic hypothesis suggests that OAB arises from generalized, efferent nerve-mediated excitation of the detrusor muscle in which there is loss of tonic inhibition, resurgence of primitive spinal reflexes, and sensitization of afferent nerves [15]. The myogenic hypothesis suggests that OAB results from increased likelihood of spontaneous excitation within the smooth muscle of the bladder [16, 17]. This is supported by findings of patchy denervation in bladders with OAB, which leads to upregulation of surface membrane receptors, altering membrane potential and increasing the likelihood of contraction [18]. Finally, the integrative hypothesis suggests that a multitude of triggers can generate small, focused, microcontractions, which propagate throughout the bladder, ultimately resulting in coordinated, global bladder contractions [19]. These small contractions, also called micromotions, may be involved in the generation of the sensation of urgency [20].

The exact mechanism for how neuromodulation affects OAB symptoms is not completely understood. Evidence suggests that neuromodulation most likely activates the somatic sacral afferent axons, causing inhibition at the spinal and supraspinal levels, and thereby suppresses interneuronal transmissions involved in both the storage and emptying reflexes in the bladder [21–24].

Management of OAB

Guidelines for the treatment of overactive bladder have been published by the AUA [25]. Since OAB is bothersome but not life threatening, observation/non-treatment may be an acceptable plan for some patients, given adequate discussion of the risks and benefits of the available treatment options.

First-line treatment for OAB involves conservative management with behavioral, lifestyle, and environmental modification. This can include various combinations of diet and fluid intake modifications, changes in voiding habits, and pelvic floor rehabilitation. Although conservative management strategies may not result in complete symptom relief, they can improve quality of life by significantly reducing urinary urgency, frequency, and incontinence episodes [26–29].

When conservative management fails, second-line treatments include antimuscarinics and beta-3-adrenoceptor agonists. There is no compelling Level 1 evidence demonstrating superior efficacy for one antimuscarinic medication over another [30–32]. However, patients who do not experience adequate symptom relief with one antimuscarinic may have a better response to another of the same class [33–35]. The main barrier to antimuscarinic therapy is poor compliance. The attrition rate is 24–50% at 1 year, which is primarily a consequence of the side effects (dry mouth, constipation, dry eyes, and impaired cognitive function) [36, 37]. Extended release formulations offer the advantage of reduced side effects and should preferentially be prescribed over immediate release formulations [38]. Additionally, frail and/or elderly patients are particularly susceptible to the cognitive side effects of antimuscarinics [39]. Quaternary ammonium compounds such as trospium, which have minimal entry into the CNS, are less likely to cause confusion and disorientation [35].

Beta-3 adrenoceptor agonists also promote detrusor smooth muscle relaxation and bladder filling. The only currently available beta-3 agonist is mirabegron, which significantly reduces the frequency of voids and incontinence episodes per day [39–41]. The typical side effects of anticholinergics are not seen with mirabegron [42]. This may be especially advantageous for those patients at risk for cognitive impairment, although this side effect has not been directly studied in any trial comparing mirabegron and anticholinergics [43].

The third-line treatments for OAB include onabotulinumtoxinA, percutaneous tibial nerve stimulation (PTNS), and sacral neuromodulation (SNM). Intravesical onabotulinumtoxinA significantly reduces incontinence episodes and urgency [44–46]. The risks include acute urinary retention, straining to void, gross hematuria, UTI, and general weakness [47, 48]. PTNS is an option for patients with moderately severe baseline levels of incontinence and frequency. The literature demonstrates that PTNS can improve incontinence, frequency, nocturia, and quality of life, with the benefit of minimal adverse events [49–51]. SNM can be offered to patients with severe or refractory OAB who are willing and able to undergo surgery. Success rates range from 62 to 90%, with overall improvement in quality of life and significant reduction in voids and incontinence episodes per day [52–54]. Risks include pain at the implant site, lead migration, infection, undesirable sensations, and adverse changes in bowel function.

Sacral Neuromodulation for OAB: A Brief History

In 1981, Tanagho and Schmidt initiated a small case series of SNM demonstrating improvement in medication-refractory OAB symptoms [55]. This was followed by a large, multicenter trial demonstrating significant improvement in episodes of urgency, urge incontinence, and voids per day in patients with medication-refractory OAB. FDA approval of SNM for the treatment of refractory urge incontinence was obtained in September 1997, and the indications were later broadened to include refractory urgency and frequency of micturition [56].

The majority of the early literature examining SNM for OAB demonstrated reasonable success rates (62–90%), but also reported frequent adverse events, including pain at the stimulator site or lead site (up to 34% of patients), lead migration (8.6% of patients), infection/irritation (14.3% of patients), electric shock (7.9% of patients), and need for surgical revision (30–40%) [52–54]. The rates of adverse events and surgical revision in these series were significantly higher than those reported in modern studies primarily due to the fact that abdominal placement of the intermittent pulse generator, which is associated with increased rates of surgical revision, was standard technique prior to 2001. Additionally, the lead was placed through an open sacral incision, as compared with the modern, minimally invasive approach using a tined lead under fluoroscopic guidance.

Advances in surgical technique have led to a reduction in adverse events. Scheepens and colleagues were among the first to relocate the generator to a subcutaneous gluteal pocket, an innovation that reduced the number of incisions from 3 to 2 and more than halved the rate of pain-related adverse events to 10% [57]. The advent of the self-anchoring tined lead reduced the number of technical failures and improved success rates of the testing phase significantly, from 60 to 80% [58, 59]. Hijaz and Vasavada reported that the tined lead reduced the incidence of lead migration to less than 1%, compared with a prior rate of 8.4% [60]. The overall surgical revision rate utilizing the tined lead was 12.2% for stage I and 20% for stage II, compared with historical rates of 33–40% [52–54].

Recent publications continue to reveal a decline in high-grade complications with further advancement and minimization of surgical intervention. Modern trials report surgical revision rates of 3–16% as compared to a prior average of 42% [61, 62].

Currently, SNM has been implanted in over 200,000 patients worldwide and continues to be a popular and efficacious option for patients suffering from refractory overactive bladder symptoms [63].

Patient Selection, Evaluation, and Counseling

Patient Selection and Contraindications

An appropriate candidate for SNM has failed both conservative behavioral therapy and an adequate trial of medications. Alternatively, patients who refuse or harbor contraindications to pharmacotherapy may proceed directly to SNM. There are no defined clinical factors, urodynamic or otherwise, which predict a favorable response to SNM. Currently, a trial of stimulation is the only reliable means of predicting success with a fully implanted SNM.

There are several basic clinical factors that must be considered. Patients must be reasonably compliant and possess the mental and physical capacity necessary to manage their device settings and judge the clinical outcome of the stimulation trial. There is no maximum age limit although patients greater than 55 years of age experience lower success rates [64]. Patients with degenerative disorders or congenital anatomic disorders of the spine or sacrum may have foraminal stenosis or abhorrent anatomy, precluding access to the sacral nerves.

Contraindications may include necessity of future MRI and pregnancy. Because magnetic fields produce currents in electrodes, there is a theoretic risk of damage to the pulse generator. Currently, all available literature demonstrates that MRI may be safely performed in patients with an InterStim® device with no incidence of adverse events, provided that the device has been completely turned off and is out of the isocenter of the MRI scanner (outside of the magnet bore) [65–67]. Despite this, manufacturer recommendations allow only for an MRI of the head, if the device is turned off and a 1.5-Tesla magnet or lower is used [68].

SNM is still contraindicated in pregnancy due to the theoretical potential for teratogenicity or abortion. Whether or not sacral neuromodulation can induce abortion or fetal malformation is not known. Yaiesh and colleagues found no impact on the rate of preterm labor, pregnancy complications, or postnatal effects on either mother or offspring [69]. Women with an indwelling SNM device who become pregnant are recommended to deactivate their devices until delivery.

Patient Counseling

Patients should be aware that SNM carries a relatively frequent incidence of adverse events, including pain at the stimulator site or lead site (7–10%), undesirable change in stimulation (12%), lead migration (1%), infection (3%), and need for surgical revision (3–16%) [61, 62, 70]. SNM patients should understand that, although the majority of studies demonstrate high rates of durable efficacy, they are predominantly small, single cohort, prospective studies with an AUA/SUFU evidence strength recommendation of grade C. Finally, patients should be aware that the devices have a finite lifespan and will require periodic replacement for battery depletion or mechanical deterioration, and that the length of time between replacements will vary between patients (mean 62.5 months) [71].

Patient Evaluation

In addition to a history and physical examination, a urinalysis is routinely performed [72]. Urine cytology can be obtained at the discretion of the clinician, but should be considered in patients at risk for urothelial carcinoma (e.g., smokers). Use of a voiding diary is critical to document and establish an objective measure of the patient's urinary complaints. This should be utilized throughout the patient's evaluation, from baseline pre-assessment through the trial phase, which will be used to evaluate the patient's candidacy for permanent implantation (>50% improvement in symptoms).

There are no established urodynamic findings predictive of a favorable response to sacral neuromodulation [73]. Therefore, urodynamic evaluation should be performed on a selected basis or in complicated patients to provide further objective data to complement the voiding diary. Cystourethroscopy is also an optional adjunctive preoperative study that can reveal anatomic anomalies such as urethral stenosis or stricture, bladder lesions, or a urethral diverticulum which may impact the ultimate management of the patient.

Guidelines and Evidence

Guidelines

The 2014 AUA/SUFU guidelines for the treatment of OAB recommend sacral neuromodulation as a third-line option (Level C evidence), after failure of an adequate trial of first-line therapy (8–12 weeks of behavior/lifestyle changes) and second-line therapy (4–8 weeks of an antimuscarinic and/or beta 3 agonist) for OAB symptoms. The panel notes that SNM may be offered as a second-line therapy in patients who are unwilling or unable to trial pharmacotherapy [54].

Similar to the AUA, the EAU recommends conservative behavioral modification as first line, followed by pharmacotherapy. Patients with refractory symptoms should be offered SNM before bladder augmentation or urinary diversion is considered (Grade A).

The Evidence for Sacral Neuromodulation

Retrospective and Prospective Case Series

The majority of the early literature following FDA approval consisted of single group observational studies [52, 56, 57, 59, 60, 74–76]. The cohorts were primarily middle-aged females with severe, medication-refractory symptoms. Despite high rates of adverse events, these studies generally showed promising results, with significant improvement in nearly all measured parameters (voids/day, incontinence episodes/day, volume/void) and quality of life (QoL) scores. Success rates ranged from 62 to 90%. Interpretation of these results is complicated by the fact that the studies often included patients with varying indications for SNM, or patients with more than one indication for SNM (e.g., pelvic pain and sexual dysfunction in addition to OAB). These patients were frequently lumped into a single cohort in the final analysis, making it difficult to assess the impact of SNM on QoL as it relates specifically to OAB.

More recent literature continues to demonstrate success in the majority of trial participants with continually declining rates of adverse events (Table 3.1). Aboseif et al. published one of the earliest prospective trials examining SNM in 44 patients with medication-refractory OAB [74]. Seventy-seven percent of the patients experienced a 50% or greater improvement in symptoms and QoL, with a mean follow-up of 2 years. There was a significant reduction in episodes of UUI per day and pad use. Patients with frequency-urgency also showed a reduction in voids per day (from 17.9 to 8.6), with a nearly 100% increase in voided volume. Notably, patients also experienced a decrease in severity of pain. In contrast to other trials at the time, these patients underwent minimally invasive lead placement and sacral IPG implantation, likely contributing to their relatively lower rate of surgical revision at 18.7%.

Van Kerrebroeck et al., Marcelissen et al., and Groen et al. reported more modest success rates in their OAB cohorts (62%, 65%, 62%, respectively) [71, 77, 78]. These three studies are notable for an average follow-up of nearly 5 years. The three studies reported significant improvements in reduction of voids per day, reduction in pads per day, and increase in voided volume. Interestingly, Groen et al. experienced a wane in efficacy over time, from 87% success at 1 month down to 62% at the conclusion of the study at 5 years. Lastly, these three studies reported higher rates of surgical revision (40%, 33%, 39%, respectively), when compared with the contemporary literature. The most likely explanation is that these studies included patients throughout the full history and evolution of SNM surgical technique and the associated higher revision rates of early techniques.

Cardarelli et al. and Moon et al. followed their cohorts for shorter durations of 11 and 12 months, respectively [79, 80]. Cardarelli et al. reported significant decreases in UUI episodes, frequency, nocturia, and pad use as well as significant increases in voided volumes at 48 weeks post-implant. Moon et al. evaluated OAB-wet and OAB-dry patients as separate cohorts. Both groups experienced significant decreases in frequency, UUI, urgency episodes, and nocturia at statistically similar rates. OAB questionnaire scores improved as did all tested urodynamic parameters.

Randomized Trials

There is a relative paucity of randomized, prospective trials comparing SNM to other treatment modalities. Designing such a trial is challenging due to the difficulty in recruiting patients who must be prepared to accept randomization to one of two completely different treatment modalities with different risk profiles. Additionally, a truly blinded study will likely never be realized, given the ethical considerations of implanting a sham device without the potential of any actual benefit.

Despite this, there are several well-designed randomized, non-blinded trials. Schmidt et al.

Table 3.1 Prospective cohort studies examining the effectiveness of SNM for OAB

	Voids/day	UUI/day	Pads/day	Volume/void (mL)	Success rate	Surgical revision rate	Follow-up (months)	Mean age
Aboseif et al. 2002 [74]	−9.3*	−4.4*	−2.3*	+130*	77%	18.7%	24	47
Groen et al. 2011 [78]	−2.9*	−5.7*	−2.9*	+44*	62%	39%	60	48
Marcelissen et al. 2010 [71]	−2*	−3.7*	−2.3*	+32*	65%	33%	53	49
Van Kerrebroeck et al. 2007 [77]	−4.5*	−5.7*	−3.2*	+72.9*	62%	40%	60	45
Cardarelli et al. 2012 [79]	−4.8*	−2.6*	−2.1*	+63.1*	NR	14%	11	58
Al-Zahrani et al. 2011 [94]	NR	NR	NR	NR	85%	39%	51	54
Moon et al. 2013 [80]	−11.9*	−7.1*	−2.5*	+31*	NR	NR	12	54

Success in each study is defined as percent of patients reporting >50% improvement in symptoms at conclusion of study period

$*p = <0.05$

conducted the first prospective, randomized trial comparing SNM to optimal medical therapy (OMT) for 6 months [56]. This study demonstrated that daily incontinence episodes, severity of episodes, and pads per day used were significantly reduced in the SNM cohort compared to the OMT cohort. In the SNM cohort, the overall success rate was 76%, with 47% of patients becoming completely dry. This efficacy was maintained at 18 months of follow-up. The overall surgical revision rate was 33%. Complications included pain at the IPG site in 16%, infections in 19%, and lead migration in 7%.

Hassouna et al. reported on the outcomes of a similarly designed study, which randomized refractory OAB patients to either SNM implantation or OMT for 6 months [75]. The SNM cohort experienced statistically significant improvements in number of daily voids, volume per void, and degree of urgency compared to the OMT group. The devices were then turned off and urinary symptoms returned to baseline levels. The stimulators were then reactivated and prior levels of efficacy were documented at 12 and 24 months follow-up.

Weil et al. randomized 44 patients to either SNM or continuation of conservative management [76]. At 6 months follow-up, the SNM cohort demonstrated significantly lower rates of incontinence (88%), incontinence severity (24%), and pad use (90%) when compared with the corresponding control group. Additionally, SNM resulted in a 220% increase in bladder volume at first contraction and a 39% increase in maximum capacity on urodynamics. However, this study was significantly affected by attrition bias, with only 76% of the original SNM cohort being available for evaluation at the conclusion of the study.

More recently, Siegel and colleagues randomized 147 OAB refractory patients 1:1 to SNM and OMT in a prospective, multicenter, clinical trial [81]. The primary outcome was overall therapeutic success, defined as demonstrating either a ≥50% improvement in average leaks/day or voids/day from baseline or a return to normal voiding frequency (<8 voids/day). At 6 months follow-up, the study found significantly higher rates of subjective improvement in OAB symptoms (86% vs. 44%), overall therapeutic success (76% vs. 49%), and complete continence (39% vs. 21%) in the SNM group as compared to the OMT group, respectively. Additionally, the SNM cohort showed significantly greater improvement in scores assessing QoL, sexual function, and depression. The overall rate of adverse events in the SNM arm was 30.5%, compared with 27.3% in the OMT arm, which was not statistically different. One notable limitation of the study was the homogeneous nature of the study population (89% Caucasian and 93% female).

Long-Term Follow-Up of Sacral Neuromodulation for OAB

There are several recent literature reviews evaluating the long-term efficacy of SNM. Van Kerrebroeck et al. reported the results of a multicenter international trial of 163 participants with 5 years of follow-up demonstrating overall success rates for urgency-frequency at 56% and UUI at 68% [77]. Peeters et al. reviewed 217 patients who received an SNM over a 14-year span [62]. After a mean follow-up of 46.9 months, patients experienced success and cure rates of 70% and 20% for UUI, respectively, and 68% and 33% for urgency-frequency syndrome, respectively. Finally, Leong et al. assessed long-term satisfaction with SNM in 207 patients and reported that 90% of patients were satisfied with SNM at a median follow-up of 77 months [82].

SNM for OAB in Patients with Neurogenic Lower Urinary Tract Dysfunction

Currently, the only FDA-approved indications for SNM are: (1) urgency and frequency of micturition, (2) urge urinary incontinence, and (3) idiopathic or non-obstructive urinary retention. The studies that lead to FDA approval of SNM excluded patients with neurologic conditions, and SNM is not currently FDA approved to treat neurologic lower urinary tract dysfunction (LUTD) [56]. Nonetheless, this patient subset often suffers from severe urgency, frequency, and UUI, and currently available literature suggests that patients with neurogenic LUTD may benefit from SNM. In a recent meta-analysis, the success rate of SNM for neurogenic LUTD was 92% with adverse event rates and success/satisfaction rates comparable to non-neurogenic indications [83]. Although the majority of the studies was small and examined heterogeneous populations, this evidence suggests that neuromodulation is safe and effective in patients with neurogenic LUTD. This section will explore SNM in the treatment of neurogenic LUTD.

Spinal Cord Injury

In 1989, Tanagho and Schmidt reported on the ability of SNM to restore continence in patients with urgency incontinence secondary to suprasacral spinal cord injury (SCI) [84]. Since then, evidence supporting the use of SNM to treat OAB secondary to SCI has come primarily in the form of small case series. An Italian study evaluated 11 patients with incomplete spinal cord lesions and DO on urodynamics who underwent SNM for refractory neurogenic LUTD. Post-implantation, at a mean follow-up of 61 months, patients experienced significant improvements in voids per day, incontinence episodes, pads per day, mean voided volume, and nocturia [85]. On postoperative urodynamics, patients experienced an 84% increase in urodynamic bladder capacity and a 50% decrease in mean maximum detrusor pressure. A follow-up study from the same group evaluated six more SCI patients with isolated urge urinary incontinence. All patients demonstrated significant improvements in voiding diary parameters by at least 50% compared to baseline [86].

Chen and colleagues reported on the results of SNM in 23 patients with SCI and refractory OAB. Ultimately, 13 of 23 patients received permanent implantation, and the mean time between injury/disease onset and SNM test was 14.4 years. The mean rates of improvement for urgency/frequency and urinary incontinence were 64.7% and 69.2%, respectively, with all patients experiencing >50% improvement in their symptoms [87].

More recently, a review of 26 patients with OAB following SCI found no significant difference in the rate of neurogenic detrusor overactivity on pre- and post-implant urodynamics. In contrast, voids per day were significantly reduced and pads per day were significantly improved. Altogether, 94% of patients reported that they were either satisfied or very satisfied with the efficacy of their SNM device [88].

Multiple Sclerosis

Sacral neuromodulation has been studied as a potentially effective treatment for bladder disorders associated with multiple sclerosis (MS). Most patients with MS suffer from a spectrum of diverse LUTS, including detrusor overactivity, detrusor underactivity, and/or detrusor-sphincter dyssynergia. Management is complicated by progressive and often unpredictable deterioration in urinary function and by the fact that MS can disrupt both the storage and emptying phase of the micturition cycle.

As expected, studies examining SNM for MS patients are small. Minardi et al. studied a retrospective series of 25 MS patients with refractory LUTD with a mean duration of MS of 13.7 years. Ultimately, 15 of 25 patients experienced greater than 50% improvement in OAB symptoms and received a permanent SNM implant. Patients reported statistically significant improvements in incontinence episodes per day and voided volume at a mean follow-up of 49.4 months. In all of the nine patients who were on CIC, there was a significant decrease in residual volume, an increase in voided volume, and an increase in number of volitional voids per day [89].

Engeler et al. prospectively evaluated 17 patients with MS and refractory LUTS, excluding patients with unstable or rapidly progressive disease. All but one patient (94%) had a positive test phase, defined as a >70% improvement in symptoms. At 3 years, there were significant improvements in mean voided volume (from 125 to 265 mL), post-void residual (from 170 mL to 25 mL), urinary frequency (from 12 to 7 voids per day), and UUI (from 3 to 0 episodes per day). The median subjective degree of satisfaction was 80% [90].

More recently, Puccini et al. noted that the majority of studies of SNM in MS patients lacked homogeneity in their methods for evaluating outcomes and generally failed to offer an objective definition of cure. However, the authors reported that patients generally responded well to SNM and had high subjective reports of satisfaction with a mean of 85%. A notable observation was that the therapeutic effects of SNM persisted over time, even with follow-up as long as 7 years post-implantation. This suggests that the progressive nature of MS does not necessarily condemn the patient to fail SNM treatment [91].

Other Neurological Disorders (Stroke, Parkinson's Disease, Cerebral Palsy)

Scant data exists examining the impact of SNM on OAB in patients with a history of stroke, Parkinson's disease, or cerebral palsy. In general, the data shows that these patients benefit from a reduction in bothersome LUTS post-implantation at similar rates to patients without neurological disorders.

Wallace et al. reported on the results of a retrospective case series of 33 patients with neurologic disease and LUTD who underwent placement of a permanent SNM, including 6 with Parkinson disease, 13 with multiple sclerosis, and 11 others with various neurologic conditions. Incontinence episodes per 24 h decreased 68%, number of voids per 24 h decreased 43%, and nocturia decreased 70%. Overall, 93% of patients reported subjective satisfaction [92].

Peters and colleagues examined the outcomes of SNM in patients with (n = 71) and without (n = 269) a comorbid neurologic diagnosis, including 17 patients with a history of stroke, 13 patients with multiple sclerosis, 10 with Parkinson's disease, and 1 with cerebral palsy [93]. The rate of complications, revisions, and reprogramming sessions were similar between the two groups. Statistically significant improvements were seen in both groups on the OAB-q questionnaire and voiding diary variables, with the exception of incontinence episodes and incontinence severity in the neurologic disorders group. The majority of patients in both groups reported moderate or marked improvement at final follow-up.

Technique for Sacral Neuromodulation

Considerations

Once it has been established that a patient is an appropriate candidate for SNM, the implantation and surgical technique follows a two-step process. The first step is either (1) an office-based peripheral nerve evaluation (basic evaluation or PNE) using a temporary neurostimulator lead or (2) a formal staged test (advanced evaluation or Stage 1) where the permanent, tined neurostimulator lead is placed under fluoroscopic guidance in the operating room. There are particular advantages and disadvantages to each approach. The second step is dependent on which first step is utilized. In the case of a successful basic evaluation, both the permanent neurostimulator lead and pulse generator are implanted in the operating room at the same setting. In the case of a successful advanced evaluation, only the pulse generator needs to be placed since the permanent neurostimulator lead was already placed and positioned during the advanced evaluation.

Test Phase

The choice of test technique (advanced vs. basic evaluation) ultimately rests with the physician and there is no single "correct" approach. Some practices utilize a purely advanced evaluation approach whereas others will only use an advanced evaluation in cases of an equivocal basic evaluation. In our practice, we favor a staged approach utilizing the advanced evaluation given that use of the permanent neurostimulator lead for the evaluation has been shown to nearly double the response rate [95–97]. We reserve the office-based basic evaluation for selected patients who are younger, have less severe symptomatology, fewer comorbidities, or have concern regarding the invasiveness of an operating room procedure. Failure of a basic evaluation does not preclude proceeding to an advanced evaluation, and it is our practice to offer an advanced evaluation to patients who have a negative or equivocal result from a basic evaluation.

Basic Evaluation (Peripheral Nerve Evaluation)

A basic evaluation (peripheral nerve evaluation or PNE) is done in the office and is quick, convenient, and well tolerated by patients. The goal of the procedure is to place a temporary unipolar electrode in close approximation to the S3 nerve root. Typically, bilateral temporary leads are utilized and a standard Verify™ temporary pulse generator system is used to deliver the stimulation to either lead [98]. Details on this approach are provided in a separate chapter in this text, but we will discuss our own approach in comparison to the staged permanent lead placement.

The patient is placed in the prone position on the procedure table, and the lower back and buttocks are draped after prepping with a 4% chlorhexidine gluconate or iodine preparation. A grounding pad is attached to the patient's heel and connected to the hook electrode and Verify™ pulse generator unit to stimulate the nerve root. The landmarks utilized for a basic evaluation are identical to those used in an advanced evaluation. Initially, the tip of the coccyx is identified, and the midline is marked approximately 9–11 cm cephalad to this point. It is vital that the patient be positioned well so that the sacral region is relatively parallel to the operating table. This facilitates directing the 20-gauge insulated 3.5″ foramen needle into the S3 foramen. Once the midline point is identified, points 2 cm directly lateral to this on either side of the midline are marked with a skin marker. This is typically the approximate location of the S3 foramen (Fig. 3.1). It is optional to mark locations 2 cm cephalad and caudad to this point as individual anatomy will vary, and this may facilitate needle placement.

Next, the skin and subcutaneous tissues at both sites are infiltrated with local anesthesia. We use a 50/50 mixture of lidocaine and bupivacaine. Care should be taken to obtain anesthesia in the deep subcutaneous tissue but not in the foramen itself. The foramen needle is then inserted at an approximately 60° angle relative to the skin (Fig. 3.2) and down into the S3 foramen. Medial insertion of the needle in the foramen increases the chance of optimal sensation and a more tightly focused motor response [95, 99–101].

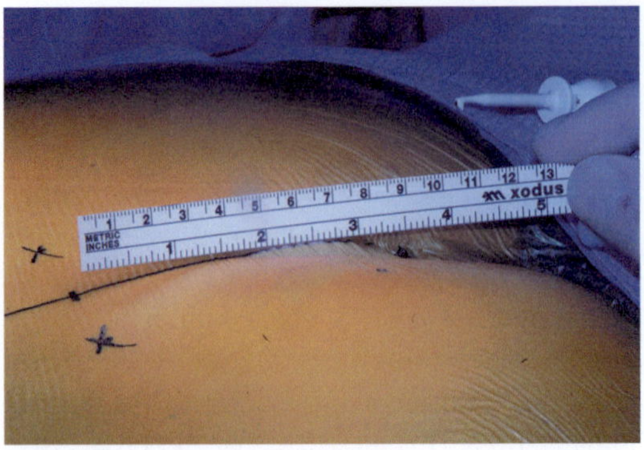

Fig. 3.1 Marking the approximate location of the S3 foramen 9–11 cm from the tip of the coccyx and 2 cm lateral to the midline

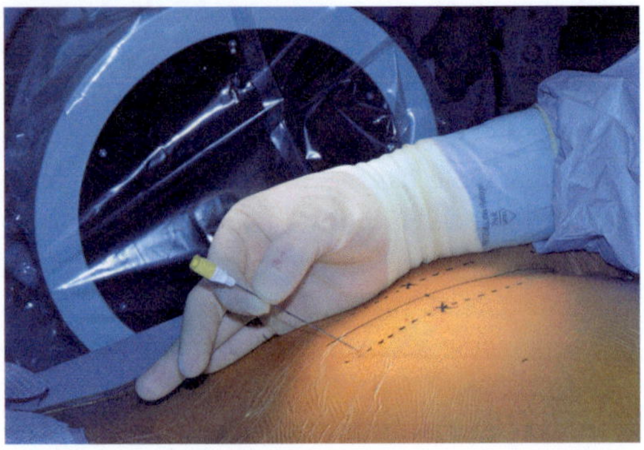

Fig. 3.2 The foramen needle is initially inserted at a 60° angle but often requires adjustment to successfully enter the S3 foramen. This subject ultimately required both angle adjustment and more cephalad placement of the needle on the skin due to flat sacral anatomy

Maintaining a needle course parallel to the midline is critical to successful placement. Frequently cannulation of the foramen requires "walking" the needle caudally or cranially on the sacrum. Longer in-and-out movement of the needle is better than short movements and is more efficient to needle placement. Additionally, individual anatomy will affect needle placement on the skin. We have found that a flat sacrum generally requires a more cephalad placement of the needle (Fig. 3.2) and at a more acute angle to the skin. Conversely, a curved sacrum often requires a more caudal needle insertion and at a less acute angle.

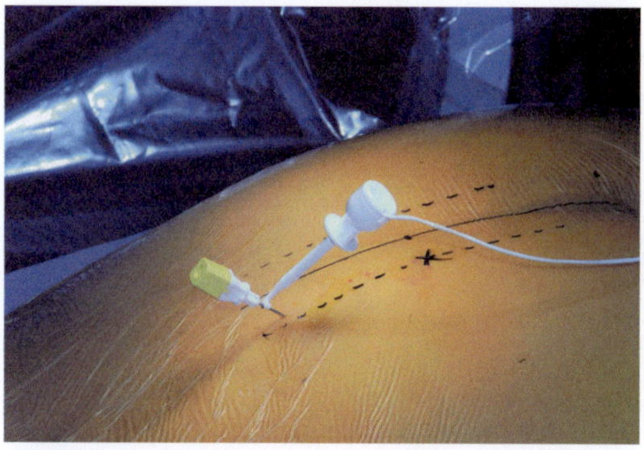

Fig. 3.3 Once in the S3 foramen, a test stimulation is performed with the hook electrode to elicit motor and sensory response in the patient

Once the foramen is cannulated, the needle is attached to the hook electrode and test stimulation is performed (Fig. 3.3). Correct needle placement will ideally result in both a motor and sensory response in the patient. If the needles are correctly positioned, there will be an inward and cephalad bellows movement of the pelvic floor muscles. Additionally, the ipsilateral hallux should contract in a plantar direction. The sensory cue is a deep "tapping" or "buzzing" sensation in the perineum. This can be described as perianal, perineal, or vaginal/labial in a female patient or the base of the penis/scrotum in a male patient. The importance of motor versus sensory response is a debated topic. Cohen et al. reported superiority of motor responses and recommended permanent electrode placement only in cases where motor responses were elicited [102]. Subsequently, Govaert et al. found an equal prognostic value of sensory or motor responses to the prediction of successful treatment [103]. Ideally, an anterior sensory location is more likely to result in a successful evaluation. In our practice, we strive to obtain both proper motor and sensory response during either temporary or permanent lead placement. We also attempt to ensure proper stimulation occurs at low voltages (ideally below 2 volts). Given that the temporary lead is not placed with fluoroscopy, we advocate testing both sides in a basic evaluation since the additional lead can aid in identification of better response for the patient on one side or the other [98].

Once the foramen needle location is satisfactory, the inner cannula is removed, and the unipolar lead is threaded through the needle. The needle is then carefully removed so as to not dislodge the lead. The leads are then secured to the patient with steri-strips and a sterile dressing is applied. One lead is initially connected to the test system, and the patient receives instruction on its use. We typically first utilize the lead that produced the better motor and sensory response during placement. The patient records daily symptoms on a voiding log.

The basic evaluation is typically carried out over 3–7 days. Our practice is to have the patient return to the office after 1 week to assess success or failure by reviewing the voiding diary and also to remove the temporary electrodes. Typically, prophylactic antibiotics are administered during the test phase while the unipolar electrode is in place. During the basic evaluation, we advise patients to avoid strenuous physical activity or excessive bending to help mitigate any chance of lead migration and subsequent lack of efficacy during the evaluation.

Advanced Evaluation (Stage 1 Permanent Lead Implantation)

An advanced evaluation is performed similarly to the basic evaluation but is done in the operating theater under fluoroscopic guidance. This affords the advantage of using the same quadripolar neurostimulator lead that resulted in a successful test for later attachment to the implanted pulse generator at Stage 2. Additionally, for patients with anxiety or limited mobility, the use of conscious sedation may ease lead placement and improve the success of the evaluation [95–97]. Though the invasiveness of the advanced evaluation is perceived by some patients to be greater than the basic evaluation, the techniques are quite similar, and it is typically well tolerated.

The patient receives an intravenous dose of appropriate antibiotics and the patient positioning is identical to the basic evaluation: prone on the operating room table, carefully padded with chest rolls and a pillow under the hips and feet such that the knees are bent. The lower back and

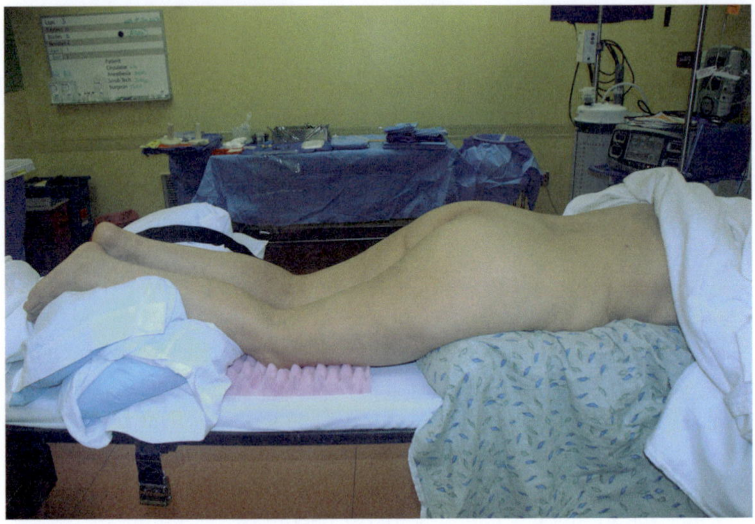

Fig. 3.4 The patient is positioned on a Jackson fluoroscopy table with chest rolls, a pillow under the hips, and pillows under the feet such that the knees are bent

buttocks are prepared in a sterile fashion. We prefer to use a Jackson fluoroscopy table which greatly facilitates efficient positioning of the fluoroscopy C-arm (Fig. 3.4).

Due the fact that the advanced trial is usually carried out over 2 weeks, we utilize a double skin preparation to minimize the possibility of infection. This consists of an initial prep with a chlorhexidine 4% solution, followed by a chlorhexidine/alcohol preparation such as ChloraPrep™. Based on surgeon preference, the use of an iodophor-impregnated barrier can also be utilized.

Landmark identification, demarcation, and local anesthesia are all delivered in an identical fashion to the basic evaluation. The addition of intravenous analgesia and amnesia improves patient comfort and relaxation throughout the advanced evaluation procedure. Good communication with the anesthesia provider is critical to avoid over sedation and resultant inability to assess sensory perception during an advanced evaluation. We have had excellent success with the use of dexmedetomidine as a continuous infusion. This allows for well-controlled anesthetic with reduced need for opioids and benzodiazepines and their associated respiratory and cardiovascular risks [104].

Placement of the foramen needles is expedited with the use of cross table and AP fluoroscopy. As noted previously, medial cannulation of the foramen is ideal to improve sensory and motor responses [99–101]. Furthermore, fluoroscopy allows for the easier identification of the S3 foramen level. This is especially true in the cross table view where the S3 foramen should be at the same cranio-caudal level as the iliac crests. Moreover, in the cross table view the S3 foramen is typically half the distance from the sacral promontory to the tip of the coccyx, and there is an anterior hillock or bump at its location (Fig. 3.5). In the AP view, the expected location of the S3 foramen is at the level of the sacroiliac joints [98].

Again, as in a basic evaluation, we advocate for cannulating both S3 foramina and testing both sides to optimize response and minimize voltage required for lead placement. The use of fluoroscopy allows for positioning of the foramen needle tips just anterior to the sacral periosteum.

Once a side has been selected for lead placement, the inner obturator is removed, a guidewire is placed through the needle, and a small skin incision is made to allow for passage of the dilator and its obturator. The depth of this placement is important to avoid a false passage for the quadripolar lead to travel away from the course of the S3 nerve. To avoid this, the radio-opaque marker on the dilator should be placed between 1/2 and 2/3 of the way across the width of the sacrum (Fig. 3.6). The obturator is then removed and the

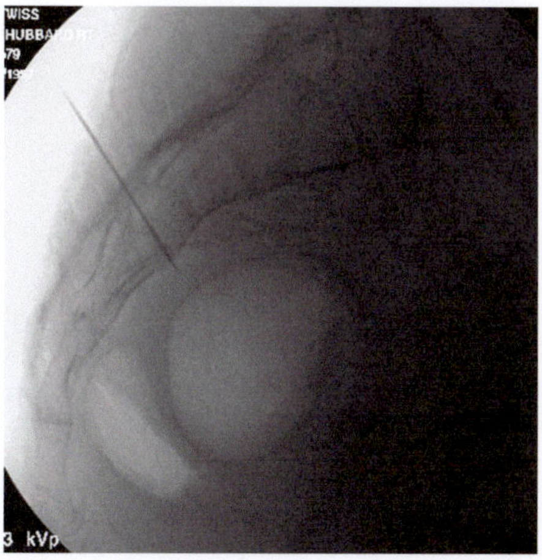

Fig. 3.5 Lateral fluoroscopy showing the foramen needle properly placed in the S3 foramen. Note that the location of the S3 foramen is roughly halfway between the sacral promontory and the tip of the coccyx and that there is a slight protuberance on the ventral surface of the sacrum at its location

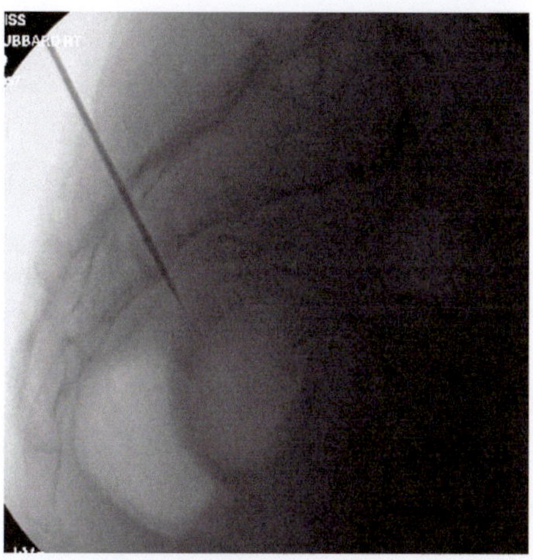

Fig. 3.6 The radio-opaque marker on the dilator is placed between 1/2 and 2/3 of the way across the width of the sacrum on lateral fluoroscopy

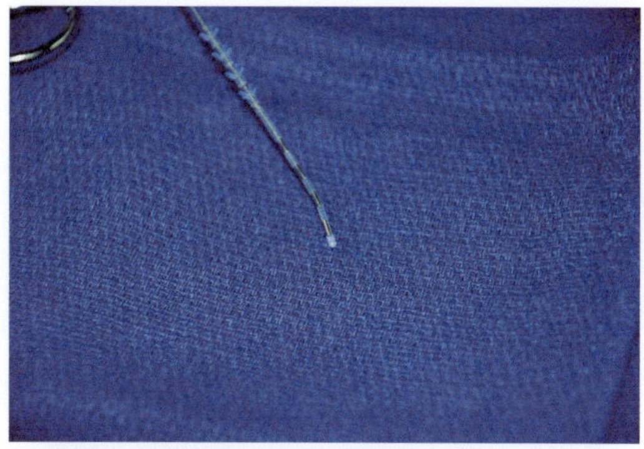

Fig. 3.7 The curved stylet angles the end of the neurostimulator lead during insertion and facilitates passage of the lead along the course of the S3 nerve

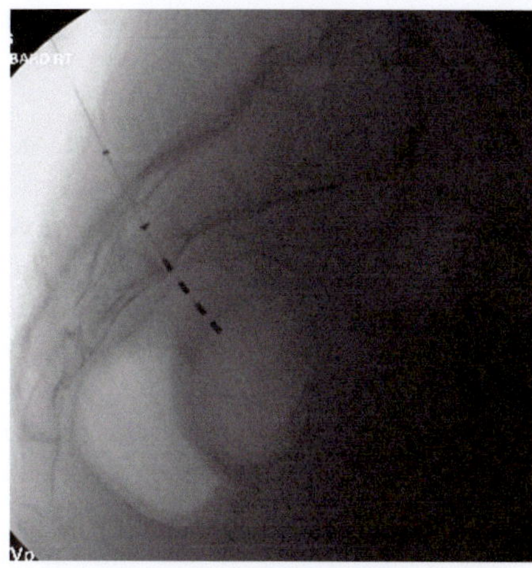

Fig. 3.8 The neurostimulator lead is first positioned with the fourth electrode just dorsal to the ventral surface of the sacrum on lateral fluoroscopy

permanent neurostimulator lead is passed through the dilator sheath. Lead insertion using a curved stylet (Fig. 3.7) as opposed to a straight stylet has been shown to improve response rates by positioning the contact points of the electrode in closer proximity to the course of the S3 nerve [105]. The lead should be inserted to the point where the fourth electrode is just dorsal to the ventral surface of the sacrum [98] (Fig. 3.8), although final location can vary as long as one has all four electrodes in contact with the nerve root.

At this point, test stimulation is again performed with the hook electrode on all four contact points of the lead. Subtle changes in response can be seen in comparison to the test stimulation done with the foramen needle. Ideally, there should be proper motor and sensory response upon stimulating each electrode [102, 103]. Once proper response has been confirmed, the dilator is slowly withdrawn while holding the electrode in place to prevent migration. It can be advantageous to have a fixed image on a second fluoroscopic screen for comparison during removal of

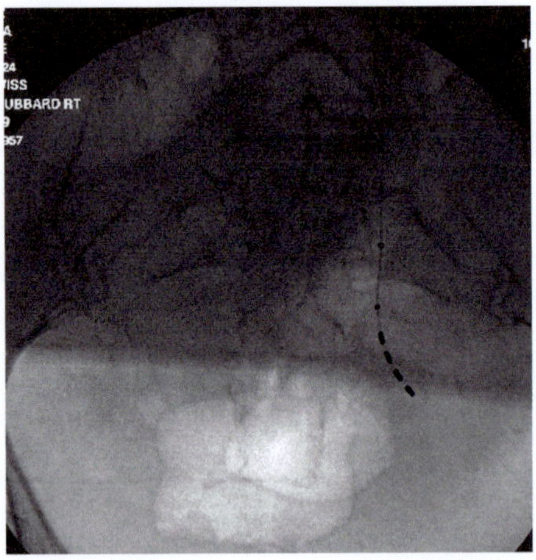

Fig. 3.9 The final AP view of the permanent neurostimulator lead showing the classic medial to lateral curve along the course of the S3 nerve

the dilator to ensure proper positioning. At this point, we perform one final test stimulation of all four contact points and record the voltage threshold associated with each electrode as reference points for initial IPG programming. The final AP position of the lead is also recorded on fluoroscopy (Fig. 3.9).

Next a separate area of skin is infiltrated with local anesthesia, and a 2–3 cm incision is made on the high lateral buttocks where the lead will be connected to the internal lead extension wire. We typically cross the midline and make the incision on the opposite side of lead placement, but an ipsilateral incision is also acceptable [95]. Electrocautery and blunt dissection is then utilized to develop a small subcutaneous pocket to accommodate the connection between the neurostimulator lead and the internal extension wire.

The tunneling device is then passed from the lead insertion incision to the gluteal incision, and the end of the neurostimulator lead passed into the gluteal incision (Fig. 3.10). The insulation boot is placed, and the extension wire is secured to the electrode using the provided torque wrench (Fig. 3.11). The insulation boot is then secured over this connection with a silk tie at either end (Fig. 3.12).

The end of the internal extension wire is then tunneled away from the gluteal incision

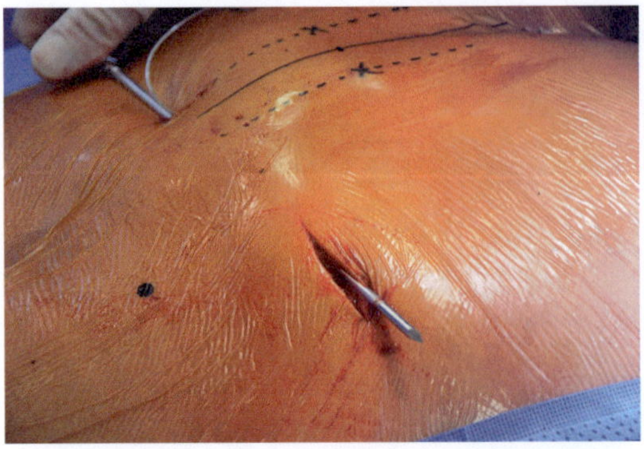

Fig. 3.10 The lead tunneling trocar is used to pass the end of the neurostimulator lead into the second incision where the internal lead extension wire will be connected

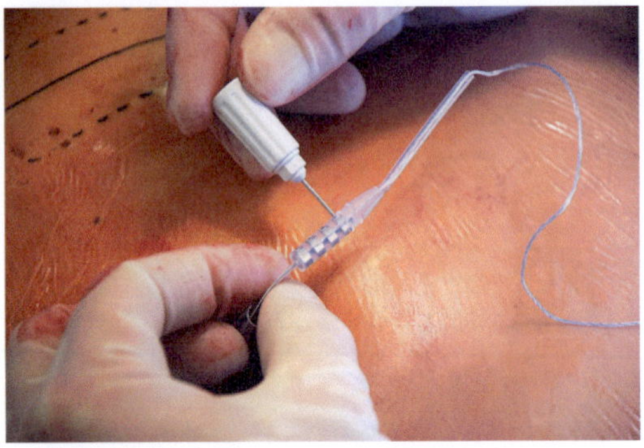

Fig. 3.11 The internal lead extension wire is connected to the neurostimulator lead by using the torque wrench to tighten all four contact screws

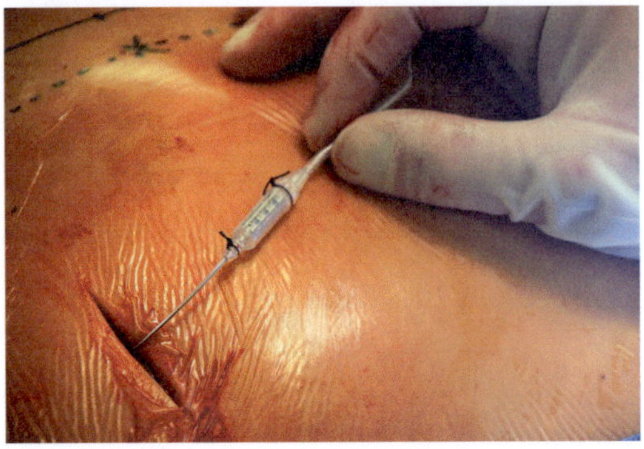

Fig. 3.12 The internal lead extension connection is sealed by covering it with the insulation boot which is fastened in place with two permanent sutures

and brought out of the skin medially in the lower back region (Fig. 3.13). The free end of the internal lead extension wire is then attached

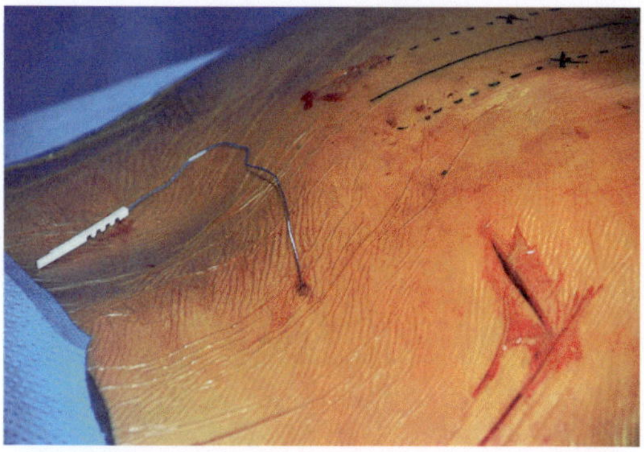

Fig. 3.13 The free end of the internal lead extension wire is tunneled out through a separate point on the skin of the lower back using the lead tunneling trocar

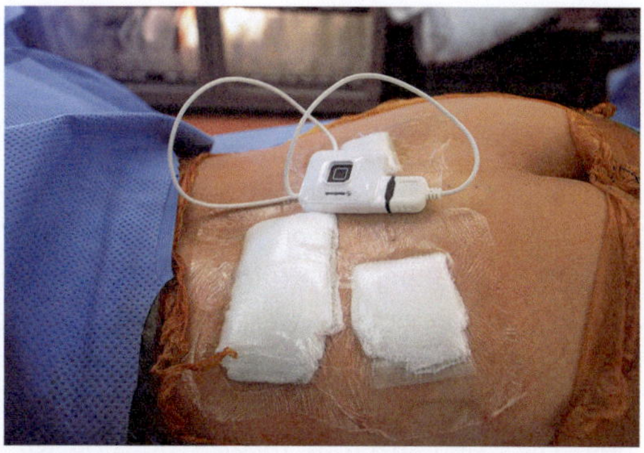

Fig. 3.15 The external lead extension wire is connected to the Verify™ external pulse generator device after all the incisions are covered with sterile dressings, and the Verify™ device is ready for programming

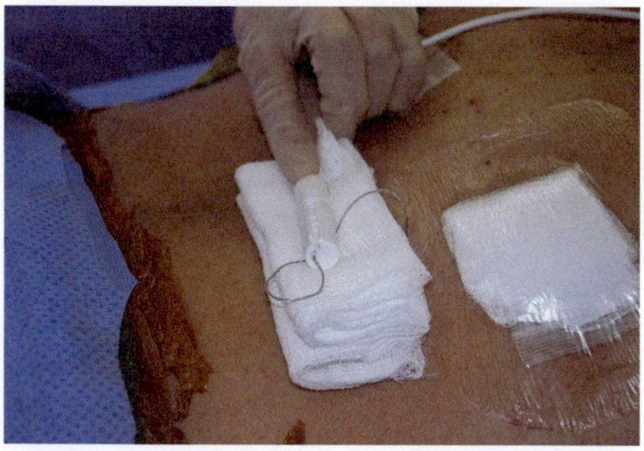

Fig. 3.14 The free end of the internal lead extension wire is connected to the Verify™ external lead extension wire, and the connection is covered with a sterile dressing

to the Verify™ external lead extension wire and a sterile dressing is applied (Fig. 3.14). The external lead extension wire connects to the Verify™ external pulse generator device (Fig. 3.15). Similar to a basic evaluation, the patient is placed on 5–7 days of prophylactic antibiotics targeted towards skin flora to decrease the likelihood of bacterial contamination of the electrode.

It is important to note that variability in sacral anatomy influences the placement, positioning, and success of either an advanced or basic evaluation. The surgeon must gain experience and knowledge over many cases to understand and adjust to these fine points of placement that can ultimately impact the likelihood of success or failure of the evaluation.

Pulse Generator Placement

The decision to proceed with placement of the pulse generator (IPG) is based on the degree of improvement in urinary frequency, urgency, and urge incontinence. If a basic or advanced evaluation is successful, then the patient proceeds to the operating room for IPG placement under either a local or general anesthetic, depending on surgeon and patient preference. If the patient underwent a successful basic evaluation, we strongly recommend that local anesthesia should be used for implantation of the permanent lead and IPG to permit sensory feedback from the patient during placement of the permanent neurostimulator lead.

Historically, three different implantable pulse generators (IPG) have been available: the InterStim® INC (Model 3023), the InterStim® II (Model 3058), and the InterStim® TWIN (Model 7427T) which can stimulate bilateral leads. This section will limit the discussion to the InterStim® II (Model 3058) pulse generator since it is the only model currently in production. Advantages of this model include smaller size of the implant itself and a streamlined, direct connection with the neurostimulator lead. Disadvantages of the Model 3058 are reduced battery capacity in comparison to the 3023 and the fact that it only connects to a single neurostimulator lead.

Pulse Generator Placement After Advanced Evaluation

The IPG placement proceeds with the same prepping and draping procedure as the advanced evaluation with dual skin prep using chlorhexidine 4% solution, followed by a chlorhexidine/alcohol preparation. The external extension wire and Verify™ device are removed prior to skin preparation. Fluoroscopy is not required for placement of the IPG after an advanced evaluation. The externalized tip of the extension wire can be prepped into the field or excluded from the field depending on surgeon preference. We typically exclude the distal end of the extension wire from the field. The previous incision from the advanced evaluation is anesthetized and the incision is opened and extended slightly to accommodate the IPG.

At this point, the connection between the permanent neurostimulator lead and the internal lead extension wire is exposed. The insulation boot covering the connection is removed and the wrench included with the IPG is used to disconnect the internal extension wire. Care needs to be taken to preserve the sterility of the incision while the internal extension wire is removed. In particular, the distal end must not contaminate the incision. In our technique, the extension wire is cut, and the proximal end is removed through the incision while the distal end (which we prep out of the surgical field) is removed by the circulating nurse.

Next, a subcutaneous pocket large enough to accommodate the IPG is developed with blunt dissection and/or electrocautery, and the IPG is attached to the neurostimulator lead using the torque wrench (Fig. 3.16). The IPG is placed into the pocket, and the incision is irrigated with antibiotic solution. The InterStim® logo etching on the IPG should be outward facing (i.e., the logo should face the surgeon) when it is placed into the pocket (Fig. 3.17). This ensures that there will be good communication between the IPG and the telemetry used to program it.

We advocate for a two-layer closure of the IPG pocket using absorbable sutures of the surgeon's preference. Steri-strips or surgical glue can then be applied, and the patient is transferred to the recovery room for device programming and patient education.

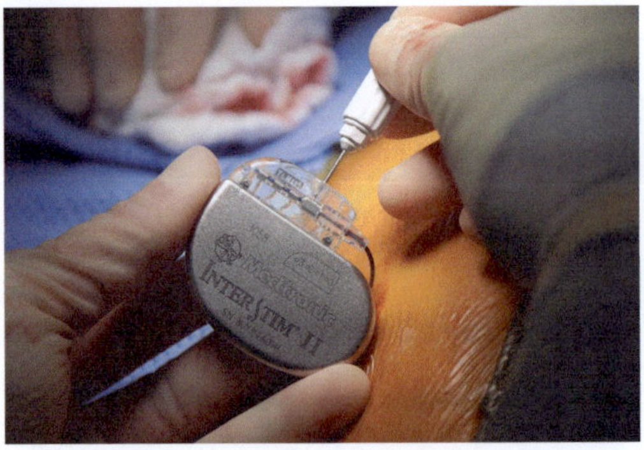

Fig. 3.16 The Model 3058 pulse generator connects directly to the free end of the neurostimulator lead by tightening the single set screw with the supplied torque wrench

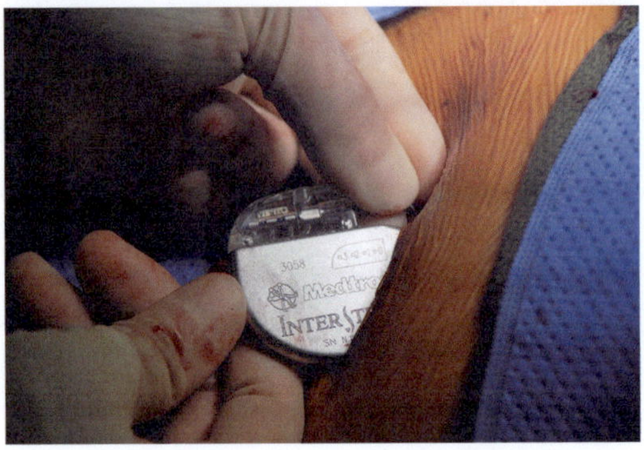

Fig. 3.17 The IPG is placed into its subcutaneous pocket with the InterStim® logo facing the surgeon to ensure good communication with the telemetry used to program the IPG

Pulse Generator Placement After Basic Evaluation

Placement of the IPG after a basic evaluation requires both insertion of the permanent neurostimulator lead under fluoroscopy and insertion of the IPG. This should be carried out with local anesthesia and sedation. The side of implantation of the permanent neurostimulator lead is selected based on the response observed during the basic evaluation. The technique for placement of the permanent lead is identical to placement of the permanent lead for an advanced evaluation without the need for connecting a lead extension wire. Instead, the IPG pocket is developed as described in the preceding section and the neurostimulator lead is tunneled into the IPG pocket. Then neurostimulator lead is connected to the IPG which is placed into the subcutaneous pocket as described above. The wound is irrigated with antibiotics and closed as described previously.

Cost-Effectiveness of SNM for the Management of OAB

The disease-specific total cost of OAB in the United States is an estimated $24.9 billion [106]. As expected, the upfront cost associated with SNM is substantial when compared to botulinum toxin A (BoNT-A), percutaneous tibial nerve stimulation (PTNS), or optimal medical therapy (OMT). However, it is also the most permanent of the interventions, offering the longest interval between repeat interventions with a decrease in overall cost expenditure over time. A US study evaluating healthcare expenditures 1 year after SNM implantation found a 73% reduction in office visit expenses from $994 to $265 per patient. There was also a significant decrease in diagnostic and therapeutic procedures leading to an additional $674 in savings per patient. Drug costs were also decreased from $693 to $483 per patient [107]. In another US study, Siddiqui et al. found that SNM was more expensive than BoNT-A ($15,743 vs. $4392) but possibly more effective (1.73 vs. 1.63 quality adjusted life years) than BoNT-A during a 2-year treatment period [108]. The ultimate conclusion was that SNM was less cost-effective than BoNT-A for refractory UUI. However, given the limited 2-year follow-up, one must consider how the additional cost of repeated BoNT-A injections over a longer time period would impact the cost-effectiveness comparison.

Three long-term European studies further explored the cost-effectiveness of SNM versus other therapies. These studies are each notable for their long evaluation period of 10 years. Autiero et al. evaluated the cost-effectiveness of SNM versus BoNT-A, PTNS, and OMT for patients with refractory OAB with respect to quality adjusted life years (QALY). At 10 years, SNM was less costly than the other therapies [109]. A study of the cost-effectiveness of SNM, BoNT-A, and OMT in refractory OAB patients within the Spanish healthcare system found that the 10-year cumulative costs of the three therapies were nearly equivalent. The QALY for SNM, BoNT-A, and OMT were 6.89, 6.38, and 5.12, respectively. Although the initial costs for SNM were higher, it was the economically preferred option in the long term given the decreasing follow-up costs and consistently greater efficacy [110]. Similarly, Bertapelle et al. assessed the cost-effectiveness of SNM and BoNT-A within the Italian healthcare system. They discovered that SNM was cost-effective at 3 years and became economically dominant (more effective and less costly) starting at 10 years post-implantation [111]. One Canadian study found that SNM was highly cost-effective when compared to either BoNT-A or OMT at 10 years of follow-up and recommended SNM as the preferred treatment option in the management of OAB refractory to conservative therapies [112].

Given the differing healthcare systems and economic climates in Europe and Canada, these results are not entirely applicable to the United States, but they do suggest that the long-term cost-effectiveness of SNM may be comparable to that of BoNT-A, PTNS, and OMT in patients with refractory OAB.

Conclusion

OAB affects a significant proportion of the adult population, and SNM is a valuable tool in the urologist's armamentarium for treating patients with refractory OAB symptoms. Although the neurophysiologic basis for SNM's therapeutic effects is not fully understood, the literature continues to support the efficacy of this treatment modality. Further work is required to decrease the rate of adverse events and optimize the cost benefit ratio of SNM therapy.

References

1. Coyne KS, Sexton CC, Bell JA, Thompson CL, Dmochowski R, Bavendam T, Chen CI, Quentin Clemens J. The prevalence of lower urinary tract symptoms (LUTS) and overactive bladder (OAB) by racial/ethnic group and age: results from OAB-POLL. Neurourol Urodyn. 2013;32:230–7.
2. Stewart WF, Van Rooyen JB, Cundiff GW, Abrams P, Herzog AR, Corey R, Hunt TL, Wein AJ. Prevalence and burden of overactive bladder in the United States. World J Urol. 2003;20(6):327–36.
3. Reynolds WS, Fowke J, Dmochowski R. The burden of overactive bladder on US Public Health. Curr Bladder Dysfunct Rep. 2016;11(1):8–13.
4. Coyne KS, Wein A, Nicholson S, Kvasz M, Chen CI, Milsom I. Comorbidities and personal burden of urgency urinary incontinence: a systematic review. Int J Clin Pract. 2013;67(10):1015–33.
5. Abrams P, Cardozo L, Fall M, Griffiths D, Rosier P, Ulmsten U, van Kerrebroeck P, Victor A, Wein A. The standardisation of terminology of lower urinary tract function: report from the standardisation sub-committee of the International Continence Society. Neurourol Urodyn. 2002;21:167–78.
6. Milsom I, Coyne KS, Nicholson S, Kvasz M, Chen CI, Wein AJ. Global prevalence and economic burden of urgency urinary incontinence: a systematic review. Eur Urol. 2014;65(1):79–95.
7. Milsom I, Kaplan SA, Coyne KS, Sexton CC, Kopp ZS. Effect of bothersome overactive bladder symptoms on health-related quality of life, anxiety, depression, and treatment seeking in the United States: results from EpiLUTS. Urology. 2012;80(1):90–6.
8. Birder L, Andersson KE. Urothelial signaling. Physiol Rev. 2013;93:653–80.
9. Birder L, de Groat W, Mills I, Morrison J, Thor K, Drake M. Neural control of the lower urinary tract: peripheral and spinal mechanisms. Neurourol Urodyn. 2010;29:128–39.
10. Andersson KE, McCloskey KD. Lamina propria: the functional center of the bladder? Neurourol Urodyn. 2014;33:9–16.
11. Janig W, Morrison JF. Functional properties of spinal visceral afferents supplying abdominal and pelvic organs, with special emphasis on visceral nociception. Prog Brain Res. 1986;67:87–114.
12. Habler HJ, Janig W, Koltzenburg M. Activation of unmyelinated afferent fibres by mechanical stimuli and inflammation of the urinary bladder in the cat. J Physiol. 1990;425:545–62.
13. Fall M, Lindstrom S, Mazieres L. A bladder-to-bladder cooling reflex in the cat. J Physiol. 1990;427:281–300.
14. Juszczak K, Ziomber A, Wyczolkowski M, Thor PJ. Urodynamic effects of the bladder C-fiber afferent activity modulation in chronic model of overactive bladder in rats. J Physiol Pharmacol. 2009;60:85–91.
15. de Groat WC. A neurologic basis for the overactive bladder. Urology. 1997;50:36–52.
16. Brading AF, Turner WH. The unstable bladder: towards a common mechanism. Br J Urol. 1994;73:3–8.
17. Brading AF. A myogenic basis for the overactive bladder. Urology. 1997;50:57–67.
18. Mills IW, Greenland JE, McMurray G, McCoy R, Ho KM, Noble JG, Brading AF. Studies of the pathophysiology of idiopathic detrusor instability: the physiological properties of the detrusor smooth muscle and its pattern of innervation. J Urol. 2000;163:646–51.
19. Drake MJ, Mills IW, Gillespie JI. Model of peripheral autonomous modules and a myovesical plexus in normal and overactive bladder function. Lancet. 2001;358:401–3.
20. Coolsaet BL, Van Duyl WA, Van Os-Bossagh P, De Bakker HV. New concepts in relation to urge and detrusor activity. Neurourol Urodyn. 1993;12:463–71.
21. Sukhu T, Kennelly MJ, Kurpad R. Sacral neuromodulation in overactive bladder: a review and current perspectives. Res Rep Urol. 2016;8:193–9.
22. Yoshimura N, de Groat WC. Patch clamp analysis of afferent and efferent neurons that innervated the urinary bladder of the rat. Soc Neurosci Abstr. 1992;18:127.
23. Yoshimura N, de Groat WC. Neural control of the lower urinary tract. Int J Urol. 1997;4:111.
24. Leng WW, Chancellor MB. How sacral nerve stimulation neuromodulation works. Urol Clin North Am. 2005;32:11–8.
25. Gormley EA, Lightner DJ, Burgio KL, Chai TC, Clemens JQ, Culkin DJ, Das AK, Foster HE Jr, Scarpero HM, Tessier CD, Vasavada SP, American Urological Association. Society of Urodynamics, Female Pelvic Medicine & Urogenital Reconstruction: diagnosis and treatment of overactive bladder (non-neurogenic) in adults: AUA/SUFU guideline. J Urol. 2012;188(6 Suppl):2455–63.
26. Fantl JA, Wyman JF, McClish DK, Harkins SW, Elswick RK, Taylor JR, Hadley EC. Efficacy of bladder training in older women with urinary incontinence. JAMA. 1991;265(5):609–13.
27. Jarvis GJ. A controlled trial of bladder drill and drug therapy in the management of detrusor instability. Br J Urol. 1981;53(6):565–6.
28. Goode PS, Burgio KL, Locher JL, Umlauf MG, Lloyd LK, Roth DL. Urodynamic changes associated with behavioral and drug treatment of urge incontinence in older women. J Am Geriatr Soc. 2002;50(5):808–16.
29. Kaya S, Akbayrak T, Beksac S. Comparison of different treatment protocols in the treatment of idiopathic detrusor overactivity: a randomized controlled trial. Clin Rehabil. 2011;25(4):327–38.
30. Arruda RM, Castro RA, Sousa GC, Sartori MG, Baracat EC, Girão MJ. Prospective randomized

comparison of oxybutynin, functional electrostimulation, and pelvic floor training for treatment of detrusor overactivity in women. Int Urogynecol J Pelvic Floor Dysfunct. 2008;19(8):1055–61.
31. Burgio KL, Locher JL, Goode PS, Hardin JM, McDowell BJ, Dombrowski M, Candib D. Behavioral vs drug treatment for urge urinary incontinence in older women: a randomized controlled trial. JAMA. 1998;280(23):1995–2000.
32. Song C, Park JT, Heo KO, Lee KS, Choo MS. Effects of bladder training and/or tolterodine in female patients with overactive bladder syndrome: a prospective, randomized study. J Korean Med Sci. 2006;21(6):1060–3.
33. Wyndaele JJ, Goldfischer ER, Morrow JD, Gong J, Tseng LJ, Guan Z, Choo MS. Effects of flexible-dose fesoterodine on overactive bladder symptoms and treatment satisfaction: an open-label study. Int J Clin Pract. 2009;63(4):560–7.
34. Zinner N, Noe L, Rasouliyan L, Marshall T, Seifeldin R. Impact of solifenacin on resource utilization, work productivity and health utility in overactive bladder patients switching from tolterodine ER. Curr Med Res Opin. 2008;24(6):1583–91.
35. Zinner N, Kobashi KC, Ebinger U, Viegas A, Egermark M, Quebe-Fehling E, Koochaki P. Darifenacin treatment for overactive bladder in patients who expressed dissatisfaction with prior extended-release antimuscarinic therapy. Int J Clin Pract. 2008;62(11):1664–74.
36. Benner JS, Nichol MB, Rovner ES, Jumadilova Z, Alvir J, Hussein M, Fanning K, Trocio JN, Brubaker L. Patient-reported reasons for discontinuing overactive bladder medication. BJU Int. 2010;105(9):1276–82.
37. Wagg A, Compion G, Fahey A, Siddiqui E. Persistence with prescribed antimuscarinic therapy for overactive bladder: a UK experience. BJU Int. 2012;110(11):1767–74.
38. Dmochowski RR, Sand PK, Zinner NR, Staskin DR. Trospium 60 mg once daily (QD) for overactive bladder syndrome: results from a placebo-controlled interventional study. Urology. 2008;71(3):449–54.
39. Herschorn S, Barkin J, Castro-Diaz D, Frankel JM, Espuna-Pons M, Gousse AE, Stolzel M, Martin N, Gunther A, Van Kerrebroeck P. A phase III, randomized, double-blind, parallel-group, placebo-controlled, multicentre study to assess the efficacy and safety of the beta(3) adrenoceptor agonist, mirabegron, in patients with symptoms of overactive bladder. Urology. 2013;82(2):313–20.
40. Nitti VW, Auerbach S, Martin N, Calhoun A, Lee M, Herschorn S. Results of a randomized phase III trial of mirabegron in patients with overactive bladder. J Urol. 2013;189(4):1388–95.
41. Chapple CR, Kaplan SA, Mitcheson D, Klecka J, Cummings J, Drogendijk T, Dorrepaal C, Martin N. Randomized double-blind, active-controlled phase 3 study to assess 12-month safety and efficacy of mirabegron, a beta(3)-adrenoceptor agonist, in overactive bladder. Eur Urol. 2013;63(2):296–305.
42. Warren K, Burden H, Abrams P. Mirabegron in overactive bladder patients: efficacy review and update on drug safety. Ther Adv Drug Saf. 2016;7(5):204–16.
43. Perk S, Wielage RC, Campbell NL, Klein TM, Perkins A, Posta LM, Yuran T, Klein RW, Ng DB. Estimated budget impact of increased use of mirabegron, a novel treatment for overactive bladder. J Manag Care Spec Pharm. 2016;22(9):1072–8.
44. Brubaker L, Richter HE, Visco A, Mahajan S, Nygaard I, Braun TM, Barber MD, Menefee S, Schaffer J, Weber AM, Wei J, Pelvic Floor Disorders Network. Refractory idiopathic urge urinary incontinence and botulinum A injection. J Urol. 2008;180(1):217–22.
45. Flynn MK, Amundsen CL, Perevich M, Liu F, Webster GD. Outcome of a randomized, double-blind, placebo controlled trial of botulinum A toxin for refractory overactive bladder. J Urol. 2009;181(6):2608–15.
46. Kuo HC. Bladder base/trigone injection is safe and as effective as bladder body injection of onabotulinumtoxinA for idiopathic detrusor overactivity refractory to antimuscarinics. Neurourol Urodyn. 2011;30(7):1242–8.
47. Orasanu B, Mahajan S. The use of botulinum toxin for the treatment of overactive bladder syndrome. Indian J Urol. 2013;29(1):2–11.
48. Kuo Y, Kuo H. Adverse events of intravesical onabotulinumtoxinA injection between patients with overactive bladder and interstitial cystitis—different mechanisms of action of Botox on bladder dysfunction? Toxins (Basel). 2016;8(3).
49. Peters KM, Macdiarmid SA, Wooldridge LS, Leong FC, Shobeiri SA, Rovner ES, Siegel SW, Tate SB, Jarnagin BK, Rosenblatt PL, Feagins BA. Randomized trial of percutaneous tibial nerve stimulation versus extended-release tolterodine: results from the overactive bladder innovative therapy trial. J Urol. 2009;182(3):1055–61.
50. Sancaktar M, Ceyhan ST, Akyol I, Muhcu M, Alanbay I, Mutlu Ercan C, Atay V. The outcome of adding peripheral neuromodulation (Stoller afferent neuro-stimulation) to anti-muscarinic therapy in women with severe overactive bladder. Gynecol Endocrinol. 2010;26(10):729–32.
51. Burton C, Sajja A, Latthe PM. Effectiveness of percutaneous posterior tibial nerve stimulation for overactive bladder: a systematic review and meta-analysis. Neurourol Urodyn. 2012;31(8):1206–16.
52. Siegel SW, Catanzaro F, Dijkema HE, Elhilali MM, Fowler CJ, Gajewski JB, et al. Long-term results of a multicenter study on sacral nerve stimulation for treatment of urinary urge incontinence, urgency-frequency, and retention. Urology. 2000;4(56):87–91.
53. Everaert K, Kerckhaert W, Caluwaerts H. A prospective randomized trial comparing the 1-stage with the

2-stage implantation of a pulse generator in patients with pelvic floor dysfunction selected for sacral nerve stimulation. Eur Urol. 2004;45:649–54.
54. National Guideline Clearinghouse (NGC). Guideline summary: Diagnosis and treatment of overactive bladder (non-neurogenic) in adults: AUA/SUFU guideline. In: National Guideline Clearinghouse (NGC) [Web site]. Rockville (MD): Agency for Healthcare Research and Quality (AHRQ); 2014 May 01. [cited 2016 Dec 01]. https://www.guideline.gov
55. Tanagho EA, Schmidt RA. Bladder pacemaker: scientific basis and clinical future. Urology. 1982;20(6):614–9.
56. Schmidt RA, Jonas U, Oleson KA, Jankgnegt RA, Hassouna MM, Siegel SW, et al. Sacral nerve stimulation for treatment of refractory urinary urge incontinence. Sacral Nerve Stimulation Study Group. J Urol. 1999;162(2):352–7.
57. Scheepens WA, Weil EH, van Koeveringe GA, Rohrmann D, Hedlund HE, Schurch B, et al. Buttock placement of the implantable pulse generator: a new implantation technique for sacralneuromodulation—a multicenter study. Eur Urol. 2001;40(4):434–8.
58. Hetzer FH. Fifteen years of sacral nerve stimulation: from an open procedure to a minimally invasive technique. Color Dis. 2011;13(2):1–4.
59. Spinelli M, Giardiello G, Arduini A, Van den Hombergh U. New percutaneous technique of sacral nerve stimulation has high initial success rate: preliminary results. Eur Urol. 2003;43(1):70–4.
60. Hijaz A, Vasavada S. Complications and troubleshooting of sacral neuromodulation therapy. Urol Clin North Am. 2005;32:65–9.
61. Siddiqui NY, JM W, Amundsen CL. Efficacy and adverse events of sacral nerve stimulation for overactive bladder: a systematic review. Neurourol Urodyn. 2010;29(Suppl 1):S18–23.
62. Peeters K, Sahai A, De Ridder D, Van Der Aa F. Long-term follow-up of sacral neuromodulation for lower urinary tract dysfunction. BJU Int. 2014;113(5):789–94.
63. Bladder and Bowel Community. Sacral Nerve Stimulation (Sacral Neuromodulation Therapy); [cited 2017 Jan 22]. https://www.bladderandbowelfoundation.org.
64. Amundsen CL, Romero AA, Jamison MG, Webster GD. Sacral neuromodulation for intractable urge incontinence: are there factors associated with cure? Urology. 2005;66(4):746–50.
65. Elkelini MS, Hassouna MM. Safety of MRI at 1.5Tesla in patients with implanted sacral nerve neurostimulator. Eur Urol. 2006;50(2):311–6.
66. Chermansky CJ, Krlin RM, Holley TD, Woo HH, Winters JC. Magnetic resonance imaging following InterStim®: an institutional experience with imaging safety and patient satisfaction. Neurourol Urodyn. 2011;30(8):1486–8.
67. Alsyouf M, Keheila M, Marinone M. Magnetic resonance imaging of the ankle performed on an InterStim patient. Can J Urol. 2016;23(1):8168–70.
68. MRI guidelines for InterStim Therapy Neurostimulation Systems. 1st ed. Medtronic, 2017; [2017 Jan 15]. https://professional.medtronic.com.
69. Yaiesh SM, Al-Terki AE, Al-Shaiji TF. Safety of sacral nerve stimulation in pregnancy: a literature review. Neuromodulation. 2016;19:770–9.
70. Noblett K, Benson K, Kreder K. Detailed analysis of adverse events and surgical interventions in a large prospective trial of sacralneuromodulation therapy for overactive bladder patients. Neurourol Urodyn. https://doi.org/10.1002/nau.23076. [Epub ahead of print].
71. Marcelissen TA, Leong RK, de Bie RA. Long-term results of sacral neuromodulation with the tined lead procedure. J Urol. 2010;184:1997–2000.
72. Wein AJ, Kavoussi LR, Partin AW, Peters CA. Campbell-Walsh Urology. 12th ed. Philadelphia, PA: Elsevier; 2016.
73. Groenendijk PM, Lycklama à Nyeholt AA, Heesakkers JP, van Kerrebroeck PE, Hassouna MM, Gajewski JB. Urodynamic evaluation of sacral neuromodulation for urge urinary incontinence. BJU Int. 2008;101(3):325–9.
74. Aboseif S, Tamaddon K, Chalfin S, Freedman S, Kaptein J. Sacral neuromodulation as an effective treatment for refractory pelvic floor dysfunction. Urology. 2002;60(1):52–6.
75. Hassouna MM, Siegel SW, Nyeholt AA. Sacral neuromodulation in the treatment of urgency-frequency symptoms: a multicenter study on efficacy and safety. J Urol. 2000;163:1849–54.
76. Weil EH, Ruiz-Cerdá JL, Eerdmans PH. Sacral root neuromodulation in the treatment of refractory urinary urge incontinence: a prospective randomized clinical trial. Eur Urol. 2000;37(2):161–71.
77. van Kerrebroeck EV, van Voskuilen AC, Heesakkers JP, et al. Results of sacral neuromodulation therapy for urinary voiding dysfunction: outcomes of a prospective worldwide clinical study. J Urol. 2007;178:2029–34.
78. Groen J, Blok BF, Bosch JL. Sacral neuromodulation as treatment for refractory idiopathic urge urinary incontinence: 5-year results of a longitudinal study in 60 women. J Urol. 2011;186(3):954–9.
79. Cardarelli S, D'Elia C, Cerruto MA, Curti P, Ostardo E, Signorello D, et al. Efficacy of sacral neuromodulation on urological diseases: a multicentric research project. Urologia. 2012;79(2):90–6.
80. Moon KH, Han JY, Kim JH, Lee HN, Lee KS, Lee JG, SJ O, Yoon HN, Choo MS. Prospective trial of sacral neuromodulation for refractory overactive bladder syndrome in Korean patients. Low Urin Tract Symptoms. 2013;6(3):175–9.
81. Siegel S, Noblett K, Mangel J, Griebling TL, Sutherland SE, Bird ET, et al. Results of a prospective, randomized, multicenter study evaluating sacral neuromodulation with InterStim therapy compared to standard medical therapy at 6-months in subjects with mild symptoms of overactive bladder. Neurourol Urodyn. 2015;34(3):224–30.

82. Leong RK, Marcelissen TA, Nieman FH. Satisfaction and patient experience with sacral neuromodulation: results of a single center sample survey. J Urol. 2011;185(2):588–92.
83. Kessler TM, La Framboise D, Trelle S, et al. Sacral neuromodulation for neurogenic lower urinary tract dysfunction: systematic review and meta-analysis. Eur Urol. 2010;58:865–74.
84. Tanagho EA, Schmidt RA, Orvis BR. Neural stimulation for control of voiding dysfunction: a preliminary report in 22 patients with serious neuropathic voiding disorders. J Urol. 1989;142:340–5.
85. Lombardi G, Del Popolo G. Clinical outcome of sacral neuromodulation in incomplete spinal cord injured patients suffering from neurogenic lower urinary tract symptoms. Spinal Cord. 2009;47(6):486–91.
86. Lombardi G, Nelli F, Mencarini M, Del Popolo G. Clinical concomitant benefits on pelvic floor dysfunctions after sacral neuromodulation in patients with incomplete spinal cord injury. Spinal Cord. 2011;49:629–36.
87. Chen G, Liao L. Sacral neuromodulation for neurogenic bladder and bowel dysfunction with multiple symptoms secondary to spinal cord disease. Spinal Cord. 2015;53:204–8.
88. Wöllner J, Krebs J, Pannek J. Sacral neuromodulation in patients with neurogenic lower urinary tract dysfunction. Spinal Cord. 2016;54(2):137–40.
89. Minardi D, Muzzonigro G. Sacral neuromodulation in patients with multiple sclerosis. World J Urol. 2012;30:123–8.
90. Engeler DS, Meyer D, Abt D. Sacral neuromodulation for the treatment of neurogenic lower urinary tract dysfunction caused by multiple sclerosis: a single-centre prospective series. BMC Urol. 2015;15:105.
91. Puccini F, Bhide A, Elneil S, Digesu GA. Sacral neuromodulation: an effective treatment for lower urinary tract symptoms in multiple sclerosis. Int Urogynecol J. 2016;27(3):347–54.
92. Wallace PA, Lane FL, Noblett KL. Sacral nerve neuromodulation in patients with underlying neurologic disease. Am J Obstet Gynecol. 2007;197(1):96.e1–5.
93. Peters KM, Kandagatla P, Killinger KA, Wolfert C, Boura JA. Clinical outcomes of sacral neuromodulation in patients with neurologic conditions. Urology. 2013;81(4):738–43.
94. Al-zahrani AA, Elzayat EA, Gajewski JB. Long-term outcome and surgical interventions after sacral neuromodulation implant for lower urinary tract symptoms: 14-year experience at 1 center. J Urol. 2011;185:981–6.
95. Spinelli M, Weil E, Ostardo E. New tined lead electrode in sacral neuromodulation: experience from a multicentre European study. World J Urol. 2005;23(3):225–9.
96. Peters KM, Carey JM, Konstandt DB. Sacral neuromodulation for the treatment of refractory interstitial cystitis: outcomes based on technique. Int Urogynecol J Pelvic Floor Dysfunct. 2003;14:223–8.
97. Scheepens WA, Van Koeveringe GA, De Bie RA, et al. Long-term efficacy and safety results of the two-stage implantation technique in sacral neuromodulation. BJU Int. 2002;90:840–5.
98. Medtronic: Manuals and Technical Resources; [cited 2017 Jan 15]. http://professional.medtronic.com/products/interstim-II-sacral-nerveneurostimulator/manuals-and-technical-resources/index.htm.
99. Benninghoff D. Anatomy. Urban & Fischer Verlag: München; 2003.
100. Amend B, Matzel KE, Abrams P, de Groat WC, Sievert KD. How does neuromodulation work. Neurourol Urodyn. 2011;30(5):762–5.
101. Swinn MJ, Schott GD, Oliver SE. Leg pain after sacral neuromodulation: anatomical considerations. BJU Int. 1999;84:1113–5.
102. Cohen BL, Tunuguntla HS, Gousse A. Predictors of success for first stage neuromodulation: motor versus sensory response. J Urol. 2006;175:2178–80.
103. Govaert B, Melenhorst J, Van Gemert WG, Baeten CG. Can sensory and/or motor reactions during percutaneous nerve evaluation predict outcome of sacral nerve modulation? Dis Colon Rectum. 2009;52:1423–6.
104. Candiotti KA, Bergese SD, Bokesch PM, Feldman MA, Wisemandle W, Bekker AY. Monitored anesthesia care with dexmedetomidine: a prospective, randomized, double-blind, multicenter trial. MAC Study Group. Anesth Analg. 2010;110(1):47–56.
105. Jacobs SA, Lane FL, Osann KE, Noblett KL. Randomized prospective crossover study of InterStim lead wire placement with curved versus straight stylet. Neurourol Urodyn. 2014;33(5):488–92.
106. Onukwugha E, Zuckerman I, et al. The total economic burden of overactive bladder in the United States: a disease-specific approach. Am J Manag Care. 2009;15(4 Suppl):S90–7.
107. Aboseif SR, Kim DH, Rieder JM. Sacral neuromodulation: cost considerations and clinical benefits. Urology. 2007;70(6):1069–74.
108. Siddiqui NY, Amundsen CL, Visco AG, Myers ER, Wu JM. Cost-effectiveness of sacral neuromodulation versus intravesical botulinum A toxin for treatment of refractory urge incontinence. J Urol. 2009;182(6):2799–804.
109. Autiero SW, Hallas N, Betts CD, Ockrim JL. The cost-effectiveness of sacral nerve stimulation (SNS) for the treatment of idiopathic medically refractory overactive bladder (wet) in the UK. BJU Int. 2015;116(6):945–54.
110. Arlandis S, Castro D, Errando C, Fernández E, Jiménez M, González P, et al. Cost-effectiveness of sacral neuromodulation compared to botulinum neurotoxin a or

continued medical management in refractory overactive bladder. Value Health. 2011;14(2):219–28.
111. Bertapelle MP, Vottero M, Popolo GD, Mencarini M, Ostardo E, Spinelli M, et al. Sacral neuromodulation and Botulinum toxin A for refractory idiopathic overactive bladder: a cost-utility analysis in the perspective of Italian Healthcare System. World J Urol. 2015;33(8):1109–17.
112. Hassouna MM, Sadri H. Economic evaluation of sacral neuromodulation in overactive bladder: a Canadian perspective. Can Urol Assoc J. 2015;9(7–8):242–7.

Neuromodulation for Non-obstructive Urinary Retention

4

C. R. Powell

Introduction

Non-obstructive urinary retention can be a challenging condition to treat. The prevalence of lower urinary tract symptoms (LUTS) in adult subjects residing in the USA, the UK, and Sweden is surprisingly high according to data from the 2009 EPILUTS project. LUTS is a widely encompassing term that includes urinary retention, and 72.3% of male respondents reported "at least sometimes" being bothered by one of the LUTS listed, while 76.3% of women reported being bothered [1].

Urinary Retention

LUTS imply that there are bothersome symptoms, but chronic urinary retention can be asymptomatic as well. In addition to this, it is difficult to estimate the prevalence of urinary retention in the USA and elsewhere since there is no standardized, generally agreed upon definition for urinary retention [2]. The most exact definition comes from the International Continence Society (ICS). This organization notes several important parameters to consider: (1) the ability of patient to release any urine (complete or partial), (2) duration (acute or chronic), (3) symptoms (painful or silent), (4) mechanism (obstructive or non-obstructive), and (5) urodynamic findings (high or low pressure) [3]. The key feature is that the patient is unable to empty the bladder to completion, but the amount remaining in the bladder that would define urinary retention, also called post-void residual (PVR) ranges from 100 to 1000 mL [4–7]. One other important feature is the degree of urinary obstruction present, determined not only by the urinary flow rate, but also by the voiding pressure. These two parameters, taken together, form the basis for nomograms to determine the severity of obstruction, such as the Schaefer and Abrams-Griffiths nomograms, useful in men suspected of urinary obstruction [8]. Women suspected of urinary obstruction can be categorized by female-specific nomograms, such as the Blaivas-Groutz nomogram, which can serve as a method to measure severity of urinary obstruction in women [9, 10].

Acute urinary retention, as the term implies, has not been present for long, and is often initially managed with a temporary urinary catheter until more definitive therapy can be planned, or until the acute process responsible for the urinary retention subsides with time. Chronic urinary retention, on the other hand, is often not painful and can be present for months or even years before coming to the attention of caregivers. In the worst cases, this can lead to hydrone-

C. R. Powell (✉)
Department of Urology, Indiana University School of Medicine, Indianapolis, IN, USA
e-mail: crpowell@iupui.edu

J. P. Gilleran, S. A. Alpert (eds.), *Adult and Pediatric Neuromodulation*,
https://doi.org/10.1007/978-3-319-73266-4_4

phrosis, recurrent urinary tract infection, sepsis, or renal failure [11]. One useful way to categorize causes of urinary retention is to make a distinction between patients having high risk features and low risk features. This concept was formalized in the 2016 American Urological Association (AUA) white paper on chronic urinary retention and underscores the idea that some patients with chronic urinary retention can be safely monitored without intervention while others cannot [4]. The degree of risk can be associated with certain causes, and so some of these are discussed below. In particular, some of the neurologic causes discussed below are more commonly associated with high risk features [11].

In addition to categorizing urinary retention by risk, it is also commonly categorized as either obstructive (implying a fixed anatomical blockage) or non-obstructive, and this helps determine therapy. In cases of obstructive urinary retention, relieving the obstruction remains the key philosophy of therapy. This distinction is best made with a urodynamic study. Figure 4.1 demonstrates an example of an obstructed voiding pattern, with a coordinated, relaxed urinary sphincter, high voiding pressures, and low flow. For cases of non-obstructive urinary retention the two approaches are to relax the bladder outlet **or** to increase the intravesical pressure with extrinsic (Valsalva straining) or intrinsic (detrusor muscle) compression. One therapy that has been very successful at relaxing the bladder outlet is neuromodulation, but some recent evidence suggests sacral neuromodulation in particular might also work by increasing detrusor muscle tone of the bladder.

The most common anatomic cause for obstructive urinary retention in men with benign prostatic hyperplasia (BPH) is bladder outlet obstruction, and the most straight forward treatment is to relieve the obstruction [5, 12]. Bladders that do not exhibit damage from long standing severe obstruction often recover function following surgical resection of the prostate, such as with transurethral resection of the prostate (TURP), holmium laser ablation of the prostate (HOLEP), or any one of the many other treatments addressing the prostate. Women, when found to have anatomic cause for obstruction, such as a midurethral sling (MUS), urethral stricture, or pelvic organ prolapse, will often benefit from relief of the obstructing anatomy, such as incision of the sling [13], although this is a much rarer phenomenon. Other causes of urinary retention include trauma, cancer, and particularly neurologic conditions.

Addressing the concerns of the patients suffering from urinary retention who do not exhibit obvious anatomic causes of urinary retention, however, can pose a challenge to clinicians. This is also known as non-obstructive urinary retention. Neuromodulation has been found to be effective in some of these cases, and situations where neuromodulation is most effective, as well as the literature supporting its use will be explored in this chapter.

Causes of Urinary Retention

It is most important to consider the cause of non-obstructive urinary retention before a plan for therapy can be considered. Causes of non-obstructive urinary retention vary widely, and a complete history and physical, serum creatinine, renal ultrasound, and urodynamic study are often helpful in determining the cause of non-obstructive urinary retention. After the history and physical exam, the urodynamic study is the most useful piece of information.

Idiopathic Causes of Non-obstructive Urinary Retention

Functional bladder outlet obstruction in children such as dysfunctional elimination syndrome (DES) [14], Hinman's syndrome, and bladder bowel dysfunction might be caused by neurologic dysfunction, but these conditions by definition are not associated with a known neurologic disorder, making them idiopathic. If urodynamic studies demonstrate **high pressure** or what some experts consider "high risk" features such as **hydronephrosis**, **chronic kidney disease stage**

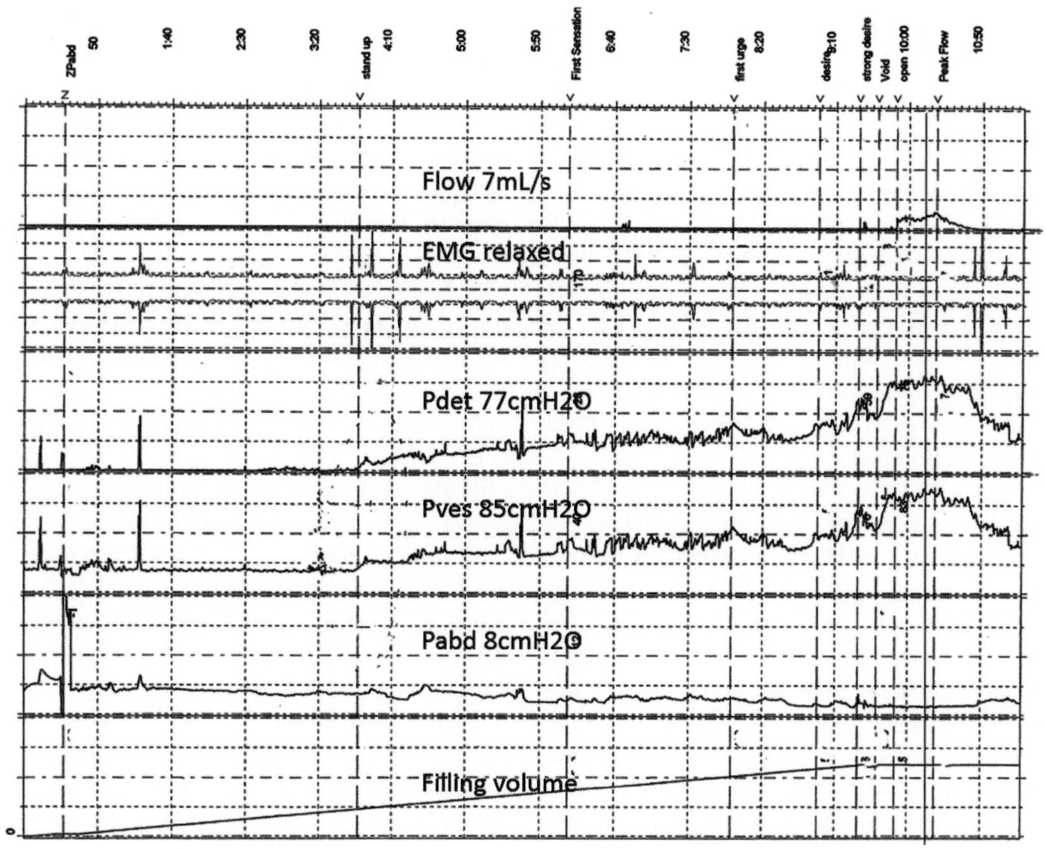

Fig. 4.1 Urodynamic tracing of a patient with anatomic bladder outlet obstruction secondary to benign prostatic hyperplasia. Note the elevated voiding pressure, low flow, and relaxed EMG tracing

3 (CKD 3), **recurrent UTI, hospitalization for urosepsis, incontinence with perineal changes**, or **decubitus ulcers**, the AUA white paper panel advocates intervention [4]. If low pressures and no high risk features are present, the panel advises that no intervention is warranted. Patients with primary functional bladder outlet obstruction may benefit from intermittent catheterization and medication, such as oxybutynin to reduce urgency or alpha-blockers such as tamsulosin to aid in emptying [15]. Similarly, non-invasive, non-pharmacologic therapies such as biofeedback have been noted to be effective and often considered first-line therapy for children with DES [16, 17]. When these measures fail to relieve the non-obstructive urinary retention, sacral neuromodulation (SNM) has been demonstrated to be effective by multiple investigators [18–21]. The largest series, describing outcomes in 105 children with DES, reports improvement for constipation in 79% (defined as at least 50% improvement), nocturnal enuresis in 66%, while 88% experienced improvement in urinary incontinence [19]. This study includes children with non-obstructive urinary retention, but these patients were not categorized in such a way to extract the outcomes from that indication alone. Groen and colleagues examined two children with DES and noted a reduction in PVR as well as seven children they labeled with Fowler's syndrome, in which five responded, 1/3 previously dependent on CIC was able to stop CIC, and two partial responders, as well as two failures [21]. It is important to note that SNM is not yet standard of care for children. It is not FDA approved for use in patients under 18 years of age, and the reoperation rate was 56%. Re-operations were necessary for "device malfunction" which includes lead migration, broken wires, dislocation of the device, and depleted battery. The authors included resolution of symptoms as a reason to "re-operate" so the device can be removed [19]. An understanding of the relationship between DES, childhood voiding syndromes, and Hinman's syndrome is evolving, and so the term "bladder-bowel dysfunction" is now recommended by the International Children's Continence Society (ICCS) to describe these syndromes, which include non-obstructive urinary retention as well as bowel dysfunction [22, 23].

Fowler's syndrome, like bladder-bowel dysfunction, DES, and Hinman's syndrome, includes uncoordinated and inappropriate urinary sphincter contraction as a cause of non-obstructive urinary retention, but the syndrome usually refers to dysfunction in the adult population [24]. An urodynamic tracing is shown in Fig. 4.2 exhibiting elevated vesical pressures, non-relaxing EMG tracing, and low flow that is typical of Fowler's syndrome. Sacral neuromodulation was first approved for non-obstructive urinary retention in adults by the US Food and Drug Association in 1999, 2 years after it was initially approved for urinary urgency and frequency [25]. First-line therapy for Fowler's syndrome includes biofeedback, selective alpha-blocker medication such as tamsulosin, and clean intermittent self-catheterization (CIC), but SNM has proven very effective for cases that do not respond to these measures. De Ridder and colleagues noted a 75% persistent benefit 5 years after undergoing SNM for non-obstructive urinary retention due to Fowler's syndrome compared with 50% of a matched cohort having non-obstructive urinary retention from other causes. They also noted that patients who were screened and found to be positive for somatization or depression did not predict for success or failure. SNM has a long track record of success in the treatment of non-obstructive urinary retention [26]. Table 4.1 lists a summary of some significant studies published in this area, specifically addressing SNM studies with ten or more subjects. As early as 1989 Tanagho and colleagues noted success in treating these patients by performing dorsal rhizotomy and stimulating S3 (third Sacral Foramen) and S4 ventral (motor) nerve roots. An example of intra-operative lead placement relative to the bony landmarks can be seen in Fig. 4.3. Although this is not the minimally invasive technique now used routinely to achieve SNM with commercial stimulators, it proved the concept and paved the way for the current technique [40]. The mechanism by which SNM works to relieve functional bladder outlet obstruction is unclear, but evolving evidence suggests it works centrally in the spinal cord reflex centers as well as in the brain. Studies utilizing functional magnetic resonance imaging (fMRI) demonstrated decreased activity in the brainstem of women suffering from Fowler's syndrome and enhanced limbic cortical activity during full bladder cycles compared with normal controls. When SNM was applied and the affected subjects were re-imaged, the brainstem activity rose to normal levels and the limbic cortical activity decreased to normal levels, suggesting a central-acting mechanism of action [41]. Further insight can be gained by looking at the work of DasGupta and Fowler who subjected 30 women to urodynamic studies before SNM and after SNM was applied. They noted that the sphincter activity remained elevated and unchanged, as did maximum urethral closure pressure, and only detrusor pressure increased to improve flow and decrease post-void residual in women affected by Fowler's syndrome [42]. Investigators from Italy explored a novel method to screen patients for SNM that may provide some additional insight. They stimulated sacral nerves under anesthesia and used urodynamic catheters to determine if a detrusor contraction was elicited. If it was not, the investigators determined the subject had detrusor acontractility and SNS was abandoned. By selecting patients in this way, the authors noted that 65% had no bladder contraction, but since they were not implanted it is not clear if they would have done well regardless of the negative screening test. Moreover, those testing positive for the screen did not all undergo SNM implantation, with only 12/24 receiving generators. Follow-up at 12–48 months revealed 67% with

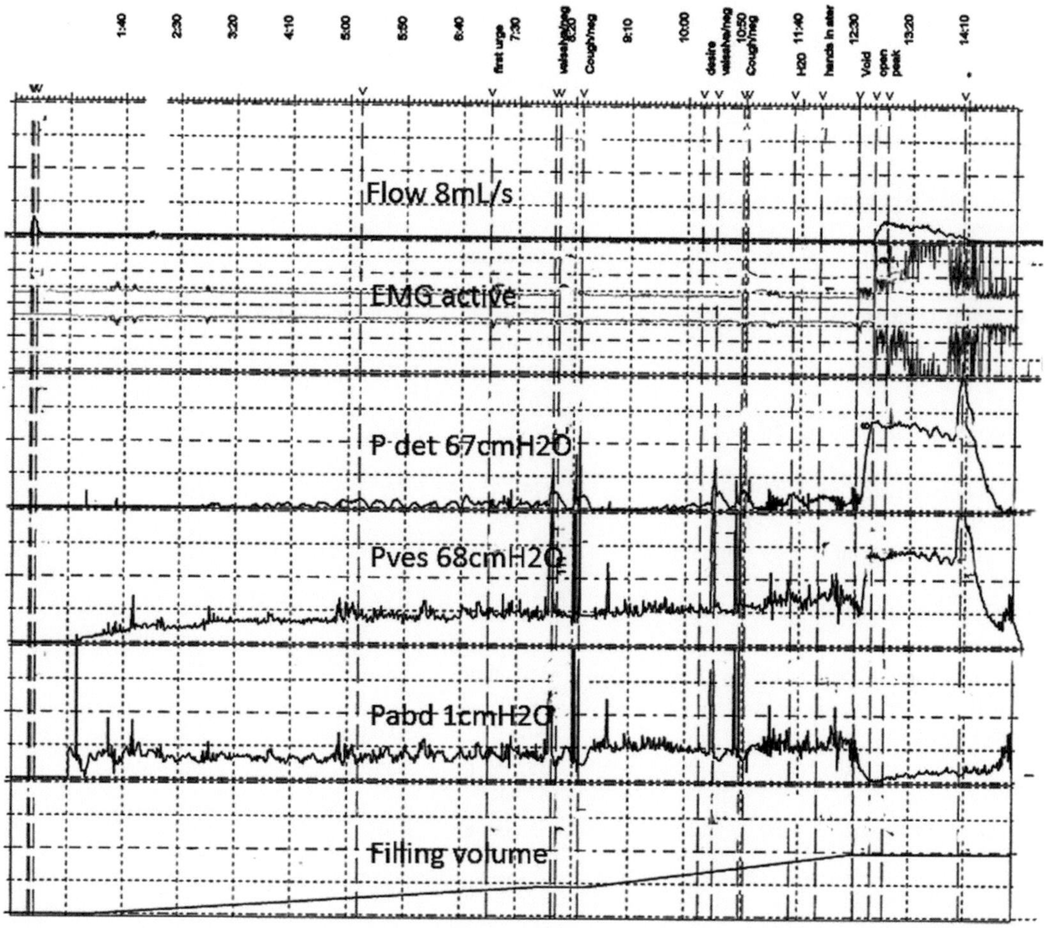

Fig. 4.2 Urodynamic tracing of a patient with Fowler's syndrome. It is important to note that this EMG tracing is created by patch electrodes and not a needle electrode as described by the original investigators. One can see the activity, elevated Pves and Pdet, as well as low flow characteristic of this type of non-obstructive urinary retention

no need to catheterize, voiding well, and 25% with the need to perform CIC 1–2 times per day. One patient was explanted [43]. This does not seem to provide any advantage over the traditional staged trial, when compared with the next investigation below.

Although not specifically enrolling patients with Fowler's syndrome, the most robust evidence for the effectiveness of SNM for non-obstructive urinary retention comes from a randomized controlled trial (RCT) involving 68 patients screened from 177 patients presenting at multiple centers in which the controls all demonstrated non-obstructive urinary retention, randomized to a 6-month delay in SNM implantation. Subjects were able to stop all catheterizing by the 6-month follow-up in 69% of cases, and an additional 14% (83% total) were able to reduce the PVR by 50% or more. Those randomized to the SNM group experienced a reduction in PVR of 270 mL compared with the 6-month delay subjects (controls) and a mean increase in voided volume of 104 mL [29]. This work was later validated by Datta and colleagues who reviewed their series of 60 patients who received SNS for non-obstructive urinary retention, 50% of whom were able to stop catheterizing, while 72% were voiding spontaneously with a mean PVR of 100 mL [35]. Similar results were described by White and colleagues

Table 4.1 Reports in the literature including prospective RCTs and retrospective case reviews having >10 subjects describing outcomes using sacral neuromodulation to treat non-obstructive urinary retention

Reference	*n* =	Follow-up period (month)	Reduction in PVR	Reduction in CIC per day	Etiology of retention
Shaker J Urol 98 [27]	20	15	78 mL to 5 mL	NA	Idiopathic
Grunewald Rest Neuro Neurosci 99 [28]	43 (21)	43	578 mL to 113 mL	(13/21) "voided without residual"	NA
Jonas J Urol 01[29]	68	18	333 mL to 109 mL	4.9 to 2.7	NA
Aboseif BJU Int 02 [25]	20	24	315 mL to 60 mL	17/20 stopped CIC	NA
Everaert BJU Int 03 [30]	13	31	582 mL to 56 mL	9/13 stopped CIC	Post-hysterectomy
Dasgupta BJU Int 04 [31]	26	37	NA to 75 mL	NA	NA
Van Voskuilen Euro Urol 06 [32]	149 (42)	70.5	NA	NA	NA
Van Voskuilen BJU Int 07 [33]	49 (10)	15.5	298 mL to 112 mL	5.4 to 1.2	NA
DeRidder Euro Urol 07 [26]	62	43.4	NA	NA	Fowler's in 30 idiopathic in 32
Van Kerrebroeck J Urol 07 [34]	163 (18)	60	380 mL to 109 mL	5.3 to 1.9	NA
Datta BJU Int 08 [35]	60	48	NA	30/60 stopped CIC	NA
White Urology 08 [36]	28	40	333 mL to 87 mL	4.3 to 1	Idiopathic
Denzinger Neuromod 12 [37]	20	12	350 mL to 135 mL	4 to 1	Idiopathic (12) neurogenic (8)
Lombardi Spinal Cord 14 [38]	36	50	353 mL to 100 mL	3.6 to 0.7	Spinal cord injury
Engeler BMC Urology 15 [39]	14	36	170 mL to 25 mL	NA	Multiple sclerosis

Series reporting on mixed populations having indications for SNM other than non-obstructive urinary retention will be reported in (parentheses)

NA signifies not given by the authors in the manuscript

with 70% implantation rate, all of whom were still experiencing 50% improvement at a mean of 40 months' follow-up and 55% were able to stop catheterizing altogether. 14.3% had to be explanted, despite good outcomes, for infection, need for MRI, and pain, suggesting these patients require close follow-up after implantation [36]. Gross and colleagues performed a meta-analysis of non-obstructive urinary retention treated with SNM including the previously mentioned RCT by Jonas as well as 13 case series and noted a mean decrease in PVR of 236 and a mean increase in voided volume of 344 favoring SNM. It should be noted that only seven studies reported PVR. Pain at the implant site was noted in 10.3% while lead migration occurred in 4.8% [44]. In a more contemporary retrospective report, Denzinger and colleagues report a 90% implantation rate following a test phase which yielded a reduction in PVR from 350 mL to 135 mL which they report did not reach statistical significance, but a reduction in the number of catheterizations from 4 to 1 which was significant [37]. The authors note that a pre-operative PVR of <400 mL is predictive of success (86% compared with 33%).

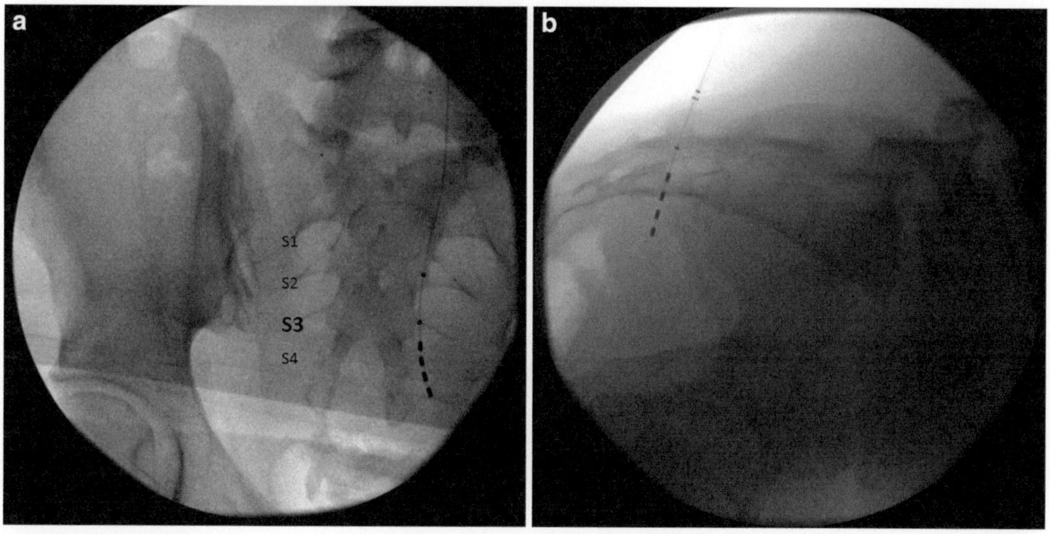

Fig. 4.3 Anterior-posterior (**a**) and lateral (**b**) films of a typical sacral neuromodulation lead going through the S3 foramen on the left

Neurogenic Causes of Non-obstructive Urinary Retention

In addition to idiopathic causes of non-obstructive urinary retention, such as pediatric DES, bladder–bowel dysfunction, as well as adult conditions such as Fowler's syndrome, SNM has been successfully used to treat LUTS caused by certain neurologic conditions such as Parkinson's disease, spinal cord injury, multiple sclerosis, cerebrovascular accident, and diabetes mellitus. Despite having been FDA approved only for non-neurogenic causes of LUTS, SNM appears to be effective for neurogenic causes of LUTS as well [45]. International guidelines recommend additional measures such as periodic renal ultrasound, serum creatinine, and urodynamic studies be performed on patients with neurogenic voiding dysfunction because many of these patients are at risk for deteriorating renal and even bladder function [46].

Spinal cord injury (SCI) is one controversial area where SNM was once thought to be ineffective and now has been proven modestly effective when other options have failed [45]. Recently, authors have reported a 42.5% response rate in a group of men with complete and incomplete SCI and urinary retention. This is lower than the success rates for other causes of non-obstructive urinary retention. The status of the SCI, ASIA score, and preoperative PVR did not appear to predict successful response to stage 1 SNM test lead, but those who did respond experienced a decrease in PVR from 353 to 100 and reduction in CIC from 3.5 times per day to 0.67 [38]. Kessler and colleagues performed a meta-analysis on the effectiveness of SNM for neurogenic causes of LUTS and noted that 67/119 (56%) had a successful test stimulation and progressed to implantation of the generator, while 65/89 (73%) experienced continued success following generator placement. This may not compare favorably to the overall pooled success rate of 92% following implantation for all indications, but still offers a reasonable chance for success in a challenging population [47]. Wollner and colleagues examined 50 SCI subjects at a spine rehabilitation facility in Switzerland and noted nine with urinary retention. Following successful implantation with a SNM generator, the median PVR decreased from 370 mL to 59 mL. Interestingly, when urodynamic studies were repeated no significant decrease in urodynamic proven neurogenic detrusor overactivity was noted although the patients reported significant improvements in urinary frequency and urge incontinence [48].

Sacral Neuromodulation as a Catalyst for Neurologic Remodeling

Some evidence exists suggesting neurologic remodeling is possible with early SNM. The assertion is that neuromodulation has the ability to remodel the brain and possibly repair damaged or dysfunctional pathways, perhaps through repurposing pathways that remain intact. One disease state where this may be particularly beneficial is acute spinal cord injury. Sacral neuromodulation has been used in patients with neurogenic bladder after spinal cord injury early during the spinal shock period, when the bladder is atonic (detrusor underactivity), which often improves with time. This was suggested in a recent investigation by Sievert and colleagues who performed urodynamic studies on ten patients who received early bilateral S3 leads. SNM occurred within 2.9 months of the injury and urodynamics confirmed an adynamic detrusor. Six patients who refused SNM were also included as control patients, but were not randomized to that group nor blinded. The controls demonstrated lower bladder capacity (294 cc vs. 582 cc) and more urinary tract infections (3.8 UTIs per year vs. 0.5) over 26 months of follow-up [49]. It is notable that erectile function and bowel function were also improved in the early neuromodulation group.

In addition to acute spinal cord injury patients, children may also exhibit neurologic remodeling. Reinberg and colleagues note this phenomenon in their experience in children with dysfunctional elimination syndrome, in which 11% (13 of 118 children) are able to be explanted with continued resolution of symptoms at an average of 40.9 months follow-up [50]. More investigation is needed as none of these were controlled studies, but rather retrospective reviews. Critics might argue that clinical evidence should be used to generate hypotheses that should then be tested with animal studies. Apart from SNM, pudendal neuromodulation has been noted in dogs to have a protective effect on the bladder if instituted within a month of a surgically induced spinal cord injury, but not if therapy is delayed 6 months after the injury, further supporting the hypothesis that early neuromodulation might provide benefit [51].

Brindley Finetech Stimulator

Introduced in 1978, this therapy for patients with neurogenic voiding dysfunction secondary to complete spinal cord injury has enjoyed moderate success at a limited number of centers. Typically, patients suffer both urge urinary incontinence and non-obstructive urinary retention. The continence comes from the surgical rhizotomy of the dorsal root of the sacral nerves and the ability to void comes from stimulation of the afferent anterior roots of S2, S3, and S4 using a surgically implanted cuff electrode. The most recent report is from Krasmik and colleagues from Germany who found that 107/137 (78%) of enrolled patients who received the rhizotomy and sacral anterior root stimulation (SARS) with a Brindley Finetech stimulator were still using it after 14.8-year follow-up. They noted 62% were continent with 80 surgical revisions, and a mean PVR of 96, suggesting that surgical revision is very common over the lifetime of the device, and improvements in PVR appear modest [52].

Another recent report from the Netherlands compared SARS with matched spinal cord injured controls. 53% of the 46 patients who responded reported being continent to urine, compared with 14% of 28 patients who did not undergo the procedure. The afferent stimulation has a modest effect on voiding efficiency, as 37% of those with the stimulator reported they no longer used it for volitional voiding, but 33% of them still enjoyed improved continence secondary to the rhizotomy. The UTI rate for the Brindley stimulator group was 50% (at least 1 per year) compared with 64% for the controls, 86% of whom were managed with CIC. Those still using it reported significantly higher quality of life scores (Qualiveen) [53]. MRI has been safely used in spinal cord injury patients who have undergone this therapy but one device began to malfunction and had to be explanted [54].

Cerebral vascular accident (CVA) is classified as a supra-pontine neurologic injury and as such typically causes loss of inhibition and detrusor overactivity, often leading to urge incontinence, but seldom leading to urinary retention [55]. One paper in the literature describes the use of posterior tibial nerve stimulation (PTNS) in a RCT involving 24 men, all of whom suffered a CVA, who were randomized to PTNS twice per week or "general advice and stretching" for 6 weeks. PTNS-treated patients experienced significant reductions in urgency (−34%), nocturia (−41%), and urge urinary incontinence (−25%); however, these differences all failed to improve upon the control group at 6 weeks and at 1 year [56]. Although the subjects did not suffer from non-obstructive urinary retention, the work demonstrates a role for PTNS in supra-pontine neurogenic voiding dysfunction.

Multiple sclerosis (MS) can be characterized by four subtypes—relapsing, remitting is the most common, affecting approximately 85% of patients, but a significant number will convert to secondary progressive MS, about 10% will have primary progressive, and the fourth and least common category is progressive relapsing MS [57]. It is common, with a prevalence of 100 per 100,000 Americans. Over 75% of MS patient suffer LUTS, making it one of the most frequent neurologic causes of LUTS [58]. This makes predicting the effects of MS on the bladder of affected individuals difficult and adds heterogeneity to study subjects. Detrusor underactivity (DU) affects 25% and detrusor sphincter dyssynergia (DSD) affects approximately 35%, making non-obstructive urinary retention a significant problem in this patient group [57]. Neuromodulation has been studied in this group by multiple authors. Engeler and colleagues treated 16 of 17 subjects with SNM and noted a reduction in urinary frequency from 12 to 7 voids per day, PVR decreased from 170 mL to 25 mL, and voided volume increased from 125 mL to 265 mL. It should be noted that although the authors did report that 16 of 17 enrolled patients with MS had "incomplete voiding," only five were reported to perform CIC and the median PVR for all 17 subjects was 83 mL [39]. One concern raised by some experts is the progressive nature of MS, and the future need for MRI, which is incompatible with SNM for most regions of the body [59]. The manufacturer (Medtronic Inc., Minnesota USA) has posted a safety advisory update, noting that MRI of the head (only) is safe for InterStim® II model 3058 and certain InterStim® 3023 devices [60]. Posterior tibial nerve stimulation is another form of neuromodulation used to treat LUTS, but unlike SNM, it has not been approved by the US Food and Drug Administration (FDA) for treatment of urinary retention. Gobbi and colleagues found PTNS improved urinary frequency in MS from 9 to 6 voids per day. Nocturia decreased from 3 to 1 episode per night, and post-void residual from 98 cc to 45 cc. Quality of life was improved in most domains assessed immediately after 12 weeks of PTNS therapy, but not the domain related to urinary retention [61]. Other investigators examining the role of PTNS in MS noted an increase bladder capacity before uninhibited contractions were seen from 124 to 217 cc. Maximum capacity increased from 199 to 266 cc [62]. Some authors have described a similar technique not requiring needles called transcutaneous posterior tibial nerve stimulation (TPTNS) used for multiple sclerosis with 82% of 70 subjects reporting "improvement of OAB" at 30 days and 83% at 90 days. The subjects underwent daily 20 min sessions at home. The endpoint was the absence of all of the following: >8 voids per day, >1 nocturia episode, and >3 urinary incontinence episodes weekly [63]. Although the endpoint was not a traditional one, this therapy can be applied daily at home and appears effective, but is not equal to sacral neuromodulation. The evidence at this time does not support either PTNS or TPTNS for urinary retention.

Myelomeningocele is a common congenital neurogenic cause for non-obstructive urinary retention. SNM has been used with some limited success in this population in children, but not in the context of a well-designed, prospective RCT. Investigators in China noted 6/9 patients with myelomeningocele in their series of 23 subjects suffering neurologic voiding dysfunction were able to successfully undergo SNM generator implantation, with 5/6 demonstrating preoperative detrusor sphincter dyssynergia (DSD). After implantation 5/6 showed improvement in urinary frequency, 5/6 had improvement in constipation, and 4/6 experienced an improvement in urge urinary incontinence [64]. Investigators in Iran have demonstrated efficacy treating myelomeningocele using a neuromodulation technique known as interferential electrical stimulation. This was performed by a physical therapist using two adhesive electrodes on the pubic symphysis and two beneath the buttocks, near the ischial tuberosities, through which a 0–50 mAmp current was passed at 1–20 Hz. They randomized 20 subjects age 3–16 years with myelomeningocele to treatment three times weekly for 6 weeks and performed sham procedure on ten control subjects. All subjects had elevated bladder pressure at capacity >40 cm H2O and urodynamic proven detrusor overactivity. They were all treated with CIC and anticholinergic medication throughout the study period. Most importantly, DSD was noted to decrease from 18/19 subjects to 7/19 post-procedure, suggesting this therapy might significantly improve the main cause of urinary retention in this patient population. Compliance improved temporarily 2 weeks following the end of the stimulation period (from 9.7 to 12.7 mL/cm H2O) but the benefit was lost at the 6-month follow-up. PVR also improved and remained improved at 6 months (113 mL to 51 mL, and then 49 at 6 months) [65].

Hemilaminectomy and Ventral Root Microanastomosis, the Xiao Procedure

Another novel and innovative method to apply neuromodulation to patients is nerve re-routing, using the existing intact nervous system to bypass deficient areas. Xiao and colleagues continue to garner significant attention after describing their work re-routing lumbar to sacral nerve roots allowing patients with spinal cord injury to increase bladder capacity and stimulate voiding by merely scratching a dermatome over the appropriate area [66]. This was done in 20 patients with myelomeningocele, with 85% gaining "satisfactory bladder control and continence within 8 to 12 months" [67]. This procedure has been reproduced in the USA with patients having neurogenic bladder secondary to myelomeningocele. Seven of nine subjects noted improved storage and volitional voiding by scratching a dermatome. Two patients were able to stop catheterizing; however, no patient was able to achieve complete urinary continence. Unfortunately, 89% had some degree of muscle weakness, and one demonstrated persistent foot drop at 12 months' follow-up, which is a challenge since many patients with myelomeningocele often suffer compromised mobility at baseline [68]. This innovative technique has been replicated with only modest success outside of the originating institution and its partner hospitals. The foot drop, initially seen in 25% of subjects in the early Chinese experience has been reduced to 5% in the more contemporary Chinese series by taking less of the L5 nerve root. Investigators in Denmark had less success, with 10/10 patients still requiring CIC after the procedure, with only some improvement in urge urinary incontinence during follow-up urodynamic studies [69]. The remarkable success rate noted by the Chinese investigators (85%) has not been reproduced in the North American or Denmark series. The significant risk and morbidity must be weighed against that of comparable options for these patients who fail conventional management such as clean intermittent self-catheterization, anticholinergics, botox, and sacral neuromodulation. Once these options are exhausted, bladder augmentation, continent catheterizable channel, and possibly sling are often considered. These carry significant morbidity as well. Dr. Xiao reports that over 2840 patients with myelomeningocele or SCI have undergone the Xiao procedure at three medical centers in China [70]. This innovative therapy will likely remain available under investigative protocols until other investigators can reliably replicate these results. The author has offered to host interested surgeons at his home institution, maintaining that the patients require careful selection and the complex procedure has a steep learning curve [70].

Detrusor Underactivity as a Cause for Urinary Retention

Detrusor underactivity (DU) has enjoyed significant attention recently, as an under-diagnosed condition that may be responsible for a significant number of cases of urinary retention. Specifically, DU can be caused by myogenic failure of the detrusor muscle [71] or neurogenic impairment, such as with diabetes mellitus (DM) [72] or sacral spinal cord injury [38]. Rademakers and colleagues have developed the first nomogram to predict success in men suffering from DU, called the Maastricht-Hannover nomogram combining urodynamic findings suggestive of bladder outlet obstruction with contractility, and found that only 20% of men scoring in the tenth percentile or below will respond to SNM for non-obstructive urinary retention while those in the 10–25th percentile have an 86% response rate [71]. The nomogram incorporates Watts factor (Wmax) and bladder outlet obstruction index (BOOI) [73]. The authors define "success" as having no need to perform CIC. As understanding of DU evolves, many new pharmacologic targets are emerging alongside a more refined understanding of the role of SNM [74].

Behavioral causes of urinary retention can include mental retardation, autism, and Alzheimer's dementia. These are challenging causes of retention with multiple factors and not easily remedied with neuromodulation. At this time, it is thought that this population may not benefit from neuromodulation.

The Future of Neuromodulation for Non-obstructive Urinary Retention

Improvements to the Existing SNM System

Although non-obstructive urinary retention has been treated successfully with neuromodulation and SNM in particular, improvements are needed. The limited battery life and need for surgical revision remain two problems with the current SNM system, called InterStim®, marketed by Medtronic ™. A rechargeable system claiming a 15-year battery life has received permission in June 2016 to begin post-marketing testing in Europe and might advance treatment in this area [75, 76].

Others have speculated that incorporating real-time bladder feedback into neuromodulation will reduce unnecessary stimulation cycles and improve battery life [77], and in fact this has been demonstrated in some animal studies. Investigators stimulated the pudendal nerve on demand after a bladder "event" and increased bladder capacity while reducing stimulation time by 67%, saving power and lengthening battery life. Using the pudendal nerve electroneurogram as a trigger, however, reduced the reliability of the technique, as 2 of the 6 cats tested did not exhibit a bladder "event" despite obvious leakage from the urethra [78]. Using information recorded from nerves in vivo has been difficult due to migration of nerve electrodes, scarring at the interface, damage to the nerve caused by the electrode itself, and poor signal-to-noise ratio, making it difficult to distinguish bladder sensory information from other information such as unrelated muscle contraction [79]. Using real-time biologic information to guide stimulation is known as closed-loop feedback. One problem with closed-loop feedback remains sensing a bladder "event" to prevent incontinence, or sensing bladder fullness in the case of non-obstructive urinary retention. Investigators have been able to sense roughly how full a bladder is using information from afferent nerves, but the technique of electrode implantation is very complex and time consuming, while the resolution, durability, and reliability are poor [80]. Another approach is to use actual bladder pressure, similar to what is done during the urodynamic study. Pressure sensing technology performs poorly over extended periods of time when implanted in animals, and, over the long term, unpredictable shifts in pressure measurement have hampered this endeavor. To this end, investigators have developed an implantable pressure sensor that does not absorb fluid from surrounding tissues, as this has been a problem in prior attempts to sense pressure in vivo. This is known as sensor drift, and although promising, this work is in very early stages [81].

Conclusion

Neuromodulation has many forms. Direct electrical stimulations to nerve roots, nerve ganglia, and peripheral nerves have all been described. Sacral neuromodulation has been particularly successful at providing patients suffering from non-obstructive urinary retention some relief, but other forms have also provided benefit. As technology improves and understanding of these conditions evolves, new SNM technologies and possibly neuromodulation incorporating bladder feedback information may allow more patients to avoid end-stage therapies such as urinary diversion or chronic Foley catheter dependency.

References

1. Coyne KS, Sexton CC, Thompson CL, Milsom I, Irwin D, Kopp ZS, et al. The prevalence of lower urinary tract symptoms (LUTS) in the USA, the UK and Sweden: results from the Epidemiology of LUTS (EpiLUTS) study. BJU Int. 2009;104:352–60.
2. Brasure M, Fink H, Risk M. Chronic urinary retention: comparative effectiveness and harms of treatments. In: Quality AfHRa, editor. Rockville, MD: Agency for Healthcare Research and Quality; 2014.
3. WIKI. Urinary Retention. ICS Wiki: International Continence Society; 2016.
4. Stoffel J, Lightner D, Peterson A, Sandhu J, Suskind A, Wei J. Non-neurogenic chronic urinary retention: consensus definition, management strategies, and future opportunities. AUA White Paper. Linthicum, MD: American Urological Association; 2016.
5. Lower urinary tract symptoms in men: management. United Kingdom: National Institute for Health and Care Excellence; 2015.
6. Oelke M, Speakman MJ, Desgrandchamps F, Mamoulakis C. Acute urinary retention rates in the general male population and in adult men with lower urinary tract symptoms participating in pharmacotherapy trials: a literature review. Urology. 2015;86:654–65.
7. Kaplan SA, Wein AJ, Staskin DR, Roehrborn CG, Steers WD. Urinary retention and post-void residual urine in men: separating truth from tradition. J Urol. 2008;180:47–54.
8. Lim CS, Abrams P. The Abrams-Griffiths nomogram. World J Urol. 1995;13:34–9.
9. Blaivas JG, Groutz A. Bladder outlet obstruction nomogram for women with lower urinary tract symptomatology. Neurourol Urodyn. 2000;19:553–64.
10. Cormier L, Ferchaud J, Galas JM, Guillemin F, Mangin P. Diagnosis of female bladder outlet obstruction and relevance of the parameter area under the curve of detrusor pressure during voiding: preliminary results. J Urol. 2002;167:2083–7.
11. Powell C. Not all neurogenic bladders are the same: a proposal for a new neurogenic bladder classification system. Transl Androl Urol. 2016;5:12–21.
12. Selius BA, Subedi R. Urinary retention in adults: diagnosis and initial management. Am Fam Physician. 2008;77:643–50.
13. Kasturi S, Hale DS. "J" cut of sling for postoperative voiding dysfunction following synthetic midurethral slings. Int Urogynecol J. 2011;22:933–6.
14. Feng WC, Churchill BM. Dysfunctional elimination syndrome in children without obvious spinal cord diseases. Pediatr Clin N Am. 2001;48:1489–504.
15. Costantini E, Lazzeri M, Bini V, Zucchi A, Fioretti F, Frumenzio E, et al. Open-label, longitudinal study of tamsulosin for functional bladder outlet obstruction in women. Urol Int. 2009;83:311–5.
16. Desantis DJ, Leonard MP, Preston MA, Barrowman NJ, Guerra LA. Effectiveness of biofeedback for dysfunctional elimination syndrome in pediatrics: a systematic review. J Pediatr Urol. 2011;7:342–8.
17. Kajbafzadeh AM, Sharifi-Rad L, Ghahestani SM, Ahmadi H, Kajbafzadeh M, Mahboubi AH. Animated biofeedback: an ideal treatment for children with dysfunctional elimination syndrome. J Urol. 2011;186:2379–84.
18. McGee SM, Routh JC, Granberg CF, Roth TJ, Hollatz P, Vandersteen DR, et al. Sacral neuromodulation in children with dysfunctional elimination syndrome: description of incisionless first stage and second stage without fluoroscopy. Urology. 2009;73:641–4; discussion 4.
19. Dwyer ME, Vandersteen DR, Hollatz P, Reinberg YE. Sacral neuromodulation for the dysfunctional elimination syndrome: a 10-year single-center experience with 105 consecutive children. Urology. 2014;84:911–7.
20. Stephany HA, Juliano TM, Clayton DB, Tanaka ST, Thomas JC, Adams MC, et al. Prospective evaluation of sacral nerve modulation in children with validated questionnaires. J Urol. 2013;190:1516–22.
21. Groen LA, Hoebeke P, Loret N, Van Praet C, Van Laecke E, Ann R, et al. Sacral neuromodulation with an implantable pulse generator in children with lower urinary tract symptoms: 15-year experience. J Urol. 2012;188:1313–7.
22. Chase J, Austin P, Hoebeke P, McKenna P. The management of dysfunctional voiding in children:

a report from the Standardisation Committee of the International Children's Continence Society. J Urol. 2010;183:1296–302.
23. Yeung CK, Shei-Dei Yang S, Hoebeke P. Development and assessment of lower urinary tract function in children. In: Wein AJ, editor. Campbell-Walsh Urology. 11th ed: Elsevier; 2013. p. 3121–33.
24. Fowler CJ, Christmas TJ, Chapple CR, Parkhouse HF, Kirby RS, Jacobs HS. Abnormal electromyographic activity of the urethral sphincter, voiding dysfunction, and polycystic ovaries: a new syndrome? BMJ. 1988;297:1436–8.
25. Aboseif S, Tamaddon K, Chalfin S, Freedman S, Mourad MS, Chang JH, et al. Sacral neuromodulation in functional urinary retention: an effective way to restore voiding. BJU Int. 2002;90:662–5.
26. De Ridder D, Ost D, Bruyninckx F. The presence of Fowler's syndrome predicts successful long-term outcome of sacral nerve stimulation in women with urinary retention. Eur Urol. 2007;51:229–33; discussion 33–4.
27. Shaker HS, Hassouna M. Sacral root neuromodulation in idiopathic nonobstructive chronic urinary retention. J Urol. 1998;159:1476–8.
28. Grunewald V, Hofner K, Thon WF, Kuczyk MA, Jonas U. Sacral electrical neuromodulation as an alternative treatment option for lower urinary tract dysfunction. Restor Neurol Neurosci. 1999;14:189–93.
29. Jonas U, Fowler CJ, Chancellor MB, Elhilali MM, Fall M, Gajewski JB, et al. Efficacy of sacral nerve stimulation for urinary retention: results 18 months after implantation. J Urol. 2001;165:15–9.
30. Everaert K, De Muynck M, Rimbaut S, Weyers S. Urinary retention after hysterectomy for benign disease: extended diagnostic evaluation and treatment with sacral nerve stimulation. BJU Int. 2003;91:497–501.
31. Dasgupta R, Wiseman OJ, Kitchen N, Fowler CJ. Long-term results of sacral neuromodulation for women with urinary retention. BJU Int. 2004;94:335–7.
32. van Voskuilen AC, Oerlemans DJ, Weil EH, de Bie RA, van Kerrebroeck PE. Long term results of neuromodulation by sacral nerve stimulation for lower urinary tract symptoms: a retrospective single center study. Eur Urol. 2006;49:366–72.
33. Van Voskuilen AC, Oerlemans DJ, Weil EH, van den Hombergh U, van Kerrebroeck PE. Medium-term experience of sacral neuromodulation by tined lead implantation. BJU Int. 2007;99:107–10.
34. van Kerrebroeck PE, van Voskuilen AC, Heesakkers JP, Lycklama á Nijholt AA, Siegel S, Jonas U, et al. Results of sacral neuromodulation therapy for urinary voiding dysfunction: outcomes of a prospective, worldwide clinical study. J Urol. 2007;178:2029–34.
35. Datta SN, Chaliha C, Singh A, Gonzales G, Mishra VC, Kavia RB, et al. Sacral neurostimulation for urinary retention: 10-year experience from one UK centre. BJU Int. 2008;101:192–6.
36. White WM, Dobmeyer-Dittrich C, Klein FA, Wallace LS. Sacral nerve stimulation for treatment of refractory urinary retention: long-term efficacy and durability. Urology. 2008;71:71–4.
37. Denzinger S, Nowrotek A, Weingart P, Burger M, Wieland WF, Rossler W, et al. Does sacral neuromodulation lead to relevant reduction in the need for intermittent catheterization? A single-center experience on patients with chronic urinary retention. Neuromodulation. 2012;15:586–91; discussion 91.
38. Lombardi G, Musco S, Celso M, Del Corso F, Del Popolo G. Sacral neuromodulation for neurogenic non-obstructive urinary retention in incomplete spinal cord patients: a ten-year follow-up single-centre experience. Spinal Cord. 2014;52:241–5.
39. Engeler DS, Meyer D, Abt D, Muller S, Schmid HP. Sacral neuromodulation for the treatment of neurogenic lower urinary tract dysfunction caused by multiple sclerosis: a single-centre prospective series. BMC Urol. 2015;15:105.
40. Tanagho EA, Schmidt RA, Orvis BR. Neural stimulation for control of voiding dysfunction: a preliminary report in 22 patients with serious neuropathic voiding disorders. J Urol. 1989;142:340–5.
41. Dasgupta R, Critchley HD, Dolan RJ, Fowler CJ. Changes in brain activity following sacral neuromodulation for urinary retention. J Urol. 2005;174:2268–72.
42. DasGupta R, Fowler CJ. Urodynamic study of women in urinary retention treated with sacral neuromodulation. J Urol. 2004;171:1161–4.
43. Bertapelle P, Bodo G, Carone R. Detrusor acontractility in urinary retention: detrusor contractility test as exclusion criteria for sacral neurostimulation. J Urol. 2008;180:215–6.
44. Gross C, Habli M, Lindsell C, South M. Sacral neuromodulation for nonobstructive urinary retention: a meta-analysis. Female Pelvic Med Reconstr Surg. 2010;16:249–53.
45. Powell CR. Neuromodulation for neurogenic bladder. In: Sandhu J, editor. Current bladder dysfunction reports: Springer; 2013. p. 282–8.
46. Drake MJ, Apostolidis A, Cocci A, Emmanuel A, Gajewski JB, Harrison SC, et al. Neurogenic lower urinary tract dysfunction: clinical management recommendations of the Neurologic Incontinence committee of the fifth International Consultation on Incontinence 2013. Neurourol Urodyn. 2016;35:657–65.
47. Kessler TM, La Framboise D, Trelle S, Fowler CJ, Kiss G, Pannek J, et al. Sacral neuromodulation for neurogenic lower urinary tract dysfunction: systematic review and meta-analysis. Eur Urol. 2010;58:865–74.

48. Wollner J, Krebs J, Pannek J. Sacral neuromodulation in patients with neurogenic lower urinary tract dysfunction. Spinal Cord. 2016;54:137–40.
49. Sievert KD, Amend B, Gakis G, Toomey P, Badke A, Kaps HP, et al. Early sacral neuromodulation prevents urinary incontinence after complete spinal cord injury. Ann Neurol. 2010;67:74–84.
50. Dwyer ME, Reinberg YE. The dysfunctional elimination syndrome in children—is sacral neuromodulation worth the trouble? J Urol. 2012;188:1076–7.
51. Chen G, Liao L, Dong Q, Ju Y. The inhibitory effects of pudendal nerve stimulation on bladder overactivity in spinal cord injury dogs: is early stimulation necessary? Neuromodulation. 2012;15:232–7; discussion 7.
52. Krasmik D, Krebs J, van Ophoven A, Pannek J. Urodynamic results, clinical efficacy, and complication rates of sacral intradural deafferentation and sacral anterior root stimulation in patients with neurogenic lower urinary tract dysfunction resulting from complete spinal cord injury. Neurourol Urodyn. 2014;33:1202–6.
53. Martens FM, Heesakkers JP. Clinical results of a brindley procedure: sacral anterior root stimulation in combination with a rhizotomy of the dorsal roots. Adv Urol. 2011;2011:709708.
54. Lopez de Heredia L, Meagher TM, Jamous MA, Hughes RJ. Long-term effect of MRI on sacral anterior root stimulator: the Stoke Mandeville experience. Spinal Cord. 2012;50:294–7.
55. Sanford MT, Suskind AM. Neuromodulation in neurogenic bladder. Transl Androl Urol. 2016;5:117–26.
56. Monteiro ES, de Carvalho LB, Fukujima MM, Lora MI, do Prado GF. Electrical stimulation of the posterior tibialis nerve improves symptoms of poststroke neurogenic overactive bladder in men: a randomized controlled trial. Urology. 2014;84:509–14.
57. Panicker JN, Fowler CJ. Lower urinary tract dysfunction in patients with multiple sclerosis. Handb Clin Neurol. 2015;130:371–81.
58. Brucker BM, Nitti VW, Kalra S, Herbert J, Sadiq A, Utomo P, et al. Barriers experienced by patients with multiple sclerosis in seeking care for lower urinary tract symptoms. Neurourol Urodyn. 2017;36(4):1208–13.
59. Tracey JM, Stoffel JT. Secondary and tertiary treatments for multiple sclerosis patients with urinary symptoms. Invest Clin Urol. 2016;57:377–83.
60. Medtronic. MRI Guidelines for InterStim Therapy neurostimulation systems. http://manualsmedtronic-com/wcm/groups/mdtcom_sg/@emanuals/@era/@neuro/documents/documents/contrib_214172pdf: Medtronic Inc.; 2016.
61. Gobbi C, Digesu G, Khullar V, El Neil S, Caccia G, Zecca C. Percutaneous posterior tibial nerve stimulation as an effective treatment of refractory lower urinary tract symptoms in patients with multiple sclerosis: preliminary data from a multicentre, prospective, open label trial. Mult Scler. 2011;17(12):1514–9.
62. Kabay S, Kabay SC, Yucel M, Ozden H, Yilmaz Z, Aras O, et al. The clinical and urodynamic results of a 3-month percutaneous posterior tibial nerve stimulation treatment in patients with multiple sclerosis-related neurogenic bladder dysfunction. Neurourol Urodyn. 2009;28:964–8.
63. de Seze M, Raibaut P, Gallien P, Even-Schneider A, Denys P, Bonniaud V, et al. Transcutaneous posterior tibial nerve stimulation for treatment of the overactive bladder syndrome in multiple sclerosis: results of a multicenter prospective study. Neurourol Urodyn. 2011;30:306–11.
64. Chen G, Liao L. Sacral neuromodulation for neurogenic bladder and bowel dysfunction with multiple symptoms secondary to spinal cord disease. Spinal Cord. 2014.
65. Kajbafzadeh AM, Sharifi-Rad L, Baradaran N, Nejat F. Effect of pelvic floor interferential electrostimulation on urodynamic parameters and incontinency of children with myelomeningocele and detrusor overactivity. Urology. 2009;74:324–9.
66. Xiao CG, MX D, Dai C, Li B, Nitti VW, de Groat WC. An artificial somatic-central nervous system-autonomic reflex pathway for controllable micturition after spinal cord injury: preliminary results in 15 patients. J Urol. 2003;170:1237–41.
67. Xiao CG, MX D, Li B, Liu Z, Chen M, Chen ZH, et al. An artificial somatic-autonomic reflex pathway procedure for bladder control in children with spina bifida. J Urol. 2005;173:2112–6.
68. Peters KM, Girdler B, Turzewski C, Trock G, Feber K, Nantau W, et al. Outcomes of lumbar to sacral nerve rerouting for spina bifida. J Urol. 2010;184:702–7.
69. Rasmussen MM, Rawashdeh YF, Clemmensen D, Tankisi H, Fuglsang-Frederiksen A, Krogh K, et al. The artificial somatoautonomic reflex arch does not improve lower urinary tract function in patients with spinal cord lesions. J Urol. 2015;193:598–604.
70. Xiao C-G. Bladder re-innervation—state of the art. Current Bladder Dysfunction Reports—Neurogenic Bladder, Zeitschrift. 2016:386–90.
71. Rademakers KL, Drossaerts JM, van Kerrebroeck PE, Oelke M, van Koeveringe GA. Prediction of sacral neuromodulation treatment success in men with impaired bladder emptying-time for a new diagnostic approach. Neurourol Urodyn. 2017;36(3):808–10.
72. Bansal R, Agarwal MM, Modi M, Mandal AK, Singh SK. Urodynamic profile of diabetic patients with lower urinary tract symptoms: association of diabetic cystopathy with autonomic and peripheral neuropathy. Urology. 2011;77:699–705.
73. Oelke M, Rademakers KL, van Koeveringe GA, et al. Unravelling detrusor underactivity: Development of a bladder outlet resistance- bladder contractility nomogram for adult male patients with lower urinary tract symptoms. Neurourol Urodyn. 2015; Epub ahead of print.

74. Juszczak K, Drewa T. Pharmacotherapy in detrusor underactivity: a new challenge for urologists and pharmacologists (from lab to clinic). Pharmacol Rep. 2016;68:703–6.
75. Cohn JA, Kowalik CG, Kaufman MR, Reynolds WS, Milam DF, Dmochowski RR. Evaluation of the axonics modulation technologies sacral neuromodulation system for the treatment of urinary and fecal dysfunction. Expert Rev Med Devices. 2017;14(1):3–14.
76. Heins S. Axionics sacral neuromodulation system receives CE mark for the treatment of urinary and fecal dysfunction. 2016.
77. Powell CR. Conditional electrical stimulation in animal and human models for neurogenic bladder: working toward a neuroprosthesis. Curr Bladder Dysfunct Rep. 2016;11:379–85.
78. Wenzel BJ, Boggs JW, Gustafson KJ, Grill WM. Closed loop electrical control of urinary continence. J Urol. 2006;175:1559–63.
79. Mathews KS, Wark HA, Warren DJ, Christensen MB, Nolta NF, Cartwright PC, et al. Acute monitoring of genitourinary function using intrafascicular electrodes: selective pudendal nerve activity corresponding to bladder filling, bladder fullness, and genital stimulation. Urology. 2014;84:722–9.
80. Mendez A, Sawan M, Minagawa T, Wyndaele JJ. Estimation of bladder volume from afferent neural activity. IEEE Trans Neural Syst Rehabil Eng. 2013;21:704–15.
81. Kim A, Powell CR, Ziaie B. An Universal packaging technique for low-drift implantable pressure sensors. Biomed Microdevices. 2016;18:32.

5 Peripheral Nerve Evaluation

Karen Noblett and Neha Talreja Sudol

Introduction/Background

Sacral neuromodulation (SNM) was initially approved by the US Food and Drug administration in 1997 for refractory urinary urgency incontinence (UUI). It was subsequently approved for non-obstructive urinary retention (UR) and urinary urgency-frequency in 1999, and refractory chronic fecal incontinence in 2011. During this time, more than 200,000 patients worldwide have received the Medtronic InterStim® sacral nerve stimulation system [1]. The widespread use of SNM has led to advances in patient selection, device quality, and placement technique.

One of the unique aspects of SNM is that patients are allowed to undergo a trial period to evaluate whether the therapy is efficacious and provides adequate symptom relief. As such, SNM consists of two phases: an initial test phase: where the patient trials the therapy to determine efficacy, followed by a second phase. The second phase consists of either implantation of the implantable pulse generator (IPG) if the trial was successful or removal of the lead wire if unsuccessful.

The initial phase is known as a test stimulation and includes an acute and subchronic period to evaluate for a successful response prior to permanent placement of the device. Prior to the development of the tined lead in 2002, the acute period was conducted with a peripheral nerve evaluation (PNE). Currently, the test stimulation can be performed with either a PNE or with a staged approach using the tined lead.

In this chapter, we will discuss peripheral nerve evaluation in detail, including patient selection, advantages and disadvantages, recommended technique, and clinical outcomes.

Patient Selection

Candidates for SNM are those with refractory UUI, urinary urgency-frequency, OAB, non-obstructive UR, and fecal incontinence. The American Urology Association recommends SNM as a third tier option for urinary dysfunction, after behavioral modifications and pharmacological therapy, which are tier one and two therapies, respectively [2]. Additionally, The American Society of Colorectal Surgeons recommends SNM for the treatment of chronic fecal incontinence [3]. For patients with urinary

K. Noblett (✉) · N. T. Sudol
Department of Obstetrics and Gynecology, Division Female Pelvic Medicine and Reconstructive Surgery, University of California, Irvine, Orange, CA, USA
e-mail: knoblett@uci.edu; nehat@uci.edu

J. P. Gilleran, S. A. Alpert (eds.), *Adult and Pediatric Neuromodulation*,
https://doi.org/10.1007/978-3-319-73266-4_5

retention, the only other currently available management options are clean intermittent catheterization (CIC) and suprapubic catheter placement. These options can be extremely difficult to manage for some patients, thus SNM is an excellent alternative that requires minimal maintenance by the patient.

An ideal candidate for PNE is one who is comfortable undergoing a procedure under local anesthesia and who is able to tolerate the potential mild discomfort related to the procedure. Patients with heightened levels of anxiety or a low pain threshold may benefit from a staged procedure in the operating room. However, provider compassion and a good bedside manner can alleviate this to some extent [4]. Additionally, body habitus, vertebral shape or history of prior back surgery may play a role in patient selection. For example, bony landmarks can be difficult to identify in an obese patient or one with severe kyphosis, without fluoroscopy or ultrasound. In these instances, a two-staged procedure may lend itself better results while minimizing patient discomfort and procedure length.

Technique

Initial Test Phase

Acute Period: Peripheral Nerve Evaluation Technique

PNE refers to the percutaneous placement of a monopolar lead through the S3 foramen, followed by acute electric stimulation to assess sensory and motor response. Thereafter, the patient undergoes a sub-acute period at home, for 3–7 days, to assess whether they are a responder or not.

The PNE stimulation kit contains a foramen needle with stylet, percutaneous lead wire, J-hook, grounding pad, and external test stimulator. In addition, the provider should have local anesthesia, tape or Tegaderm™, and antiseptic solution available.

The patient is placed in prone position and the buttocks are exposed in order to visualize the perineum and anus for evaluation of motor response. Some physicians choose to tape the buttocks laterally to maximize visualization. The upper sacrum (S1 and S2) lies in a more horizontal plane than the lower sacrum (S3–S5), which is often oriented in the frontal plane. In order to flatten the sacrum, pillows or bolsters may be placed under the lower abdomen and hip area (Fig. 5.1). The patient's toes should dangle freely to assist in motor evaluation. This can be achieved by placing them at the edge of the table or placing a pillow underneath the patient's shins, which also relieves pressure on the knees. A grounding pad is placed on the patient's thigh or foot and connected to the test stimulation cable and external test stimulator. The patient's skin is then prepped and draped in a sterile fashion from the top of the lumbar spine to the anus (Fig. 5.2). Depending on physician preference, the procedure can be performed via palpation of bony landmarks, with fluoroscopy, or with ultrasound. The PNE is generally performed bilaterally and takes anywhere from 15 to 30 min to complete.

Contraindications for PNE
Contraindications

Unable to tolerate prone position for up to 60 min
Requires >1 week for test phase (i.e., urinary retention, fecal incontinence)

Relative Contraindications

Elderly patient (i.e., severe osteoporosis)
Anticipate challenging lead placement (i.e., prior back surgery)
Morbidly obese patient

The most common and most readily available route of PNE is via palpation of bony landmarks. Important landmarks include the sciatic notch, coccyx, and sacral midline (Fig. 5.3). The sciatic notch represents the junction of the pelvis and sacrum and is anatomically in line with the S3

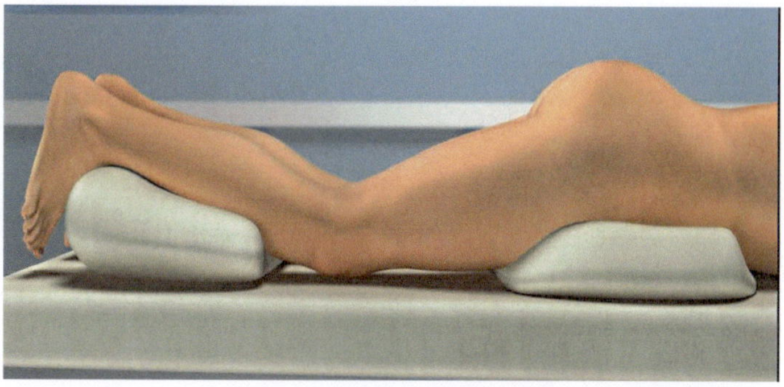

Fig. 5.1 Patient positioning: A pillow is placed under the hips to flatten the sacrum. A pillow is placed under the shins to elevate the toes. Reprinted with the permission of Medtronic, Inc. © 2017

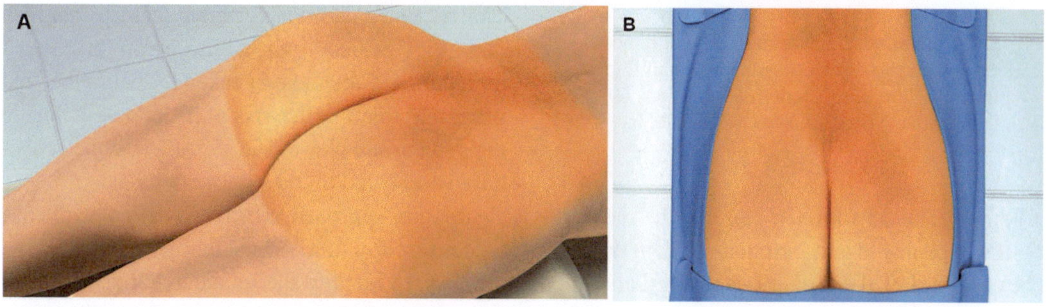

Fig. 5.2 Sterile preparation of the patient. (**a**) The skin is prepped with betadine or chlorhexidine. Prior to cleansing the skin, tap can be placed on the lateral aspect of the buttocks to expose the anus. (**b**) The lumbar back to the anus are draped in a sterile fashion. Reprinted with the permission of Medtronic, Inc. © 2017

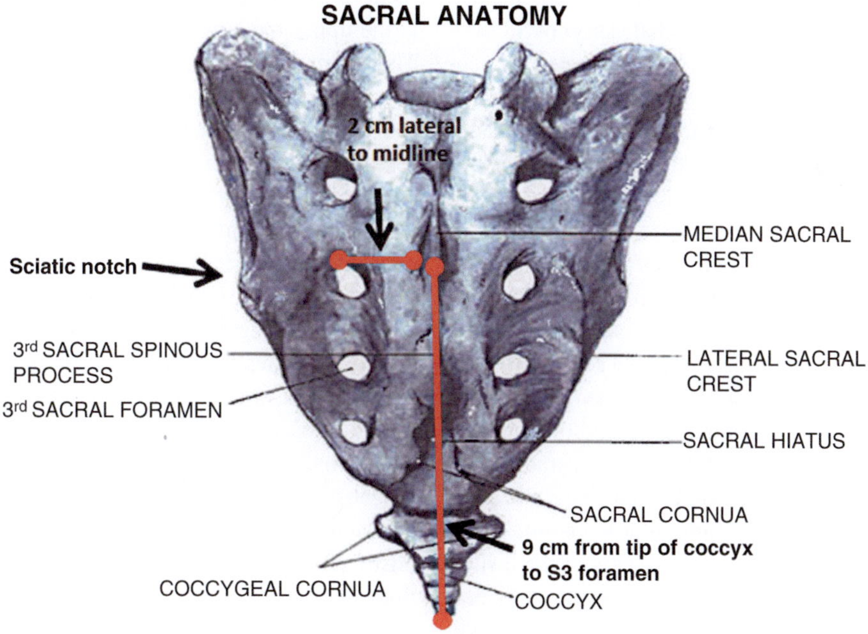

Fig. 5.3 Bony landmarks. On the dorsal sacrum, the coccyx and sciatic notch can be palpated. As highlighted by the red line, the S3 foramen can be measured 9 cm cephalad and 2 cm lateral from the coccyx. The sciatic notch is lateral and in line with the S3 foramen. Reprinted with the permission of Medtronic, Inc. © 2017

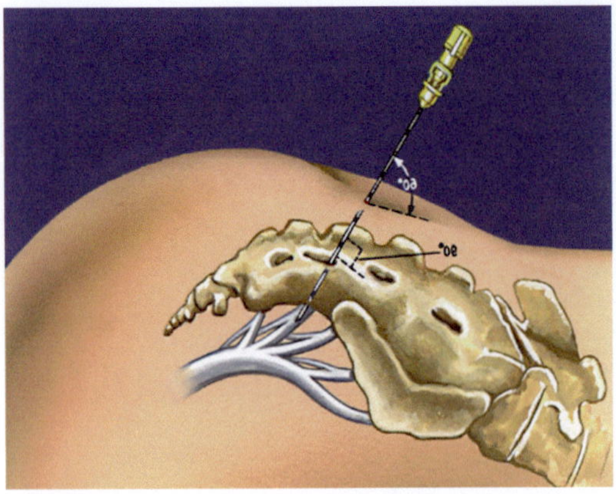

Fig. 5.4 Correct needle placement. The foramen needle correctly enters the superior-medial aspect of S3 foramen by puncturing the skin 2 cm cephalad at a 60° angle. Reprinted with the permission of Medtronic, Inc. © 2017

foramen. The S3 foramen can also be measured 9–10 cm cephalad and 2 cm lateral from the tip of the coccyx. Local anesthetic is utilized and liberally injected 2 cm cephalad to the expected S3 foramen to provide anesthesia from the skin to the bony shelf. A foramen needle (3.5 or 5 inches) is then introduced through the anesthetized skin site at an approximate 60° angle and, ideally, passed into the superior-medial aspect of S3 foramen (Fig. 5.4). The needle is then tested for sensory and motor response using a J-hook cable connected to the external test stimulator (Fig. 5.5). The needle should be able to be advanced 1–2 cm further into the foramen and still achieve an adequate response. This will ensure a parallel orientation of the lead along the nerve root and minimize the loss of response due to lead migration. The correct sensory response will result in a tingling or tapping sensation in the vagina, labia, or perineum in women; in the scrotum or base of the penis in men and/or rectum in both. Motor response should demonstrate a contraction of the levator ani muscles near the anus, which appears as a pulling in of the buttocks and anus (bellows), and plantar flexion of the ipsilateral great toe (Table 5.1). Motor response is preferred over sensory in most situations, but is not necessary to confirm correct placement, as the response can vary based on patient discomfort. In a cohort of 21 patients, Cohen et al. found that 95% of patients with greater than 50% improvement with test stimulation and subsequent permanent implant demonstrated a positive motor response [5]. Conversely, despite having a sensory response during test stimulation, 48% of the patients were not responders.

Once correct placement of the needle is confirmed, the stylet is removed and the monopolar lead wire is passed through the needle to the correct depth as determined by marks on the lead (Fig. 5.6). The needle is then removed over the lead wire, holding the position of the wire steady. The response should be tested again to confirm that the correct wire placement has been maintained. Care must be taken to secure the lead wire so as to minimize risk of dislodgment during the subchronic phase (Fig. 5.7). The same procedure is repeated on the contralateral side.

Another approach to office PNE is with the use of fluoroscopy. Initial imaging is obtained in the AP view to identify the sciatic notch, medial border of the foramen and vertical midline. The C-arm is then moved into the lateral position to visualize the S3 foramen. The PNE procedure, as discussed above, is performed. The ideal placement of the needle, as visualized on fluoroscopy, is the upper most medial border of the foramen. This is approximately 1 cm above the hillock and parallel to the fusion plate (Fig. 5.8). While sensory and motor findings are the primary means to assess correct placement, AP and lateral fluoroscopy views can further troubleshoot incorrect or suboptimal placement [6]. Specifically, they can confirm correct lead depth and that it has been placed in the upper medial aspect of the foramen.

Another imaging option to aid in identification of the sacral foramina is the use of ultrasound. Ultrasound guidance has the advantage over fluoroscopy of avoiding radiation exposure. Additionally, ultrasound is used for many other diagnostic purposes and is often more readily available than fluoroscopy. A recent study demonstrated that ultrasound was non-inferior to fluoroscopy with regard to locating the foramen during the test procedure [7]. Specifically, there was no difference between the groups in the number of needle passes required to successfully place the foramen needle. There are specific

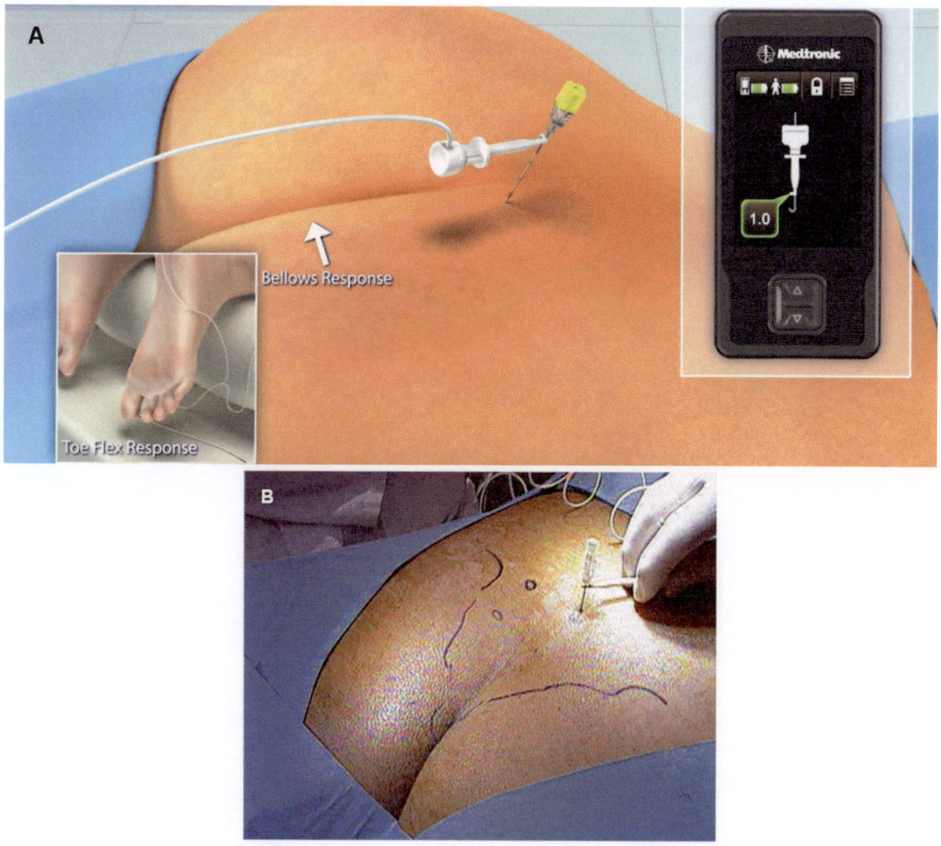

Fig. 5.5 Test stimulation with a J-hook cable. (**a**) As seen in a simple drawing, the J-hook cable is easily connected to the foramen needle to assess for the correct motor response; anal bellows and toe flexion. (**b**) Same step of the procedure as seen on a live patient. Reprinted with the permission of Medtronic, Inc. © 2017

Table 5.1 Sacral nerve motor and sensory responses

	Response		
Nerve innervation	Pelvic floor	Foot/calf/leg	Sensation
S2 Primary somatic contributor of pudendal nerve for external sphincter, leg, foot	"Clamp"[a] of anal sphincter	Leg/hip rotation, plantar flexion of entire foot, contraction of calf	Contraction of base of penis, vagina
S3 Virtually all pelvic autonomic functions and striated muscle (levator ani)	"Bellows"[b] of perineum	Plantar flexion of great toe, occasionally other toes	Pulling in rectum, extending forward to scrotum or labia
S4 Pelvic autonomic and somatic No leg or foot	"Bellows"[b]	No lower extremity motor stimulation	Pulling in rectum only

[a]Clamp: contraction of anal sphincter and, in males, retraction of base of penis. Move buttocks aside and look for anterior/posterior shortening of the perineal structures

[b]Bellows: lifting and dropping of the pelvic floor. Look for deepening and flattening of buttock groove

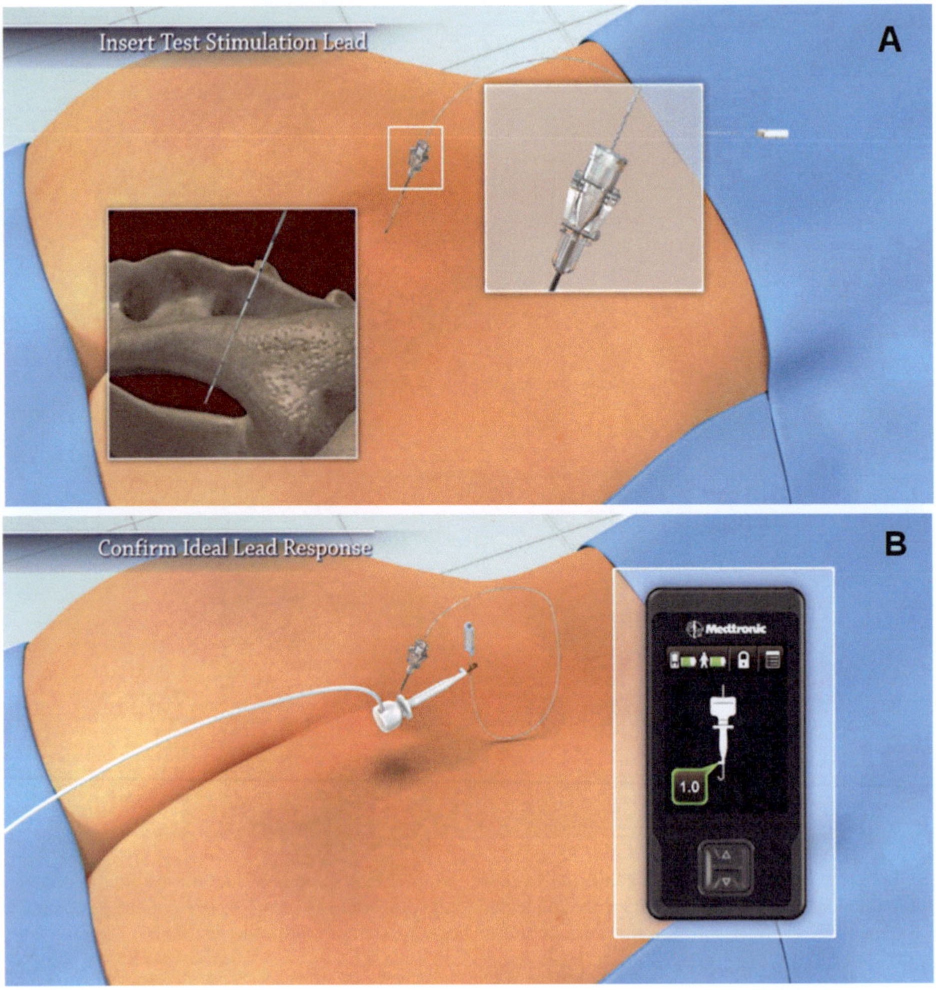

Fig. 5.6 Placing the PNE lead wire. (**a**) The stylet is removed and the PNE lead wire is advanced through the foramen needle. (**b**) The PNE lead wire should be tested to confirm correct placement. Reprinted with the permission of Medtronic, Inc. © 2017

landmarks that aid in the identification of the S3 foramen and are shown in Figs. 5.9 and 5.10.

Subchronic Phase: Home Testing

The sub-acute trial phase is generally conducted over 3–7 days after the PNE office procedure. During this period, objective data identifying change in symptoms is obtained with a voiding diary, which is then compared to baseline. A responder is defined as a patient who demonstrates a ≥50% improvement in the number of average voids/day or return to normal voiding (<8 voids/day) for patients with urinary frequency; and 50% improvement in average leaks/day in patients with urinary urgency incontinence [8]. Those meeting criteria for success are candidates for permanent implantation with the SNM. Permanent implantation is performed in the operating room with general anesthesia or under sedation with local anesthesia.

While the trial may be performed for up to 2 weeks, this can be difficult to maintain due to several restrictions and risk of infection. To avoid water damage to the electrode, the patient must not bathe or shower during the PNE trial. They are also asked to avoid strenuous exercise or

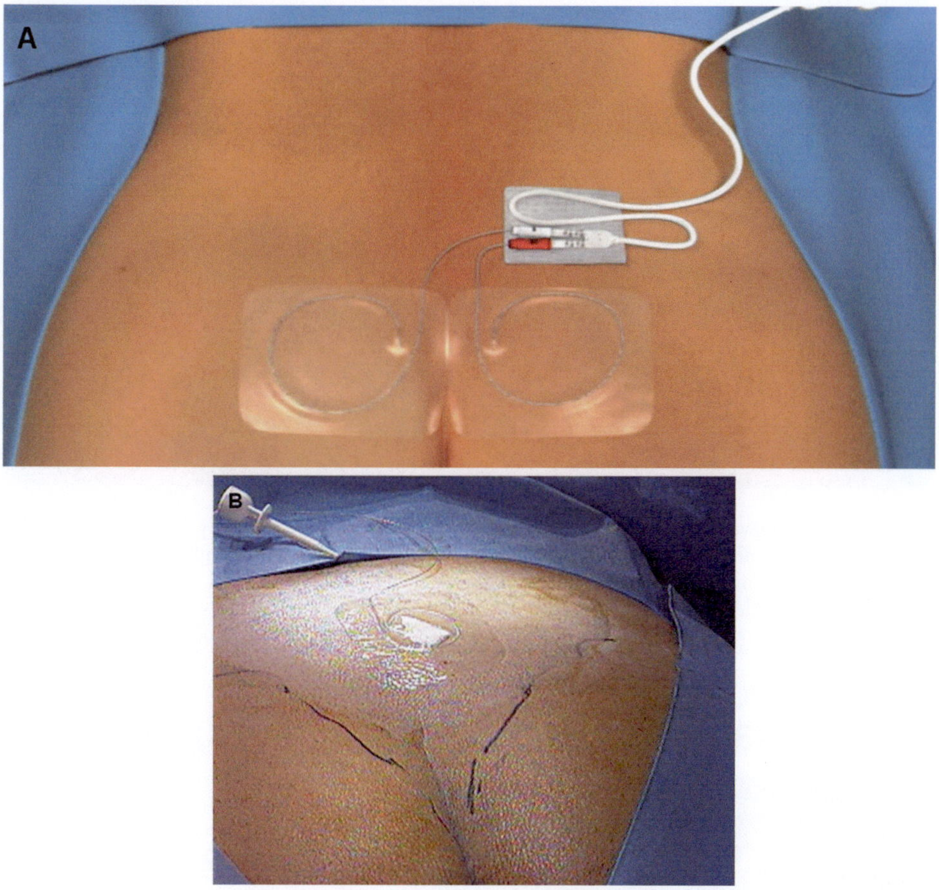

Fig. 5.7 Securing the PNE lead wire. (**a**) Technique to secure bilateral PNE wires using a surgical adhesive that water resistant, transparent, conforming tape is critical to minimize risk of migration. (**b**) Securing a unilateral PNE wire. Reprinted with the permission of Medtronic, Inc. © 2017

activity to minimize risk of lead migration. Given the percutaneous exposure of the lead, risk of infection exists. Panneck reported significant bacterial growth in 45% of PNE electrodes; however, no patient showed signs of local or systemic infection [9]. The use of antibiotics during the PNE and subchronic periods remains controversial and is left to the clinician's discretion as data is lacking to guide best practices in this area.

Advances

While PNE has several advantages (Table 5.2), reported success rates to conversion vary widely from 24 to 75% [6, 13]. Prior to 2002, PNE was the primary route to accomplish the initial testing phase. In 1997, Janknegt and colleagues proposed that non-responders were actually a result of lead displacement after PNE [6]. They hypothesized that the permanent electrode was the only stable electrode available, and prospectively enrolled 10 of 47 non-responders who initially had a good response but did not meet criteria for permanent implantation. These patients underwent placement of the permanent electrode in the operating room, of which 80% demonstrated 90% improvement in their symptoms. This was significantly better compared to their average response rate of 52% using PNE. While their results supported suspicions that lead migration during PNE was the etiology for varying responder rates, the invasive and costly nature of placing the permanent lead for initial testing limited its use in clinical practice.

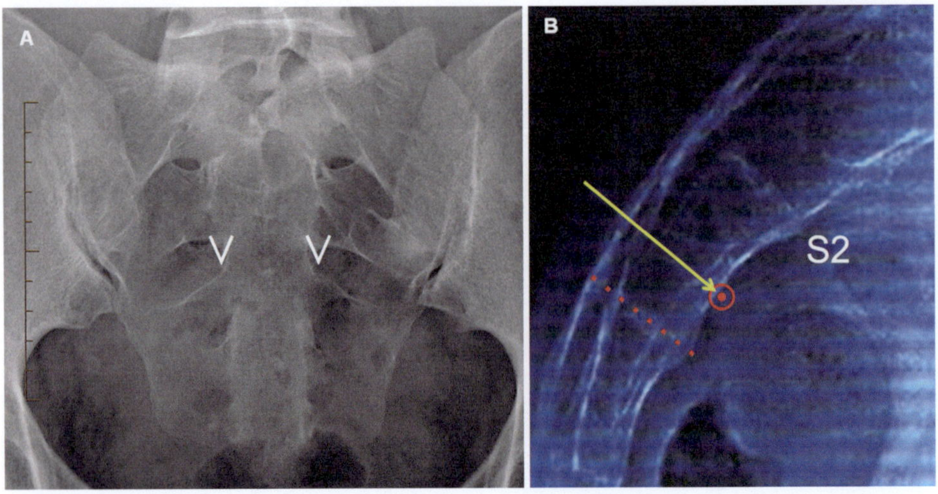

Fig. 5.8 Fluoroscopic view of landmarks. (**a**) In the AP view of the sacrum, the medial aspects of the foramen are marked. The lead wire should pass through this space. (**b**) In the lateral view, note the angle of needle placement is approximately 1 cm above the hillock and is parallel with the fusion plate. Reprinted with the permission of Medtronic, Inc. © 2017

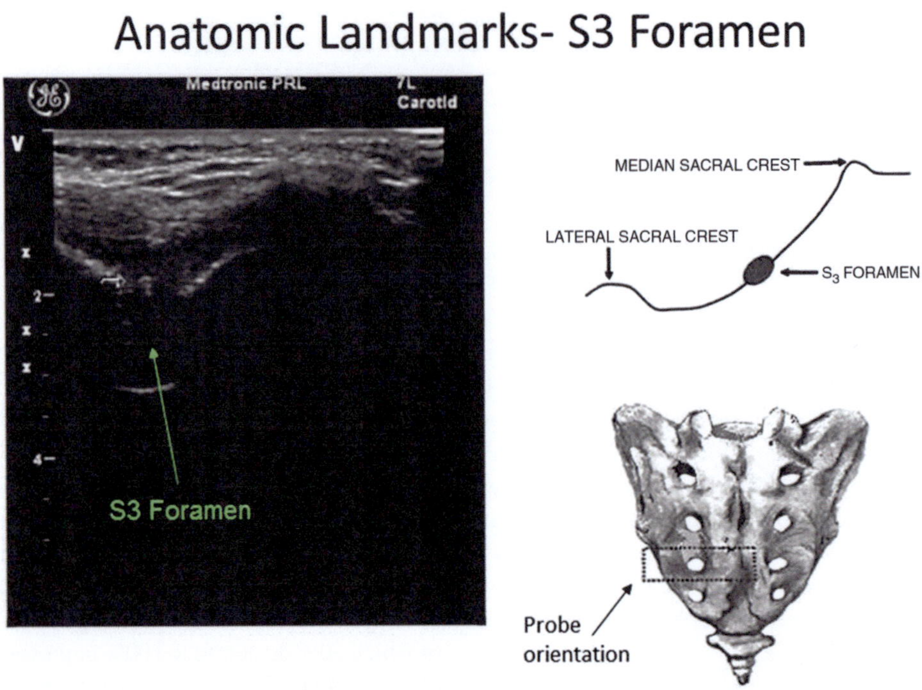

Fig. 5.9 Ultrasound view of landmarks. In the axial view, the S3 foramen can be visualized between the lateral and median sacral crest. Reprinted with the permission of Medtronic, Inc. © 2017

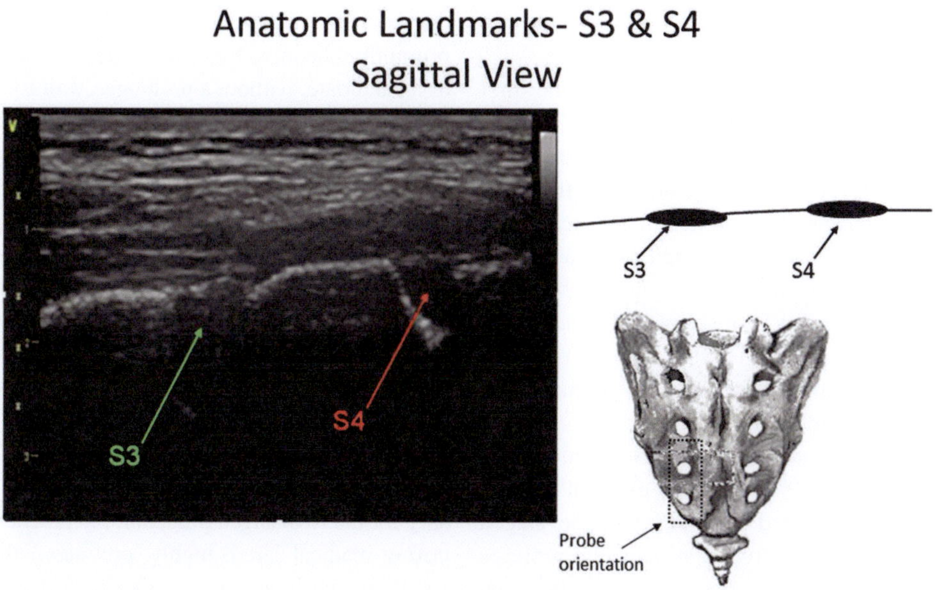

Fig. 5.10 Ultrasound view of landmarks. In the sagittal view, the S3 and S4 foramen can be visualized in the same image. Reprinted with the permission of Medtronic, Inc. © 2017

Table 5.2 Com-parison of PNE versus TLE

PNE (one-staged implant)		TLE (two-staged implant)	
Advantages	Disadvantages	Advantages	Disadvantages
Less invasive	Patient discomfort	Patient comfort	Risks of anesthesia
Less resource intensive	Risk of lead migration	Allows for longer trial period	Unreliable sensory response
Bilateral	Successful conversion 40%	Ideal for obese patients	Costly
Reliable sensory response	Unipolar lead	Tined lead already placed	
		Successful conversion 80–90%	
		Quadripolar lead	

Siegel et al. described good, long term, clinical efficacy in a large cohort of patients among 12 European centers who underwent SNM for UUI, UR or urgency-frequency [10]. Despite this, only 44% (260/581) had successful test stimulation with PNE. This highlighted the need to improve test stimulation to identify responders. Furthermore, when patients did demonstrate a positive response to PNE, as many as 28% did not see sustained results with permanent implantation [11]. Siegel cited a newly available test stimulation lead as a hopeful future direction to improve the success of PNE for identification of responders.

In 2000, a coiled permanent lead (Medtronic® Model 3057) was introduced. This lead could be placed percutaneously under local anesthesia but still had a 25% rate of lead migration, despite various locking devices to secure it to the sacrum. In 2002, Medtronic introduced a quadripolar lead with self-anchoring tines. The lead contained four cylindrical electrodes and four flexible tines to act like anchors and minimize migration. The tines were novel in that lead placement did not require a large incision or anchoring.

Spinelli and colleagues presented the first experience with the tined lead electrode (TLE) in 15 patients, of which 12 underwent permanent implantation [12]. They concluded that this two-staged, percutaneous approach under local anesthesia was superior to PNE and two-stage open with a responder rate of 80%. Furthermore, the minimally invasive nature of the tined lead maintains the ability to assess sensory response since it can be performed under local anesthesia and mitigates the need for general.

A recent advance is the development of the Medtronic Verify™ system: an external generator that can be used for PNE and the staged implant. This is a wireless system that replaces the external programmable generator (EPG) that had to be directly connected to the externalized lead. With the Verify™ system, the patient has a handheld controller that remotely connects to the EPG. Thus, it simplifies the test period by eliminating the connection wire, which many patients found to be troublesome.

Adverse Events

Adverse events (AE) related to SNM can occur with initial test stimulation or permanent implantation. While implantation site infection and cellulitis are rare, more common AEs are undesirable changes in stimulation, pain, or skin irritation at the implant site. Rarely, temporary leg weakness has been reported. While AEs are not uncommon, most are therapy or permanent device related rather than secondary to initial test stimulation with PNE.

Advantages/Disadvantages

While the PNE has been used less often in recent years, it maintains several advantages. It continues to be the least invasive approach for test stimulation, requiring only a needle stick, and no incision. Furthermore, it avoids the cumbersome aspects of going to the operating room twice for placement of the lead and subsequent IPG. Patients can be promptly scheduled for office PNE once identified as a candidate, without a prolonged wait for a surgical date and multiple pre-operative appointments for obtaining consent, lab work, and medical clearance. Additionally, the risks associated with anesthesia and hospital admission are reduced by only having one procedure in the hospital versus two. Without the use of sedation or general anesthesia, providers can rely on, both, sensory and motor response to lead placement and stimulation. In a European study comparing cost of PNE versus TLE, the cost of each kit was 210 versus 7750 pounds, respectively [14]. These costs did not include the use operating room resources necessary for the two-staged procedure. In an era where cost of medical care is highly scrutinized, the role for PNE may increase. Another consideration is that bilateral placement is the standard for PNE and as such, is acceptable for billing. This is not the case for the two-staged approach. While, PNE has a lower response rate, a bilateral test approach can increase a patient's chance for a successful response [4, 15]. Additionally, a modified technique in which the electrode is subcutaneously tunneled can improve the response rate without increasing cost [16].

Disadvantages of PNE are highlighted through the advantages of TLE (Table 5.2). After receiving a good response with the PNE lead, one runs the risk of losing that precise orientation when replacing the permanent lead in the operating room. With the current two-staged approach, the lead wire that is initially placed is maintained in the second stage for responders. Furthermore, PNE can be uncomfortable and make correct placement difficult. This can lead a physician to incorrectly conclude that the patient is not a responder. For this reason, patients who do not obtain a response to initial stimulation with PNE should be considered for a two-staged procedure.

Conclusion

The peripheral nerve evaluation remains a viable option for the testing phase of sacral neuromodulation. It is minimally invasive and carries very little risk. Although the conversion rate to permanent implant is not as high as the staged implant, careful patient selection and the use of bilateral PNE leads may lead to higher success.

References

1. InterStim® sales analysis of 2013.
2. Gormley EA, Lightner DJ, Faraday M, et al. Diagnosis and treatment of overactive bladder (non-neurogenic) in adults: AUA/SUFU guideline amendment. J Urol. 2015;193:1572–80.
3. Paquette IM, Varma MG, Kaiser AM, et al. The American Society of Colon and Rectal Surgeons' Clinical Practice guideline for the treatment of fecal incontinence. Dis Colon Rectum. 2015;58(7):623–36.
4. El-Azab A, Siegel S. Specific tips for general controversies in sacral neuromodulation. Curr Urol Rep. 2016;17:79.
5. Cohen B, Tunuguntla H, Gousse A. Predictors of success for the first stage neuromodulation: motor versus sensory response. J Urol. 2006;175:2178–81.
6. Janknegt R, Weil E, Eerdmans P. Improving neuromodulation technique for refractory voiding dysfunctions: two stage implant. Adult Urol. 1997;49:358–62.
7. Rodine P, Falkner P, Brelje T, et al. Sacral foramen localization for needle placement: diagnostic ultrasound vs. fluoroscopy. Neurourol Urodyn. 2015;34(S1):S90.
8. Siegel S, Noblett K, Mangel J, et al. Results of a prospective, randomized, multicenter study evaluating sacral neuromodulation with InterStim therapy compared to standard medical therapy at 6-months in subjects with mild symptoms of overactive bladder. Neurourol Urodyn. 2015;34:224–30.
9. Pannek J, Grigoleit U, Hinkel A. Bacterial contamination of test stimulation leads during percutaneous nerve stimulation. J Urol. June 2005;65:1096–8.
10. Siegel S, Catanzaro F, Dijkema H et al. Long-term results of a multicenter study on sacral nerve stimulation for treatment of urinary urge incontinence, urgency-frequency, and retention. Urology. 2000;56(Suppl. 6A).
11. Bosch J, Groen J. Sacral nerve neuromodulation in the treatment of patients with refractory motor urge incontinence: long-term results of a prospective longitudinal study. J Urol. 2000;163:1219.
12. Spinelli M, Giardiello G, Gerber M, et al. New sacral neuromodulation lead for percutaneous implantation using local anesthesia: description and first experience. J Urol. 2003;170:1905–190.
13. Van Kerrebroek P, Voskuilen A, Heesakkers J, et al. Results of sacral neuromodulation therapy for urinary voiding dysfunction: outcomes of a prospective, worldwide clinical study. J Urol. 2007;178:2029–34.
14. Auterio S, Hallas N, Betts N, et al. The cost-effectiveness of sacral nerve stimulation (SNS) for the treatment of idiopathic medically refractory overactive bladder (wet) in the UK. BJU Int. 2015;116(6):945–54.
15. Amend B, Khalil M, Kessler T, et al. How does sacral modulation work best? Placement and programming techniques to maximize efficacy. Curr Urol Rep. 2011;12(5):327–35.
16. Sievert KD, Nagele U, Pannek J, et al. Subcutaneous tunneling of the temporary testing electrode significantly improves the success rate of subchronic sacral nerve modulation. World J Urol. 2007;25: 607–12.

6 Use of Electromyography (EMG) in Neuromodulation

Kevin Benson

Introduction

Neuromodulation is an emerging field that offers promise for patients with a variety of pelvic floor disorders; these include recalcitrant urge-frequency syndrome, urinary retention, and fecal incontinence. The use of neuromodulation continues to grow exponentially and more indications for neuromodulation will surely follow. For neuromodulation to be effective, one has to deploy electrodes near the nerve target in a consistent fashion. Unfortunately, there is no clinical way to view the actual nerve targeted. Currently, only surrogate markers of response are used, including visual cues bellows response and great toe flexion. These markers are arbitrary and depend on personal interpretation. In many cases, adequate motor responses may not be possible due to medical disease or body habitus. Sensory responses are also used and are not consistent. These clinical responses are subjective, inaccurate, and leave room for interpretation. Recent studies show an 80% response rate to SNS [1, 2]. One reason that one in five do not respond may be due to the subjective interpretation of responses. The use of electroneurodiagnostics may aid in better use of neuromodulation. electroneurodiagnostics include electromyography (EMG), nerve conduction studies and evoked potentials. In this chapter, we will focus on the use of EMG. The use of EMG allows recording of a compound motor action potential (cMAP). The use of compound muscle action potential (cMAP) monitoring objectifies the process of neuromodulation and may increase the success of the therapy. Currently, there is a paucity of data evaluating the effectiveness of cMAP monitoring, and most experts in the field are just implementing the use of this technology in clinical practice. In time, the use of cMAP evaluation will become standard care for the application of pelvic neuromodulation. This chapter focuses on a complete review of cMAP technology and cMAP applications for pelvic neuromodulation.

Background

As the use of neuromodulation grows, so do dilemmas in its use. Many physicians struggle with optimal lead placement and often patients lack ongoing efficacy. Often it is unknown whether clinical failure of neuromodulation represents a lack of response to the therapy or a failure in optimal surgical execution. Compound motor action potential (cMAP) guidance may fill the gap, answering basic questions. Implementing

K. Benson (✉)
Female Pelvic Medicine and Reconstructive Surgery, Sanford Health, Sioux Falls, SD, USA
e-mail: kevin.benson@sanfordhealth.org

J. P. Gilleran, S. A. Alpert (eds.), *Adult and Pediatric Neuromodulation*,
https://doi.org/10.1007/978-3-319-73266-4_6

the use of electroneurodiagnostics and the use of cMAP responses intraoperatively and in the office will result in more effective delivery of neuromodulation with better patient outcomes.

Critical to executing and interpreting neuromodulation effectively is decreasing reliance on subjective findings. Patients may struggle expressing accurate sensation during testing despite pretreatment counseling. In addition, motor responses are also subjective to the observer and may not correlate with sensory response. Patients may also have physical barriers to exhibiting motor responses as well (muscle wasting, paralysis, amputation, etc.). cMAP evaluation provides an objective measure of nerve response leading to more efficient and accurate application of neuromodulation. cMAP monitoring makes up for many patient difficulties. Not only does cMAP monitoring assure more consistent application of neuromodulation therapy. Application of cMAP monitoring shortens operating time could reduce the rate of lead revisions and increases device battery life, thus leading to a more cost-effective procedure.

History of Electroneurodiagnostics

The role of electrical signaling in muscles has been researched for several 100 years. Many integral discoveries have ultimately led to the useful, commercial technology in use today. Francesco Redi is first credited with discovery of electric current in eels in the 1700s. During the 1800s, Matteucci created the first Galvanometer and described the action potential. The term electromyography was coined by Etienne Marey shortly thereafter. In 1929, Adrian and Bronk developed the concentric needle for neurorecording. The development of the recording needle electrode helped facilitate Herpert Jasper's invention of the first form of the electromyograph in 1942. The first modern, commercially available EMG came on the scene in 1950. In the 1980s, paperless systems for analysis became available. With the advent of the digital age, computer enhanced interpretation of signals became possible. Computer advancements have made data collection much less onerous and increased the value of EMG for research and clinical use. Today, the use of EMG monitoring may be as simple as using a "smart" phone. The use of EMG for the science of neuromodulation is just beginning and has not yet been adopted on a large scale. Few clinicians use electroneurodiagnostics and many are unfamiliar with its potential value.

This chapter would be remiss if not to mention the contributions to the understanding of electrophysiology of the pelvis by Drs. Tom Benson, Chet DeGroat, and Ken Peters. These pioneers have helped us understand the complex concepts of neural control of the pelvic floor.

Electroneurodiagnostics is a broad term which encompasses a variety of nerve testing including electromyography (EMG), nerve conduction testing (a form of EMG), and somatosensory evoked potentials (SSEP). Currently, only EMG testing appears to be useful in evaluating success of neuromodulation. Other electroneurodiagnostic studies (nerve conduction testing) have been used to establish some normative data for a variety of pelvic floor reflexes, most notably the clitoral-anal reflex, bulbocavernosus-anal reflex, and the pudendal-anal reflex. Studies looking at the implications of abnormal pelvic nerve studies have struggled to define a clinically meaningful difference in outcomes [3, 4].

Application of neuromodulation for pelvic floor disorders is a newly developing field and normative data is lacking. No reference studies are available. Many questions still remain as to the role for electroneurodiagnostics used in conjunction with neuromodulation.

Clinical Scenarios Where cMAP Monitoring May Be Beneficial

Mrs. Smith is a 42-year-old patient with a 5-year history of recalcitrant urinary urgency and urge-associated incontinence. In the past, she has tried a number of medications, behavioral modification, and physical therapy without success. The option of sacral neuromodulation is offered. A success rate of 80% is discussed. The patient asks what factors may influence her chance of success.

You explain to the patient that deployment of a properly placed lead is essential for success of the therapy. The use of cMAP monitoring in the operating room helps assure an efficient and successful primary surgical outcome.

Mrs. Smith is a 42-year-old patient referred to your practice after previous placement of sacral neuromodulation for recalcitrant urge-frequency syndrome. She had InterStim® device placed 3 months ago and has yet to see clinical success despite multiple reprogramming attempts. Office interrogation with cMAP determines whether reprogramming is possible or whether lead revision is necessary.

Mrs. Smith is a 42-year-old with recalcitrant urge-frequency syndrome that had a sacral neuromodulation lead placed 1 year ago and initially had excellent response; she now has lost success and is unable to return to efficacy despite normal device function and sensation. The decision is made to proceed with a trial of pudendal neuromodulation. CMAP technology is mandatory for pudendal neuromodulation as traditional responses are not measurable.

In each of the three common scenarios above, the use of cMAP evaluation leads to more efficient and cost-effective management with greater patient satisfaction. Multiple benefits are achieved through cMAP monitoring. Some potential benefits are listed below:

Potential cMAP Benefits

- Reduced operating room time
- Less reprogramming
- Improved patient satisfaction
- Longer battery life
- Reduced complications

Mechanism of cMAP

CMAP is an abbreviation for compound muscle action potential. This is a measurement of simultaneous muscle action potentials from a group of closely grouped muscle fibers.

At a basic level, cMAP is a recording (summation) of individual motor unit potentials (MUPs). An action potential is a temporary depolarization of a nerve membrane that conducts along the nerve leading to muscle contraction. An action potential has two phases: subthreshold and threshold. An adequate stimulus is needed to reach threshold which induces a change in membrane potential opening a sodium channel which triggers the voltage difference seen as an action potential [5]. In a given muscle, multiple action potentials are activated simultaneously resulting in contraction. There are a finite minimum number of action potentials required to induce muscle contraction. The strength of the muscle contraction is influenced by the number of action potentials activated. Individual action potential follows an "all-or-none" phenomenon; which states if the stimulation reaches threshold, it will create a response, if the stimulation does not meet threshold, no response will be seen. However, a muscle contraction is "graded," which requires a minimum number of motor unit potentials to create contraction and additional potentials to increase contraction strength as seen with recruitment of more individual muscle fibers.

To record cMAP, one uses a paired set of electrodes to measure neural muscle response to stimulation. In some cases, the morphology of the cMAP recording may be indicative of certain disease processes. In the case of neuromodulation, the implications of different tracing morphologies is not known. Currently, a simplistic tracing is all that is needed for clinical practice. It appears that the binary presence or absence of cMAP response is critical to clinical response to neuromodulation therapy. CMAP is used for a variety of clinical applications including measurement of nerve injury, neuropathic processes, and nerve degeneration. CMAP may be used with a variety of neural targets with neuromodulation including sacral, pudendal, and dorsal clitoral nerves. Using cMAP for measurement of neural response in conjunction with neuromodulation is novel and much remains unknown.

Mechanism of Neural Stimulation of the Pelvis

The mechanisms of pelvic neuromodulation are described in detail elsewhere in this textbook. In brief, in the case of standard pelvic neuromodulation (InterStim® therapy) stimulation is applied through a quadripolar lead deployed in the sacrum (Medtronic 3889-28). Sacral peripheral nerve stimulation in turn leads to central neural modulation through ascending pathways via the spinal cord to the level of several brain centers. Central neuromodulation and the gross muscle movement seen with stimulation are *not* analogous. For cMAP to be demonstrated, motor activation is required. The motor activation seen through dorsiflexion of the great toe or bellows response of the buttocks does not occur from direct motor stimulation, but instead through an irritative lumbosacral interneuron mechanism that induces a response resulting in distal muscle contraction. The muscle responses seen in the buttocks and great toe are analogous to pulling a hand away from a hot stove. Therefore, stimulation of pelvic nerves is not the same as direct motor activation of the clinically seen muscle contractions in the buttocks and foot. It is not known whether central nervous system responses are always coupled with motor responses, or whether motor responses are necessary to indicate potential for central nervous system (CNS) modulation. Currently, muscle responses are all that are available as a surrogate for CNS modulation.

A typical cMAP tracing represents the schematic depiction of the depolarization of a number of individual action potentials within a muscle leading to muscular contraction. As shown in Fig. 6.1, the baseline represents the resting muscle potential with a recording of "zero" (membrane potential is actually −70 μV).

Before muscle contraction can occur, an electrical stimulus is applied. This is recorded as either a positive or negative sharp deflection from baseline and is considered a "stimulation spike/artifact." Convention recommends this be a positive deflection. The direction of deflection is determined by the position of the recording electrodes. If a sponge electrode is used, this is not applicable. If the initial deflection is negative (downward), one may reverse the perianal electrode order in the connecting block (Fig. 6.2).

After electrical stimulus is applied to the muscle, if the stimulation is of sufficient intensity (threshold), depolarization occurs and muscular contraction follows.

In certain situations, measurement of latency as well as the size of the action potential (depolarization) response is possible. The significance of latency and intensity of the cMAP (action

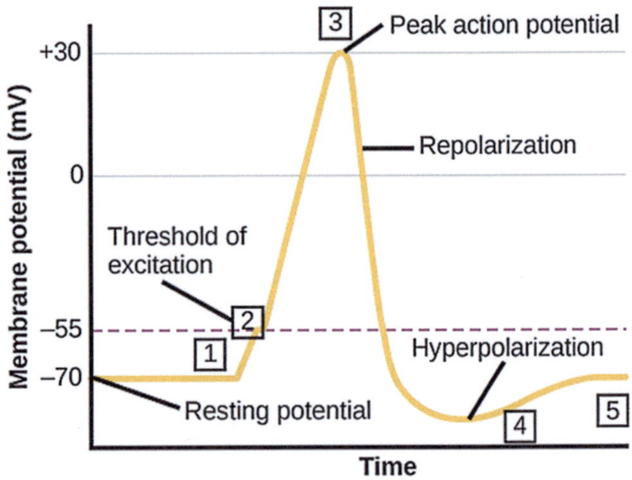

Fig. 6.1 Anatomy of an action potential [15]. Source: OpenStax College, How Neurons Communicate. October 17, 2013. OpenStax CNX Creative Commons 3.0

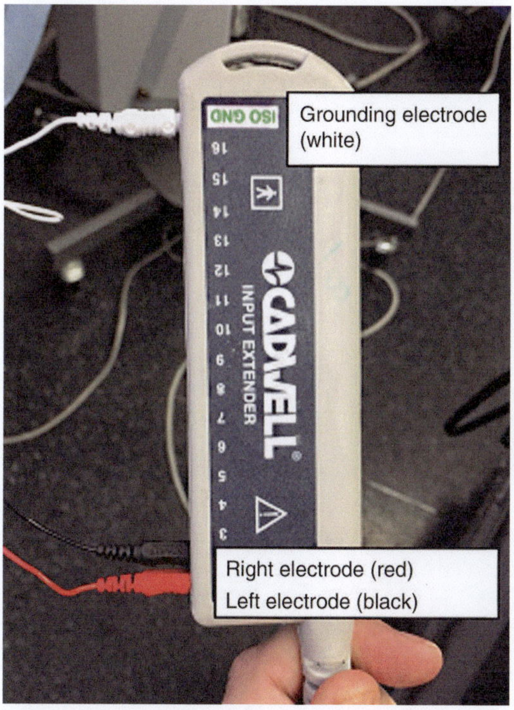

Fig. 6.2 Lead input extender connection block. Reversing the black and white electrode will change the polarity (+/−) of the stimulation artifact on the tracing

potential) response remains undetermined using current pelvic floor neuromodulation applications. At this time, one is simply documenting the presence or absence of depolarization leading to muscular contraction.

Once depolarization occurs the nerve will repolarize, hyperpolarize, and then return to the baseline resting potential and may be stimulated again.

Fig. 6.3 represents a typical real-time cMAP EMG tracing recorded during a trial of sacral neuromodulation. As depicted, both a "live" and a "captured" image are present (live seen in white and captured in pink). Further discussion of live versus captured images occurs later in this chapter. Of note, rarely does the live depicted waveform appear exactly as a textbook example and some interpretation of the image is dependent on the surgeon and operating room EMG staff.

Operating Room Staff

Most operating room-based procedures employ a neuro-technologist to help set up the EMG machinery and monitoring electrodes. The technologist often stays throughout the procedure to help interpret results. Reaching out to your hospital-based technologists is a helpful starting place in implementing EMG studies. Neurotechnologists are often employed in the department of radiology or neurology and may be known as EMG technologists or "neuro techs." Contacting your operating room coordinators to determine who helps with intraoperative cMAP procedures in your institution works well. Neurotechnologists work commonly with neurosurgeons and orthopedic surgeons on neurologic surgery cases, such as laminectomies and discectomies. Often there is a shortage of EMG technologists available and scheduling their presence in advance is a necessity for smooth case flow.

EMG Equipment

For the most part, equipment used for cMAP evaluation is readily available as standard equipment used in the operating room or office. Use of EMG equipment is commonplace for neurologists, rehabilitation physicians, and spine surgeons. Traditional EMG monitoring equipment is available through several manufacturers.

EMG equipment falls into one of two groups, a sophisticated, multichannel laptop model or a simple, single channel handheld model. A simple single channel model is ideal for clinic-based monitoring. However, laptop-based systems are more common, and available through a hospital-based format (Fig. 6.4). Handheld versions are commonly used in clinic settings by rehabilitation specialists and physical therapists for a number of therapy applications such as biofeedback. For the purposes of pelvic floor neuromodulation, a simple, single channel device is usually adequate. Often, the more robust multichannel laptop system is what is available in the OR setting, and although

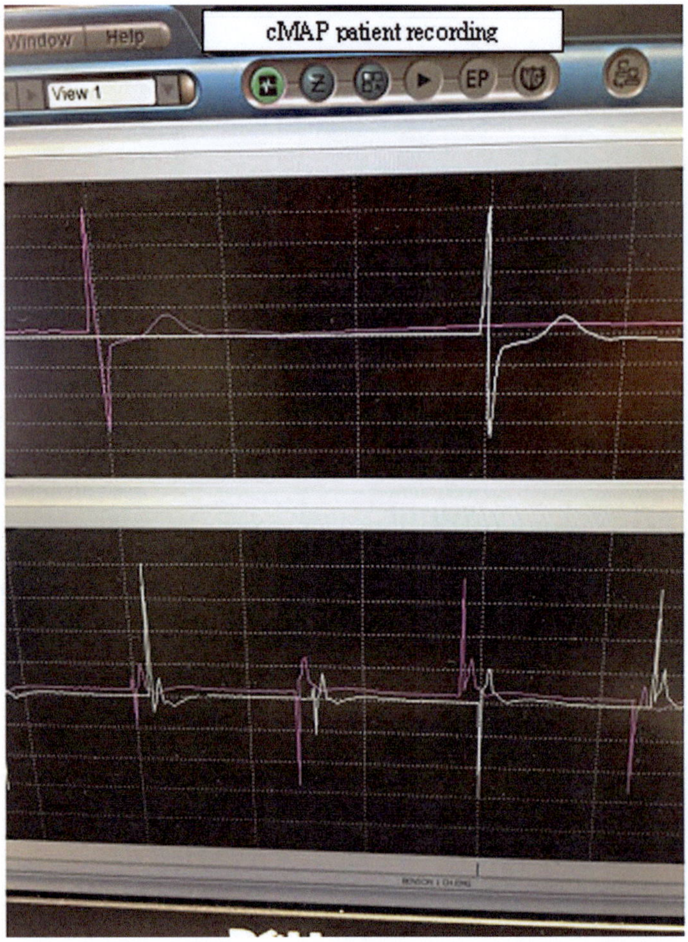

Fig. 6.3 Intraoperative cMAP recording. Note split screen. The top screen only demonstrates captured (suprathreshold) recordings. The bottom screen reveals all responses, whether of threshold or not. Actual live recording depicted in white, captured recording in pink. Initial stimulation is noted as the sharp spike. Patient response is seen following the spike

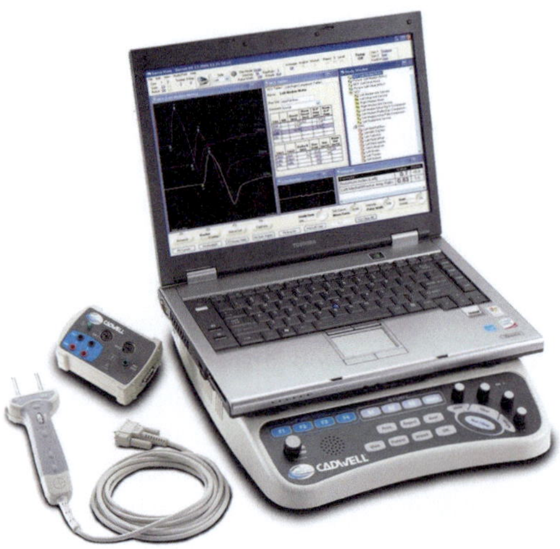

Fig. 6.4 Typical laptop-based EMG system. Photo of Sierra® Wave courtesy of Cadwell Electronics, Inc.

more cumbersome will be more likely accessible to most physicians. For the purposes of this chapter, a laptop-based device will be featured. A multichannel EMG system costs $3000.00–5000.00. Many simple handheld systems are substantially less expensive.

EMG Components

- Laptop based system (Fig. 6.4)
- Monopolar needle electrodes (Fig. 6.5)
- Sponge electrode-optional (Fig. 6.7)
- Electrode connector block (Fig. 6.2)
- Programming recording sheet (Fig. 6.9)

Equipment Settings

Equipment setup and interpretation is straightforward and can be mastered quickly. Contemporary monitoring devices have settings to help filter signals. Essentially, all filter settings are designed to narrow the signal width and decrease artifact and noise. Selection of appropriate filter settings enhances the ability to correctly identify true nerve response signals. Standard modifiable filter settings are as follows:

High frequency: Sets the device's upper frequency sensing limit, reducing signals above this value, standard setting is 1000 Hz.

Low frequency: Sets the lower limit, reducing signals below this value, standard setting is 10 Hz.

Notch filter: Eliminates noise/artifact that occurs at a set rate, such as electrical interference in standard circuits. The standard setting is 60 Hz. It is important to use an isolated circuit if possible.

Gain: This setting represents "volume" and reflects the input to output ratio. Standard gain setting is 100 μV/division.

Sweep speed: This setting represents the "analysis time" of how long a recorded event will be stored before it is visually replaced on the screen, after the triggered event has occurred. Reducing the sweep speed results in less the artifact but more missed events, increasing the sweep speed captures more information along with more artifact. 10 ms/division triggered events and 50 ms/division for live display.

Stimulation rate: Represents the rate of stimulation set by the screener box. Standard neuromodulation stimulation rates are 5–14 Hz. Lower stimulation rates result in more target separation and clearer individual wave forms.

Threshold: Reflects the minimal voltage required to create a captured event. A common setting is 100 μV. There is no standard regarding threshold, as it is dependent on each patient's anatomy and electrode placement; this setting is at the discretion of the user.

> **EMG Settings**
>
> High frequency = 1000 Hz
> Low frequency = 100 Hz
> Notch = 60 Hz
> Screener box stimulation rate = 5–15 Hz
> Sweep speed = 50 ms/division for live recording and 10 ms/division for triggered events
> Time base = 10 ms/division
> Trigger threshold = 100 mV

Time base: Represents a screen setting of increments of time elapsed per area of display. Standard setting is 10 ms/division.

Electrode Choices

Paired monopolar recording needles are used for most applications (Fig. 6.5). Monopolar needles are typically placed at 6 and 12 o'clock around the anus (Fig. 6.6). Another option is a sponge electrode (Fig. 6.7). Sponge electrodes may be placed either in the rectum or vagina. The use of a sponge electrode allows for differential recording of levator muscle and anal sphincter responses. Monopolar needles have the advantage of measuring a very precise muscular area and have the disadvantage of revealing more noise artifact. Monopolar needles also are more painful on insertion than a sponge electrode and carry the theoretical risk of skin

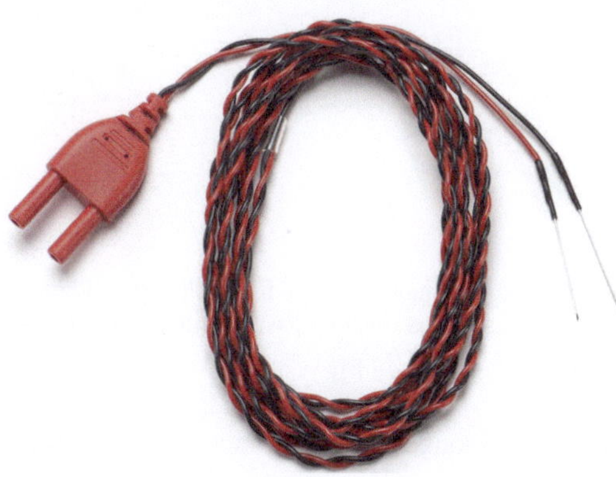

Fig. 6.5 Paired monopolar needle electrodes. Reprinted with the permission of Medtronic, Inc. © 2015

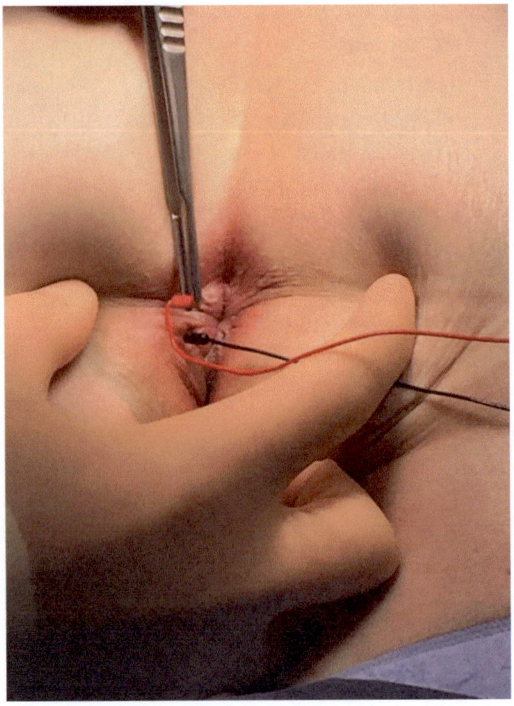

Fig. 6.6 Placement of perianal concentric needle electrodes, note forceps which should be discarded once placed to avoid contamination

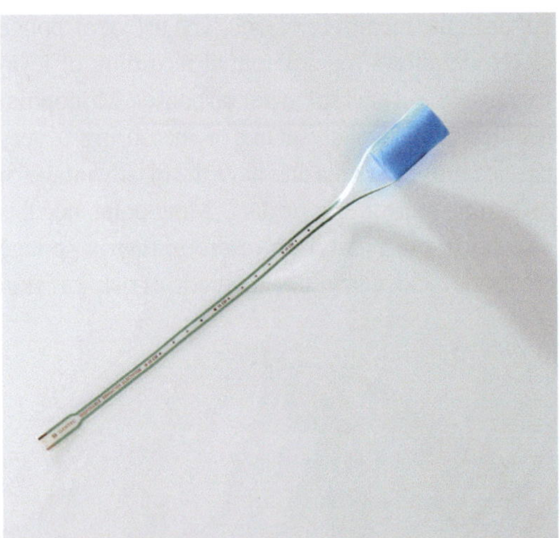

Fig. 6.7 Rectal/vaginal sponge EMG electrode. Photo of electrodes supplied in the past courtesy of Laborie/Mediwatch

infection. Sponge electrodes measure a larger area and record averaged responses. Sponge electrodes tend to show less movement artifact compared to

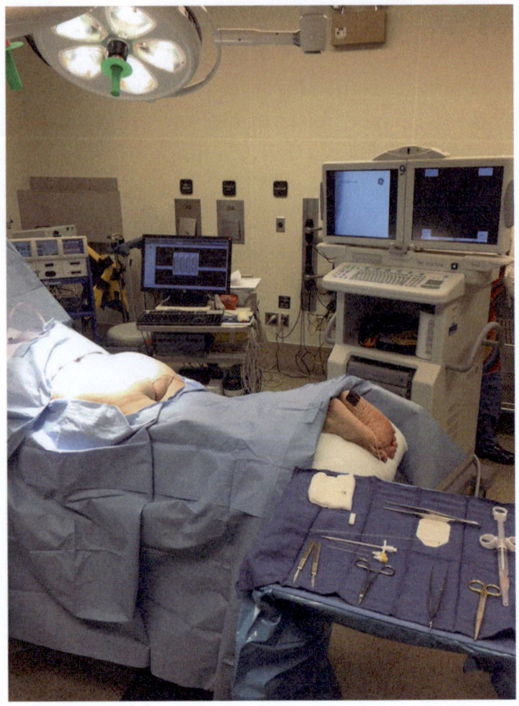

Fig. 6.8 Typical cMAP operating room setup. Note positioning of drapes to allow for anal access. Also note position of EMG display for intraoperative viewing

needle electrodes. Sponge electrodes are also more comfortable than needles. Sponge electrodes do not allow one to select a focused muscular area. For sedated patients' use of needle electrodes work well and can isolate smaller muscles with less noise artifact. For patients who are awake or in an office setting the use of a rectal or vaginal sponge electrode may be better tolerated. One may wish to experiment with both needle and sponge electrodes to find which is most feasible for their practice. Unfortunately, there is currently a paucity of sponge electrode manufacturers and thus availability is limited. The majority of monitoring uses monopolar needles.

Patient/Electrode Positioning

Patients are placed in standard prone position. Surgical drapes must be placed low enough to access the anus for placement of needle electrodes, or the vagina/anus for placement of a sponge electrode (Fig. 6.8). Care should be taken to not contaminate the surgical field during electrode placement. It is recommended to use a forceps to apply the needle electrodes and discard the instrument after placement of the electrodes (Fig. 6.6). In addition to the recording electrodes, a grounding electrode is also placed (generally on the thigh). Once the electrodes are placed an equipment test is performed. A common source of artifact is a lead that is not all the way inserted into the skin. If the baseline tracing is not flat, one should inspect the recording electrodes. Taping the electrodes to the buttock helps ensure that they will not become dislodged throughout the surgery or office evaluation.

Operational Steps

Pelvic neuromodulation using cMAP assistance is performed as standard practice dictates. The steps for successful cMAP lead monitoring:

The only additional steps required are initial recording electrode placement and lead "mapping" once the lead is placed. Once one is adept at performing cMAP interpretation, the time to perform neuromodulation is actually expedited using cMAP monitoring. One of the most valuable steps in cMAP testing is "lead mapping" described in the following chapter. Equipment needed for implementation of cMAP monitoring is listed below.

Operative Steps for cMAP Monitoring

Apply perianal electrodes-connect to input extender connector block

Apply grounding electrode-connect to input extender connector block

Assess EMG equipment for function

Perform standard neuromodulation technique monitoring for cMAP responses

Once appropriate stimulation is noted, perform cMAP bipolar lead assessment

Remove perianal electrodes and grounding electrode

CMAP Screen Display

All EMG systems utilize a monitor screen display for real-time readout. The screen is often "split" with captured image on the top and a live image below. The "captured" screen is often easier for interpretation as the only images that appear are those that reach threshold. The lower image is responses that occur. Figure 6.3 demonstrates the two readouts seen.

CMAP Lead Testing Protocol

Establishing a routine intraoperative and office protocol for recording CMAP responses is essential for consistent and effective use of cMAP technology. Recording a fixed set of anode/cathode combinations is termed "Mapping." Mapping may be performed intraoperatively or in a clinic setting. Intraoperatively, the lead may be tested once deployed. It takes just a few minutes to evaluate a number of anode/cathode setting responses. The recorded responses may be used as a reference for postoperative patient management. Knowing the objective voltage required for nerve

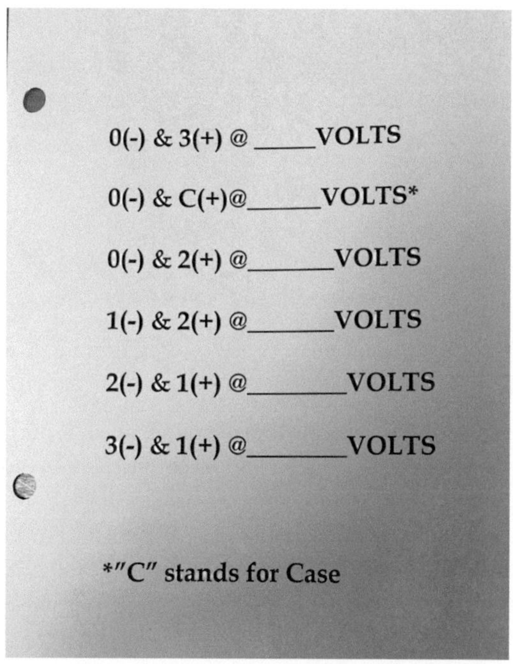
0(-) & 3(+) @ ____VOLTS

0(-) & C(+)@_____VOLTS*

0(-) & 2(+) @______VOLTS

1(-) & 2(+) @______VOLTS

2(-) & 1(+) @_______VOLTS

3(-) & 1(+) @_______VOLTS

*"C" stands for Case

Fig. 6.9 Intraoperative program recording sheet

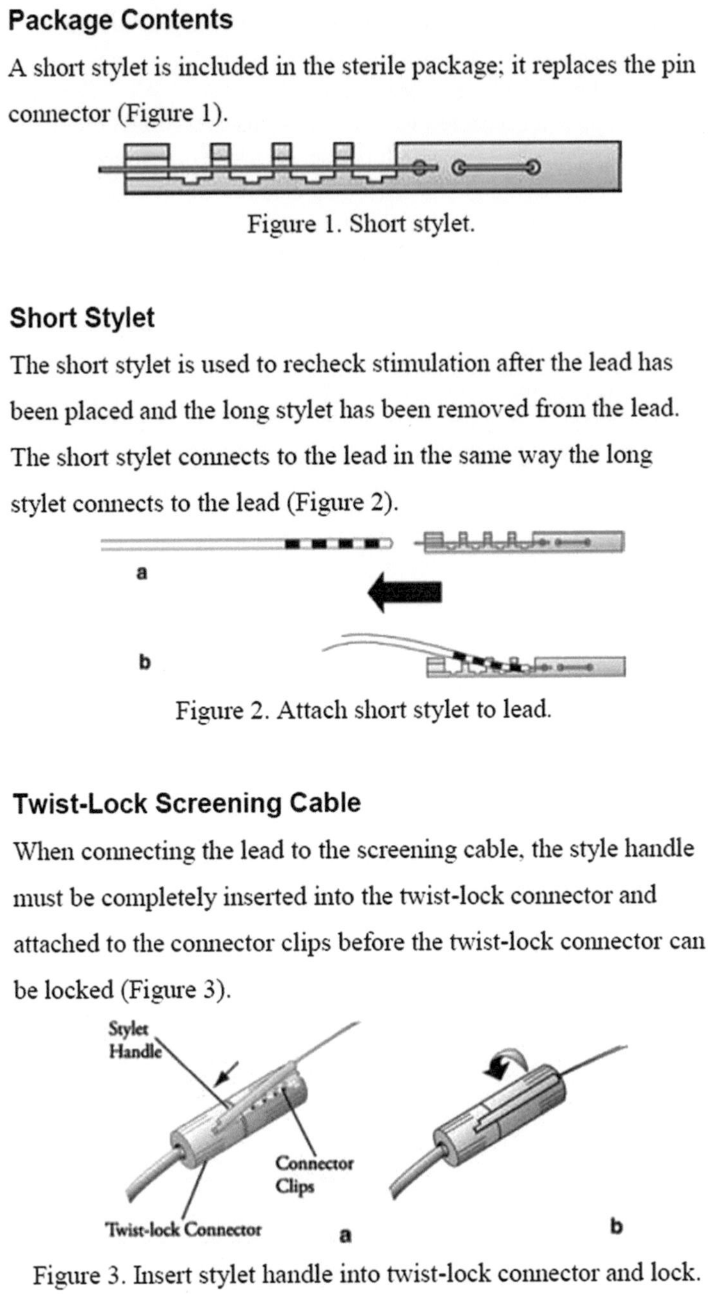
Package Contents

A short stylet is included in the sterile package; it replaces the pin connector (Figure 1).

Figure 1. Short stylet.

Short Stylet

The short stylet is used to recheck stimulation after the lead has been placed and the long stylet has been removed from the lead. The short stylet connects to the lead in the same way the long stylet connects to the lead (Figure 2).

Figure 2. Attach short stylet to lead.

Twist-Lock Screening Cable

When connecting the lead to the screening cable, the style handle must be completely inserted into the twist-lock connector and attached to the connector clips before the twist-lock connector can be locked (Figure 3).

Figure 3. Insert stylet handle into twist-lock connector and lock.

Fig. 6.10 Medtronic 3550 lead connector kit for intra operative testing. Reprinted with the permission of Medtronic, Inc. © 2015

activation is valuable for programming staff post-operatively, as patients are often uncertain as to sensory feedback.

A typical testing protocol involves a variety of bipolar (the use of an electrode as a cathode and an electrode as an anode) settings that tests the complete lead length using anode/cathode combinations (Fig. 6.9).

Bipolar Testing Protocol Anode/Cathode Combinations

0(−) & 3(+)
0(−) & 2(+)
1(−) & 2(+)
2(−) & 1(+)
3(−) & 1(+)

To facilitate bipolar testing, one needs to use the *Short Stylet* contained within the Medtronic accessory kit 3550-03 (Fig. 6.10). Contained in the 3550 kit is a small white snap-on adaptor that replaces the long stylet and connects the *Twist-lock Screening Cable* to a screener box or to the Medtronic Verify© system. Once connected, one may test a variety of anode/cathode combinations in an orderly fashion. Monopolar settings cannot be tested with this setup. Usual stimulation combinations are listed below. Once response thresholds are established for each anode/cathode combination it allows for rapid postoperative programming and postoperative patient surveillance. Knowing objective levels of stimulation is invaluable as staff can rapidly and consistently assess response without questioning the level of stimulation applied.

Applications of CMAP Monitoring

CMAP monitoring is a useful tool in a variety of settings. From original lead placement to assessing need for lead revision/replacement cMAP is beneficial. Once one incorporates the technology it is useful for all applications of neuromodulation. Listed below are some specific circumstances applicable for cMAP monitoring.

CMAP Applications

- Initial lead placement
- Reprogramming
- Lead replacement
- Lead revision
- Pudendal neuromodulation
- Dorsal genital nerve stimulation
- Subsensory programming

Initial Lead Placement

Initial cMAP lead placement guidance objectifies neural response. The use of sensory response or visual motor response to judge electrode placement allows for subjective interpretation. The use of sensory responses appears inferior to the use of motor responses in measurement of patient outcomes [6]. cMAP simplifies the process using objective measures. Many patients may not give accurate verbal information during the procedure and often visual motor responses are difficult to see due to body habitus or muscle wasting or neurologic conditions. cMAP technology helps to guide intraoperative staged lead placement and in-office percutaneous lead placement (PNE).

Reprogramming

Patients who initially respond to neuromodulation may lose efficacy over time. The cause of this loss of effectiveness is not known. Theories for loss of efficacy include lead migration and modulation of brain responses due to chronic stimulation. The former may require lead revision, the latter may respond to reprogramming. Reprogramming to positive cMAP responses may reduce the rate of lead revision and removal. A study by Everaet et al. [7] revealed that in patients with an optimal cMAP response at time of failure reprogramming or lead revision was not successful and in those with suboptimal initial cMAP response either reprogramming to positive cMAP or lead revision to positive cMAP had resumption of success. When loss of efficacy occurs, it is frustrating to both the patient and physician. Reprogramming with cMAP guidance may provide help in restoring efficacy. A recent study by Lee et al. [8] investigated 31 patients previously implanted with InterStim® therapy to determine the correlation between sensory and motor responses and whether those reprogrammed under cMAP guidance would see improvement in voiding parameters. Of the 31 patients 12 had cMAP responses at baseline. Ten of those with baseline + cMAP responses (83%) experienced >50% improvement in symptoms compared to 13 of 19 (63%) of those without baseline +cMAP. Sixteen of nineteen without baseline motor response were successfully reprogrammed to achieve cMAP. Improvements of 15–20% in nocturia, incontinence and urgency incontinence episodes were seen in the reprogrammed group. These two studies point to the potential benefit of additional objective guidance for reprogramming/lead replacement.

Lead Revision

Just as cMAP is useful with initial lead placement, it can be used to guide lead revision as well. Often the decision to revise the lead can be made more expeditiously with in-office cMAP testing. Many patients present with leads that were originally not placed with cMAP guidance and lead revision may be the first opportunity to utilize cMAP guidance.

Pudendal Neuromodulation

Pudendal neuromodulation is an emerging form of therapy which may have some advantages over traditional sacral neuromodulation. The pudendal nerve is a mixed sensory and motor nerve arising from levels S2–S4 and, as such, it is a major contributor to pelvic floor function. As outlined elsewhere in this text, this may represent a different neural target for a variety of disorders including urinary dysfunction, fecal incontinence, constipation, pudendal neuralgia, and persistent genital arousal disorder. A paucity of data exists on comparative effects of pudendal neuromodulation versus traditional sacral neuromodulation. There is evidence that it may be superior for patients that have failed sacral neuromodulation [9]. The pudendal nerve is accessible through a variety of approaches including transgluteal and transperineal. Proper lead placement requires intraoperative EMG guidance as lower extremity responses are not demonstrable. cMAP responses are robust and easy to demonstrate.

Dorsal Genital Neuromodulation

The dorsal genital nerve (DGN) is a branch of the pudendal nerve supplying sensory innervation for the clitoris and penis. Several publications show promise for neuromodulation of the target to treat a variety of conditions including overactive bladder, urinary retention, fecal incontinence, and sexual dysfunction [10–14]. The use of cMAP guidance fits nicely for this application as well.

Subsensory Programming

For many, stimulation applied to a sensory threshold may be uncomfortable or associated with radicular symptoms. Potentially, many may respond at levels below conscious awareness. Up to 25% of patients exhibit motor response before awareness of sensory feedback. CMAP may allow one to benefit from stimulation without the negative stimulation sensation. This may allow use of a previous implanted lead saving explantation.

References

1. Spinelli M, Weil E, Ostardo E, et al. New tined lead electrode in sacral neuromodulation: experience from a mulitcentre European study. World J Urol. 2005;23:225–9.
2. Peters KM, Killinger KA, Ibrahim IA, et al. The relationship between subjective and objective assessments of sacral neuromodulation effectiveness in patients with urgency-frequency. Neurourol Urodyn. 2008;26:1–4.
3. Olsen A, Ross M, Stansfield B, Kreiter C. Pelvic floor nerve conduction studies: establishing clinically relevant normative data. Am J Obstet Gynecol. 189(4):1114–9.
4. Wester C, FitzGerald MP, Brubaker L, Welgoos L, Benson JT. Validation of the clinical bulbocavernosus reflex. Neurourol Urodyn. 2003;22:589–92.
5. Daube JR, Devon IR. Clinical neurophysiology. 3rd ed. Oxford: Oxford University Press; 2009. p. 839.
6. Cohen B, Tunuguntla H, Gousee A. Predictors of success for first stage neuromodulation: motor versus sensory response. J Urol. 2006;175:2178–81.
7. Everaert K, De Ridder D, Baert L, et al. Patient satisfaction and complications following sacral nerve stimulation for urinary retention, urge incontinence and perineal pain: a multicenter evaluation. Int Urogynecol J Pelvic Floor Dysfunct. 2000;11(4):231–5;discussion 236.
8. Lee J, Osann K, Noblett K. Comparison of motor and sensory response of InterStim® for overactive bladder syndrome. Female Pelvic Med Reconstr Surg. 2013;19(6):317–21.

9. Peters KM, Killinger KA, Boguslawski BM, Boura JA. Chronic pudendal neuromodulation: expanding available treatment options for refractory urologic symptoms. Neurourol Urodyn. 2010;29:1267–71.
10. Tajkarimi K, Burnett A. The role of genital nerve afferents in the physiology of the sexual response and pelvic floor function. J Sex Med. 2011;8:1299–312.
11. Opisso E, Borau A, Rijkhoff N. Subject-controlled stimulation of the dorsal genital nerve to treat neurogenic detrusor activity at home. Neurourol Urodyn. 2013;32:1004–9.
12. Worsoe J, Fynne L, Laurberg S, Krogh K, Rijkhoff N. Electrical stimulation of the dorsal clitoral nerve reduces incontinence episodes in idiopathic faecal incontinent patients: a pilot study. Coloproctal Dis. 2012;14:349–55.
13. Goldman H, Amundsen C, Mangel J, Grill J, Bennett M, Gustafson K, Grill W. Dorsal genital nerve stimulation for the treatment of overactive bladder symptoms. Neurourol Urodyn. 2008;27(6):499–503.
14. Farag F, Martens F, Rijkhoff N, Heesakkers J. Dorsal genital nerve stimulation in patients with detrusor overactivity: a systemic review. Curr Urol Rep. 2012;13:385–8.
15. Boundless. Nerve Impulse Transmission within a Neuron: Action Potential. Boundless Biology Boundless. 2016. https://www.boundless.com/biology/textbooks/boundless-biology-textbook/the-nervous-system-35/how-neurons-communicate-200/nerve-impulse-transmission-within-a-neuron-action-potential-762-11995/. Accessed 3 May 2017.

Pudendal Neuromodulation

7

Jason P. Gilleran and Natalie Gaines

Abbreviations

AMPA	α-amino-3-hydroxy-5-methyl-4-isoxazolepropionic acid
EMG	Electromyography
GABA	Gamma ammino-butyric acid
IPG	Implantable pulse generator
IS	Ischial spine
NMDA	N-methyl-D-aspartate
OAB	Overactive bladder
PN	Pudendal nerve
PNM	Pudendal neuromodulation
PNS	Pudendal nerve stimulation
PTNS	Percutaneous tibial nerve stimulation
SNM	Sacral neuromodulation
TNS	Tibial nerve stimulation

Introduction

The pudendal nerve (PN) was first named in 1762 by Camper, its root from the Latin word *pudendus*, meaning "to be ashamed," a reference to its role in the private areas of the human body [1]. The PN innervates the anogenital region and has dual functions of both motor and sensory innervation. Because of its focused innervation of the lower urinary tract and pelvic floor, it has been proposed as an ideal site for neuromodulation in select patients. Early studies of electrostimulation using animal models from Tanagho and Schmidt [2] at the University of California, San Francisco, in the 1980s described use of the pudendal nerve as a useful target, and in 1986, Vodusek stated that "it seems quite clear that the somatic afferent input having the most consistent vesicoinhibitory influence is excitation of the pudendal nerve" [3]. However, in spite of the lumbodorsal fascia cutdown required, S3 neuroprosthesis placement remained less invasive than a pudendal nerve exposure and became standard by 1992 [4].

The pudendal nerve continues to be of notable interest to clinicians who perform neuromodulation on a regular basis. This chapter will discuss recent animal studies that have helped elucidate the unique role of the pudendal nerve and its role in neural control of the lower urinary tract and will present outcomes from clinical studies in several indications. The focus will be on pudendal neuromodulation, rather than other forms of pudendal nerve surgery, such as nerve blocks and decompression. We will also present our experience with patient selection, perioperative management, and the surgical technique when using

J. P. Gilleran (✉)
Department of Urology, Oakland University William Beaumont School of Medicine, Royal Oak, MI, USA
e-mail: jgilleran@urologist.org

N. Gaines
Urology San Antonio, San Antonio, TX, USA
e-mail: natalie.gaines@urologySA.com

J. P. Gilleran, S. A. Alpert (eds.), *Adult and Pediatric Neuromodulation*,
https://doi.org/10.1007/978-3-319-73266-4_7

the PN as an alternative to the standard sacral approach for patients with overactive bladder and/or pelvic pain.

Pudendal Nerve Anatomy

The pudendal nerve comprises contributions from the ventral, or anterior, rami of nerves from the S2, S3, and S4 foramina. Once formed, the "supralevator" portion of the PN traverses the ventral surface of the piriformis muscle within the greater sciatic foramen. From the piriformis muscle, the PN then courses behind the sacrospinous ligament and the overlying coccygeus muscle, just medial to the ischial spine. Because of the course of the nerve, the ischial spine is a clinically relevant landmark for pudendal nerve block. Knowledge of the close proximity of the PN to the ischial spine also allows for identification of the PN during sacrospinous ligament fixation, which helps to avoid ligation or injury to the nerve. The PN then exits the pelvis through the greater sciatic foramen, traveling on the posterolateral surface of the sacrospinous ligament. It enters the perineum through the lesser sciatic foramen and then enters Alcock's canal, which is located on the lateral wall of the ischioanal fossa. This canal, formed by a splitting of the obturator internus muscle fascia, contains roughly one-third of the length of the pudendal nerve and embeds the nerve in loose areolar tissue [5].

While considerable anatomic variation exists, the pudendal nerve generally has three terminal branches: the inferior rectal nerve, the dorsal nerve to the clitoris, and the perineal nerve. The inferior rectal nerve typically branches within the pudendal canal and pierces the wall of the canal medially around its midpoint; it then courses inferomedially and its branches innervate the external anal sphincter and perianal skin [6]. The dorsal nerve to the clitoris exits the pudendal canal, traveling along the inferior pubic ramus, and terminates at the clitoris. After exiting the pudendal canal, the perineal nerve branches and supplies the ischiocavernous, bulbocavernous, and superficial transverse perineal muscles as well as the external urethral sphincter and the skin of the labia [6, 7].

Pudendal Nerve Studies in Animal Models

Recent animal model studies have been essential in elucidating underlying mechanisms and effects associated with pudendal nerve stimulation. Several studies have been generated from the lab of Dr. William C. de Groat at the University of Pittsburgh, who deserves special notoriety.

Neurotransmitters

Important inhibitory neurotransmitters involved in pudendal neuromodulation include gamma aminobutyric $acid_A$, 5-HT_3, β-adrenergic, and glutamate receptors. $GABA_A$ receptor inhibition primarily works in the spinal cord via interneurons [8]. 5-HT_3 receptors rely on serotonin receptors in the sacral spinal cord, with input from the brainstem [9]. In addition, the non specific 5-HT_2 receptors also play a role in PNS inhibition of reflex bladder activity, and at the same time interact with opioid mechanisms in micturition reflex pathway [10]. β-adrenergic receptors cause reflex activation of sympathetic inhibition in the lumbar sympathetics of the spinal cord [11, 12]. Several important glutaminergic receptors include Gln-5 [13] as well as *N*-methyl-D-aspartate (NMDA) and α-amino-3-hydroxy-5-methyl-4-isoxazolepropionic acid (AMPA), which are all involved in modulating pudendal nerve stimulation's effect on bladder capacity in cats with reduced bladder capacity due to acetic acid irritation [14].

Pudendal Stimulation Compared to Tibial Stimulation

Pertinent negative studies showed that different receptors are responsible for PNS than TNS. Opioid receptors play a very minor role in

PNS inhibition of bladder overactivity but a large role in the inhibitory behavior of TNS [15–17]. Cannabinoid-1 (CB1) receptors are more associated with tibial inhibition of bladder overactivity, not PNS [18]. Lyon et al. showed that only PNS, not TNS, utilizes β-adrenergic receptors [12].

A recent neuroanatomical study from Bansal et al. isolated the nerve roots involved with tibial or pudendal nerve stimulation. The authors found that transection of the ipsilateral S2 nerve root completely inhibited the effect of pudendal nerve stimulation, thus S2 clearly has a profound effect on PNS efficacy [19].

Another difference between PNS and TNS seen in animal studies is how stimulation frequency leads to different outcomes. At low frequencies (5 Hz), PNS is inhibitory to the bladder but excitatory at high frequencies (20–30 Hz), whereas TNS is inhibitory both at low (5 Hz) and high (30 Hz) frequencies [13, 20, 21].

Pudendal Stimulation and Effect on Bladder Capacity

In a nociceptive C-fiber afferent-mediated feline model of bladder overactivity, transdermal amplitude-modulated stimulation of the pudendal nerve inhibited the spinal bladder reflex and increased bladder capacity [22]. Intraurethral stimulation of female rats with overactive bladder (OAB) using a 2.5-Hz frequency has been another means shown to improve bladder capacity [23].

In another rat model using pulsed radiofrequency (PRF) stimulation, Jen et al. showed increased bladder capacity lasting 4 h after stimulation ended [24]. Of note, PRF also was shown to cause no neural damage, as no caspase-3 activity was seen (a marker of apoptosis).

Intermittent Versus Continuous Stimulation

In feline studies, stimulation of the pudendal nerve led to sustained bladder contractions [25]. Tai et al. showed that intermittent electrical stimulation of PN was as effective as continuous stimulation in cats [13]. They proposed that intermittent stimulation could be applicable in humans and conserve battery life when using a chronic stimulator.

Mechanism of Action in Humans

Pudendal nerve stimulation, compared to sacral, modulates a much broader composition of fibers from S2, S3, and S4. This allows the PN to have a wide range of effects, since it innervates the bladder, external urethral and anal sphincters, the pelvic organs, and the pelvic floor musculature.

Centrally, pudendal stimulation leads to increased activity in the cortical regions involved with bladder control. In their study of 8 spinal cord injured patients who underwent acute pudendal stimulation while being monitored with functional MRI, Zempleni et al. reported increased activity in the right posterior insula [26].

Peripherally, a majority of pudendal afferent activity is derived from the S2 nerve root. Huang et al. provided an early description of the pudendal afferent mapping in 105 children with cerebral palsy and spasticity (but no bladder dysfunction). They found the S1, S2, and S3 roots provided 4, 60.5, and 35.5% of the overall afferent activity, respectively. The distribution was asymmetric in more than half, and in 18% was confined to a single sacral level [27].

Locally, pudendal nerve stimulation causes increased pressure in the bladder neck and external urethral sphincter. In a study of 20 spinal cord injured males, PN stimulation, delivered via the dorsal penile nerve, resulted in increased pressure in the bladder neck (via autonomic afferents) and external urethral sphincter (via somatic afferents) [28].

Patient Selection and Perioperative Counseling

The discussion on expectations, recovery, risks, and postoperative care is similar to that for sacral neuromodulation with some notable exceptions.

The most important and obvious surgical difference between sacral and pudendal is the location of the lead itself.

Rather than placed via transforaminal approach and anchored to the periosteum, the pudendal lead passes through the ischiorectal space, as explained in the surgical technique section of this chapter.

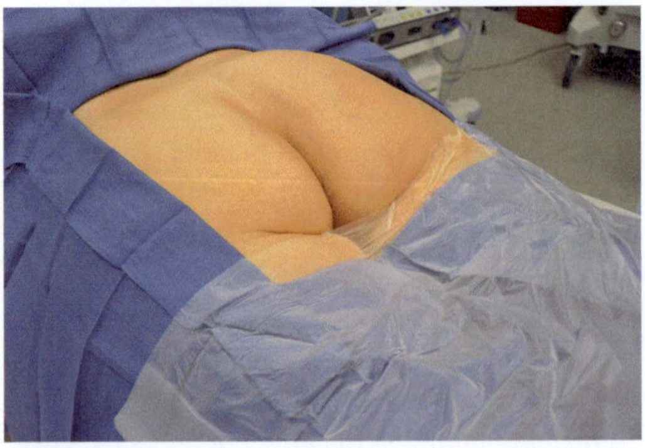

Fig. 7.1 Patient positioning for first-stage pudendal lead placement. Note that lower buttocks and upper thighs must be completely exposed and prepped, unlike sacral lead placement

Indications/Appropriate Patient Selection

The most common indication for trial of pudendal neuromodulation implant is after failed attempt to address OAB symptoms with S3 nerve root stimulation. If placement of a tined sacral lead during a first-stage procedure is unsuccessful, the patient can be offered to place a pudendal lead at the time previously saved for second-stage implantation—that is, instead of implanting the implantable pulse generator, the sacral lead can be removed and a pudendal lead placed, saving the patient an additional procedure.

Unlike SNM, PNM is not FDA approved and is currently an off-label therapy for patients with refractory lower urinary tract symptoms. Since pudendal neuromodulation utilizes some of the same sacral afferents as SNM (S3), we will annotate the surgical dictation as "placement of tined electrode to the lesser sciatic foramen at the pudendal nerve as a means of sacral neuromodulation with intraoperative monitoring of EMG programming and fluoroscopy." This clarifies the lead location but still provides a means to perform sacral neuromodulation.

Surgical Technique

Positioning, EMG Needle Placement and Draping

Patient positioning for the pudendal approach is similar to that for sacral neuromodulator implant: prone with all pressure points padded. However, one important difference between PNM and SNM is that the entire buttock and upper thigh area needs to be exposed for PNM to provide access to the lower buttock near the ischial tuberosities. Deep conscious sedation and local anesthesia is usually sufficient for patient comfort. We drape off about 10–15 cm caudal to the cleft between the buttock and upper thigh (Fig. 7.1). We use a chlorhexidine prep to cleanse the entire lumbosacral area, buttocks, and upper thigh, and the final portion of the prep includes the gluteal cleft and perianal region. Care must be taken to allow the prep to dry for 3 min before beginning the surgery. Sterile blue towels are used to surround the operative area—one placed across the mid-thigh, one on either side up the lateral thigh and flanks, then one across the mid-back. We use a 51 by 51 inch adhesive barrier (3M™ Steri-Drape™ Medium Drape with Incise Film 1060) to cover the upper thigh area transversely after placing towels.

Since pudendal nerve identification cannot be done without intraoperative neurophysiologic guidance, electromyography (EMG) needles are placed in the 3- and 9-o'clock positions next to the anal sphincter (anal sphincter electromyography), then secured with a Nexcare™ Steri-Strip™ skin closure strip at 2–3 points, after the adhesive barrier but before the surgical drape (Fig. 7.2). They are then passed off to the neurophysiology technologist to hook into the computerized oscilloscope. We recommend first double-gloving to place the needle, then immedi-

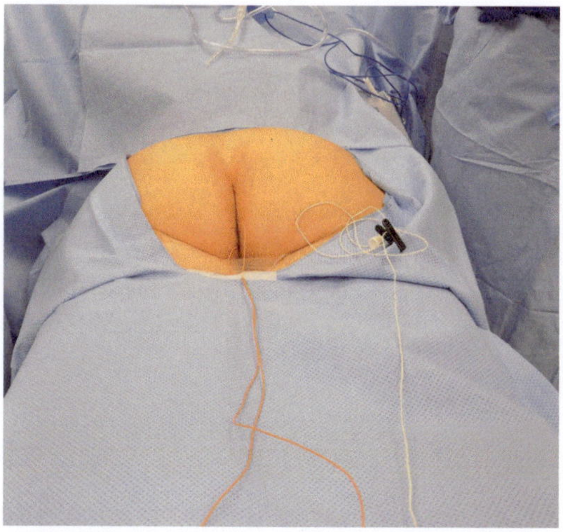

Fig. 7.2 Patient positioned with bilateral electromyography (EMG) needles placed in the external anal sphincter at 3 and 9 o'clock

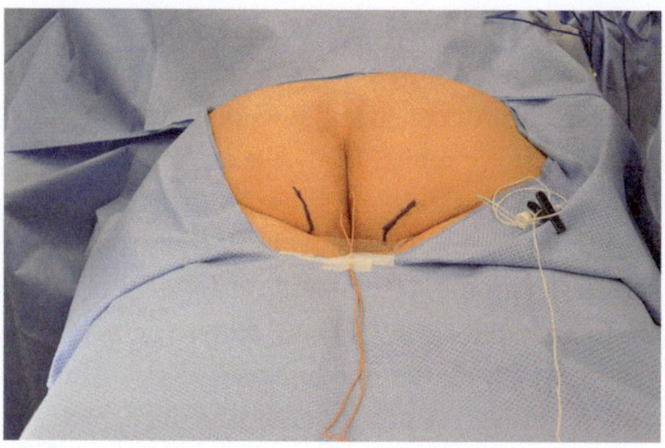

Fig. 7.3 Skin markings noting the palpable medial edges of the ischial tuberosities

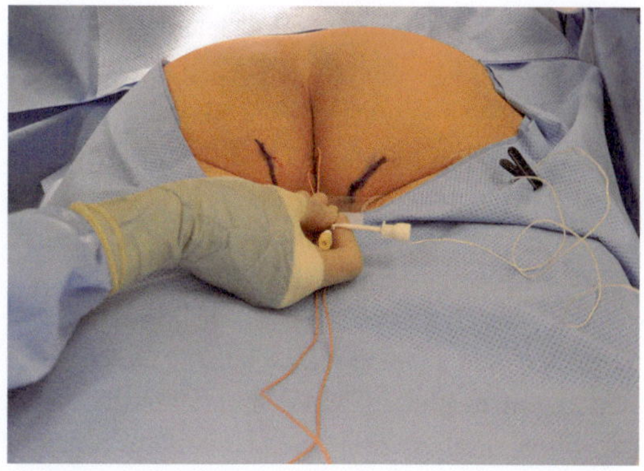

Fig. 7.4 Access to pudendal nerve through the ischiorectal fossa using a 5″ spinal needle with the stimulating cable attached and set at 5 V and 5 Hz to allow for optimal visualization of a CMAP

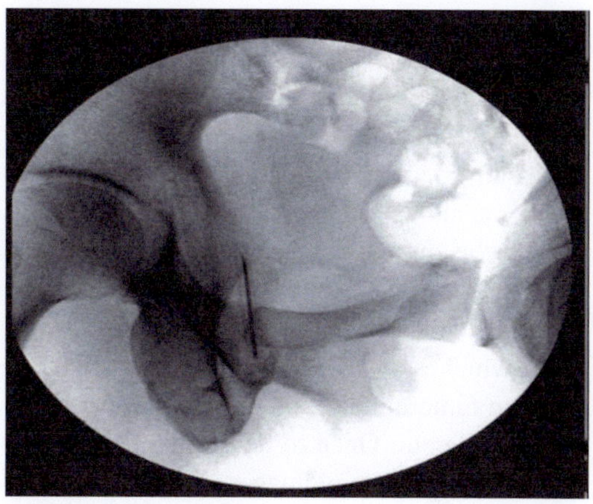

Fig. 7.5 AP view of pelvis, with needle denoting ischial spine landmark for locating pudendal nerve

ately discarding the external pair of gloves to avoid contamination from the anal region.

Pudendal Nerve Location and Landmarks

Begin with palpation of the medial aspect of each ischial tuberosity, and mark the skin to delineate this landmark (Fig. 7.3). After liberal infusion of local anesthesia to the skin just medial to these markings, insert a 5″ foramen needle with the Verify™ cable attached to provide electrical stimulation at the tip. The entry point should be near the level of the perineum, about 2–3 cm superior to the anal verge, but hugging close to the tuberosity (Fig. 7.4). The initial passes are designed to "find" the nerve, and we stimulate using 5 V at 5 Hz—a voltage higher and a frequency lower than standard sacral stimulation—to allow our EMG technician to better visualize the compound muscle action potential (CMAP). We start with AP fluoroscopy, and aim the tip of the 5″ foramen needle along the tuberosity, through the ischiorectal space, and at a slight medial-to-lateral angle. The target should be a point just medial to the ischial spine, which should be seen on AP fluoroscopy as a thin, triangular protuberance (Fig. 7.5).

Lead Placement

Once the pudendal nerve is in contact with the stimulating needle, a CMAP of variable strength is identified, often accompanied by a motor reflex of an anal sphincter spasm. Be mindful that a motor reflex can be deceptive, and it must be accompanied by a CMAP to assure accurate placement along the pudendal nerve. As the goal is to slide a quadripolar lead along the nerve, with contact on all four electrodes ideally, it is critical to align the introducer needle along the path of the nerve. To accomplish this, we will advance the needle ~1 cm deeper than the point of initial nerve contact; if the CMAP does not abolish during this passage, one can assume that the needle is oriented in the proper manner to allow lead placement.

In the event, the nerve cannot be easily found on this initial attempt, lateral view fluoroscopy may facilitate identification of proper needle passage, which should be approximately halfway between femoral head and coccyx, almost parallel to the femur. Once in the proper plane, save both the AP and lateral images in the event access is lost and one needs to repeat initial introducer needle passage.

Placement of the Tined Lead

Similar to the sacral stimulator implant, the next step is to carefully pass the directional guide wire to the appropriate depth, as shown in Fig. 7.6. With the guide wire in the same location as the introducer needle, make a 1 cm skin incision above and below the guide wire, with extreme care to avoid moving it in or out at all. Upon passing the lead introducer, reattach the lead stimulation cable to the metal portion (Fig. 7.7) to allow for stimulation upon entry of the introducer.

Once along the course of the nerve again and with stimulation of the nerve (and accompanying CMAP), slowly remove the trocar of the introducer and guide wire, leaving only the access sheath. We recommend doing this under live AP fluoroscopy to assure the radiopaque tip of the introducer does not deviate medially, which would make lead placement along the nerve very difficult. Be mindful that the CMAP will abolish upon removal of the trocar. We advise using the 41 cm straight InterStim® electrode (Model #3889-41) to allow for adequate length to reach the subcutaneous pocket at the upper buttock. Upon passing the lead, use the cable to stimulate the 0 (zero, or deepest) lead and advance deeper along the course of the nerve until the lead is passed about 1–1.5 cm or the CMAP is lost (Fig. 7.8).

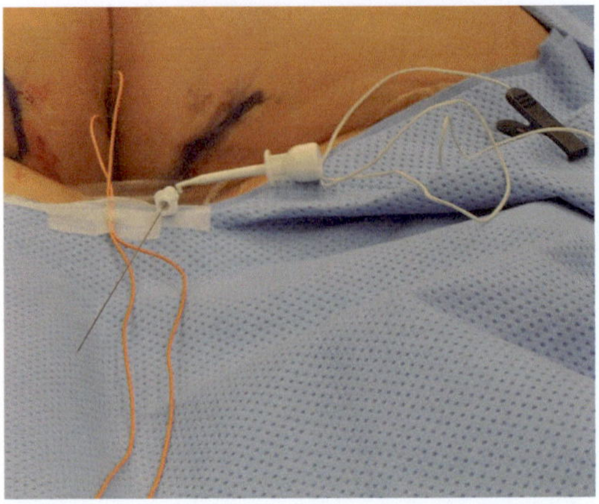

Fig. 7.6 Once spinal needle is along the course of the pudendal nerve, a bidirectional guide wire (similar to that used for sacral lead placement) is passed through the lumen, while still providing electrical stimulation

Check all four electrodes in standard fashion and record the threshold for CMAP on each (similar thresholds will be measured in bipolar fashion once connected to the external source). Ideally, one should attain CMAP on all 4 electrodes, but 3 (or in rare cases 2) may be adequate for programming and clinical efficacy. Consider repassing the trocar at a different angle if one is uncertain about adequate stimulation. Confirm final position of lead on AP and lateral fluoroscopy, as demonstrated in Fig. 7.9. Figure 7.10 shows ideal lead placement along the nerve in a cadaver model, with corresponding fluoroscopic images in AP and lateral views. If the lead is placed improperly across the nerve, one may be limited to a single electrode in contact with the PN, as shown in Fig. 7.11.

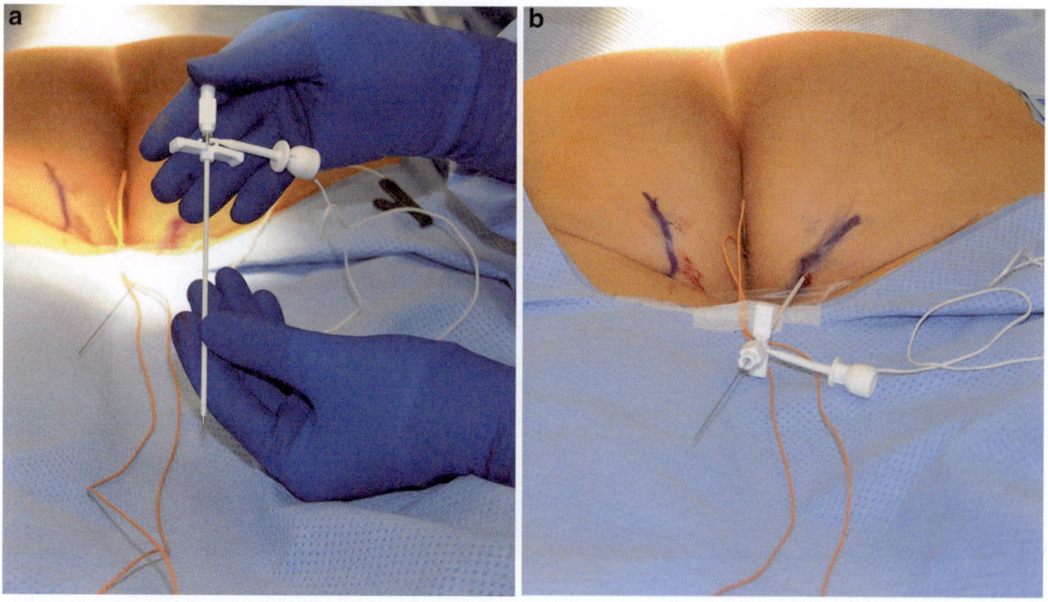

Fig. 7.7 (**a**) Stimulating needle attached to lead introducer, contacting metal of the inner obturator sheath, then (**b**) passed over bidirectional guide wire

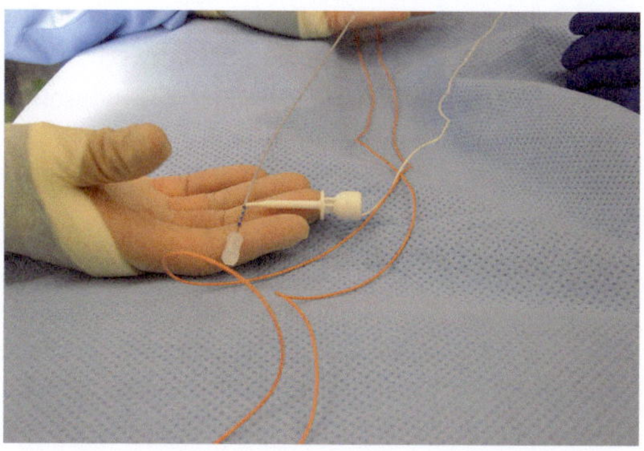

Fig. 7.8 41 cm tined lead is passed through sheath, with stimulating cable attached to deepest electrode (electrode 0), before testing all four electrodes

Lastly, repeat testing on either the deepest (0) or most superficial (3) electrode with gentle upward pressure on the bottom of the buttock to simulate the sitting position, followed by ventral pressure on the buttock to simulate the supine position.

Tunneling and Connecting to Temporary Percutaneous Extension

Once satisfied with lead position, the subcutaneous pocket is made in the ipsilateral upper buttock, identical to location for a sacral lead. The long lead tunneler is then passed from the upper to the lower buttock incision, with extreme care taken to protect the lead from damage with the sharp tip of the tunneler (if necessary, place a finger over the incision to protect the lead) (Fig. 7.12). The proximal end of the lead is passed cephalad and connected, then tunneled again, in standard fashion similar to a stage I sacral lead implant. The incisions are closed with absorbable subcutaneous or horizontal mattress suture.

Surgical Approaches

There are currently four published approaches for electrostimulation of the pudendal nerve—the posterior, perineal, the "STAR" approach, and a laparoscopic approach. While we describe the

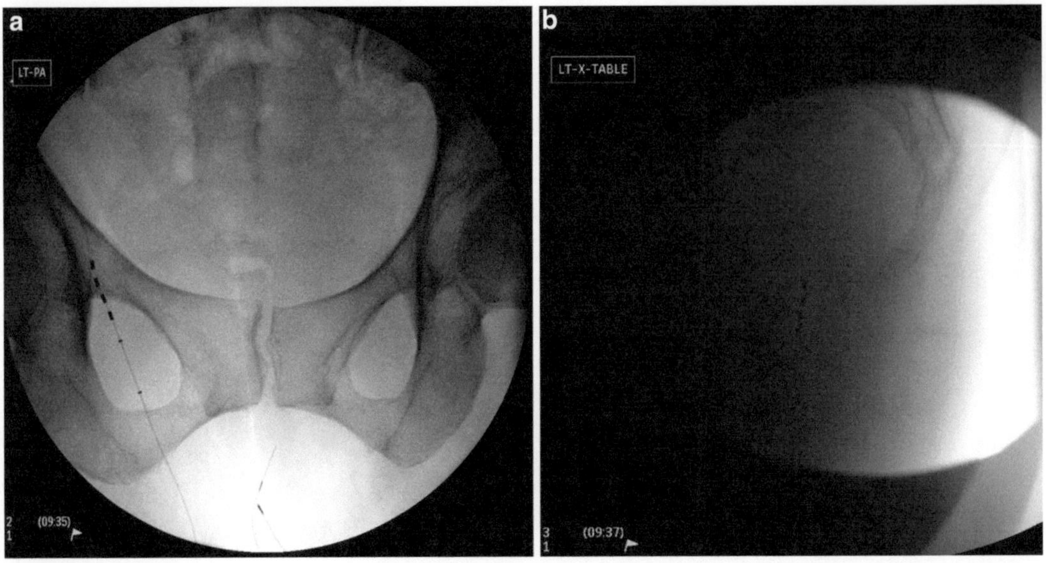

Fig. 7.9 (**a**) AP and (**b**) lateral fluoroscopic view of pudendal lead in final proper position, PN in contact with all four electrodes

perineal technique in this chapter, the other approaches have also been successful.

The posterior approach, also called the ischiorectal approach, was described in detail by Schmidt and localizes the pudendal nerve through the sacrum by palpation of external anatomical landmarks. By triangulating a horizontal plane from the greater trochanter with a vertical plane from the ischial tuberosity with a needle, one should pass through the sacrotuberous ligament, feel the ischial spine, and encounter the pudendal nerve [29]. The approach described by Spinelli in 2005 touted the benefit of the electrode contacting the PN at a more orthogonal, rather than tangential, angle [30]. Bock described a similar technique that relied on palpation with a gloved finger in the rectum [31]. While accessing the nerve reliably, these techniques may not allow for contact of all four electrodes with the PN, using the current lead in use. The surgical approach for the perineal technique is the one described at length in this chapter and was first described by Vodusek in 1988 [32].

Another technique that relies on fixed anatomical landmarks is the STAR method. STAR is an acronym where S stands for ischial spine, T for ischial tuberosity, A for acetabulum, and R for anal rim (Fig. 7.13). Heinze et al. showed that by using this method, one decreases the anatomic variability between patients and can more reliably locate the ischial spine for lead placement [33]. The anatomic basis of these approaches is summarized in Fig. 7.14 [34].

More recently, a laparoscopic approach to access the pudendal nerve for neuromodulation was described by Possover in 2014 and then by Konschake in 2016 [35, 36]. Intra-abdominally, the internal iliac artery and its anterior trunk are identified. From there, the internal pudendal artery (IPA) is located and followed to the pelvic floor, where overlying coccygeus is partially incised to expose the sacrospinous ligament (SSL). The medial portion of the SSL is opened so that the PN is now visualized in the "biligamentary tunnel" that comprises of the SSL and the sacrotuberous ligaments, and a stimulating lead is placed [35].

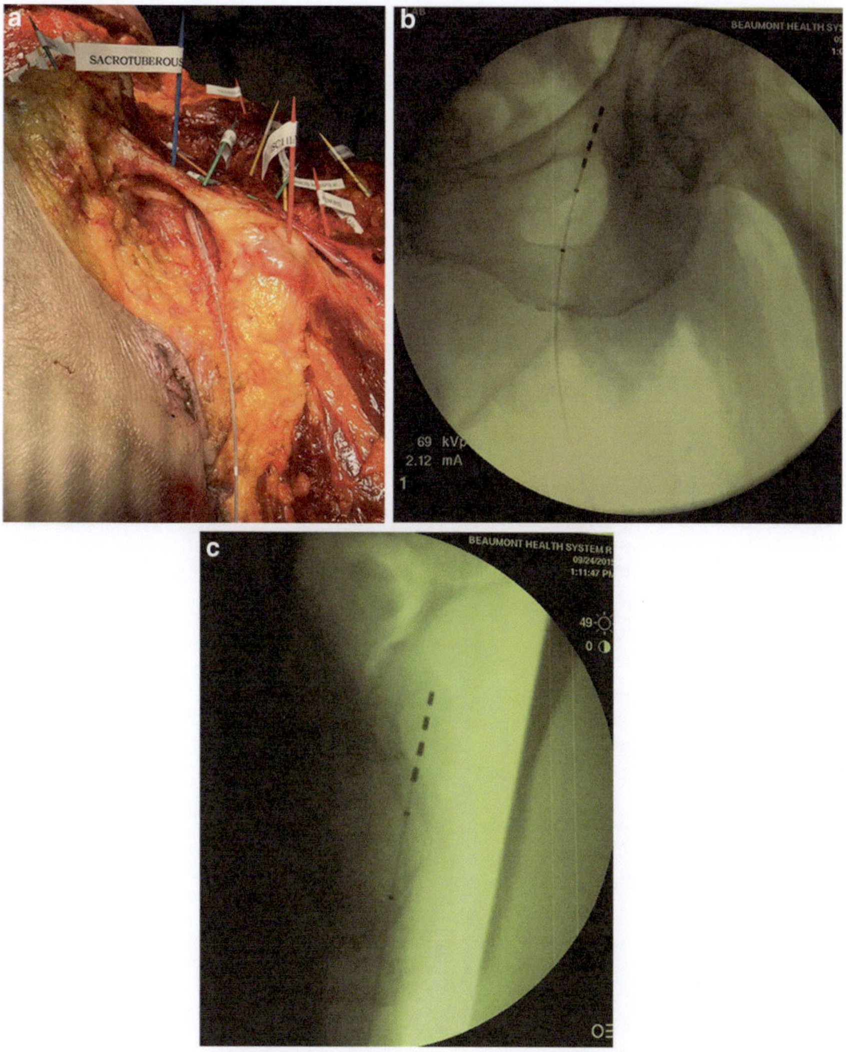

Fig. 7.10 (**a**) Cadaver model showing ideal placement of lead along the pudendal nerve. Corresponding fluoroscopy, showing (**b**) AP view, and (**c**) lateral view

Complications

Like the standard sacral neuromodulator implant, patients need adequate counseling on the risks of infection, mechânical malfunction, such as lead breakage resulting in open or closed circuits, and local complications such as exposure of lead or IPG, or pain at IPG site. Due to the unique location of the lead at the incision site, the pudendal lead is at a slightly increased risk of lead migration. The most likely mechanism of action is due to excessive or abrupt increase in pressure to the low buttock area, particularly with sitting down on a hard surface. The tined leads function like an arrowhead—they allow forward migration but resist backward movement. Since the tines are not anchored in the ischiorectal space connective tissue as they are in SNM, there is a greater risk of lead migration for PNM. Thus, we counsel patients to sit as gently as possible, particularly on the side of the lead for the first 6–8 weeks to allow the lead and tines to scar in. Table 7.1 details the studies that reported rates of

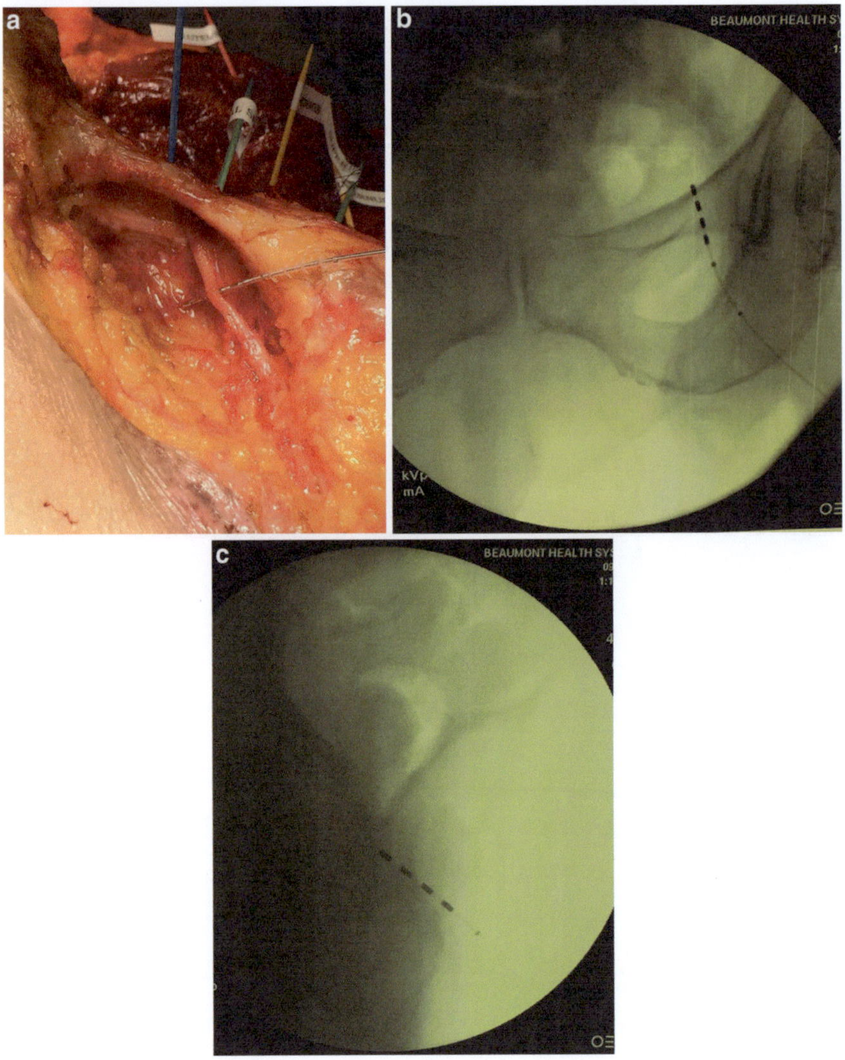

Fig. 7.11 (**a**) Cadaver model of lead "crossing" the nerve, with only one electrode in contact, (**b**) Corresponding fluoroscopic AP, and (**c**) lateral view of same lead

complications after PNM. The most common event is lead migration. When a lead is placed at the pudendal nerve no bony landmarks secure the lead in place. Peters et al. reported lead migration in 3/55 patients with PNM, two of which were revised to a sacral lead to avoid repeat migration [37].

If the lead needs to be removed, the approach is similar to removing a sacral lead. Under sedation, the insertion incision in the low buttock is anesthetized and opened. Dissection is performed to find the electrode and the electrode is grasped and pulled in a circular motion. Typically, the tines on the lead will cause resistance, so dissection may extend deep into the buttock and ischiorectal fat, but once the tines can be grasped, the lead can usually be extracted.

Outcomes

Idiopathic Overactive Bladder

Like sacral neuromodulation, PNM is effective in managing overactive bladder (OAB) and urge incontinence. In a novel randomized study, 30 subjects with various voiding dysfunctions had leads placed at both the sacral and pudendal nerve. Each lead was stimulated for 7 days (sub-chronic phase) and the patients were blinded to which stimulation was being used. Symptom improvement was assessed for each lead after the 7-day period. The patients were then allowed to choose which one they wanted attached to an for

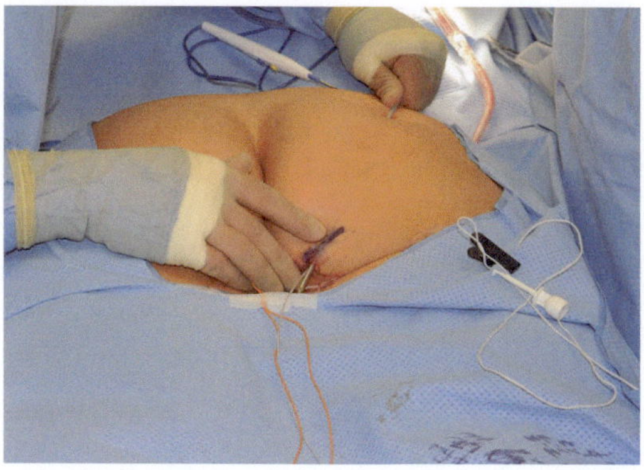

Fig. 7.12 Lead is now tunneled to upper buttock, with care taken to avoid lead trauma with sharp end of tunneler trocar

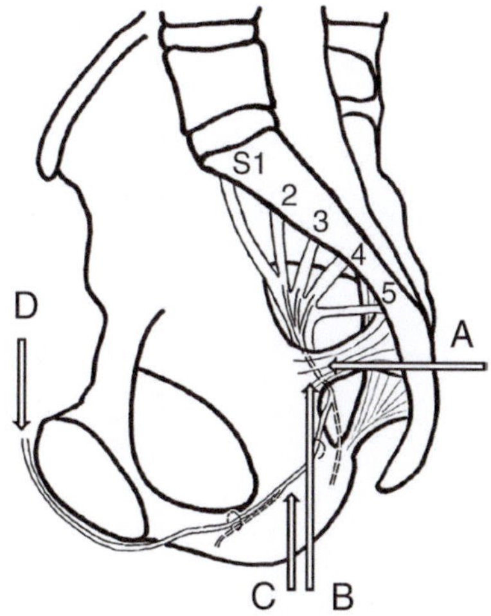

Fig. 7.14 Various approaches for electrical stimulation of pudendal nerve. A and B show access points around the ischial spine—A denotes the posterior approach and B the perineal approach. C shows where the pudendal nerve can also be reached perineally via Alcock's canal. D denotes dorsal genital nerve access. From Martens et al. [34]. Reprinted with permission from Elsevier Limited

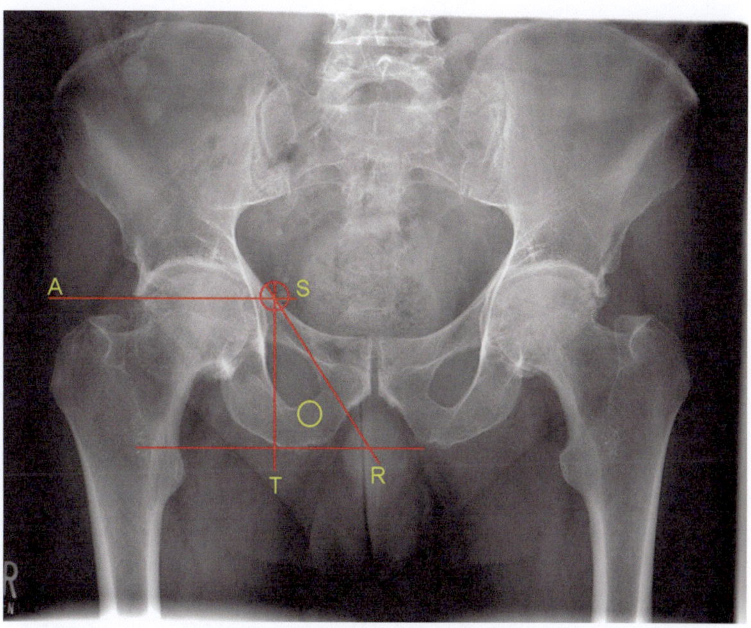

Fig. 7.13 Fixed anatomical landmarks result into a triangle on skin surface, the initials of the different landmarks add up to the STAR acronym (*S* ischial spine, *T* ischial tuberosity, *A* Acetabulum, *R* anal rim). The junction of the bisection lines serves as the starting point for needle puncture (yellow circle), the apical tip of the triangle pinpoints the spina, i.e., the anatomical area of the trunk of the PN (red circle). From Heinze et al., [33]. Reprinted with permission from Springer

Table 7.1 Complications of pudendal lead placement

	Pain at implant site	Pain at IPG site	Pain—other	Lead migration	Infection	Bowel dysfunction	Unusual reactions	Reoperations
Peters (2005)	N/R	N/R	N/R	1/19	0%	0%	N/R	N/R
Groen (2005)	0%	0%	New-onset discomfort while riding bike (resolved with new seat): 1/6	0%	Vaginal fungus (due to intraoperative antibiotics): 1/6	"Changed" bowel function (for the better): 3/6	Vaginal dryness with device "on": 1/6	N/R
Peters (2010)	N/R	N/R	2/84	3/84	1/84	N/R	0%	Second lead placed for bilateral stimulation: 2/84 IPG replaced: 2/84 Device removed: 5/84
Possover (2014)	N/R	N/R	N/R	0%	N/R	N/R	N/R	0%

N/R not reported

permanent implantation. Of the 24 patients (80%) who went on to stage II, 19 (79%) patients chose the pudendal lead versus 5 (21%) who chose the sacral lead. PNM also resulted in better overall symptom improvement than SNM (63 vs. 46%, $p = 0.02$) and was also superior to SNM for improving urgency ($p = 0.005$), frequency ($p = 0.007$), bowel function ($p = 0.049$), and pelvic pain ($p = 0.024$) [38].

Using a permanent bion® implant to the pudendal nerve near Alcock's canal, Groen et al. tested 14 and ultimately modulated 6 women with treatment-resistant urodynamic detrusor overactivity. The implanted cohort went from a mean of 6.2 incontinence episodes daily down to 2.4 and from using a mean of 5.2 pads daily to 2.8. Repeat urodynamics showed that the bladder volume at which the first involuntary detrusor contraction was seen nearly doubled—from a mean of 191 ± 152 mL to 341 ± 94 mL ($p = 0.046$) [39].

Possover et al. laparoscopically implanted tined leads to the pudendal nerve in 14 patients (12 women, 2 men) who reported at least a year of OAB and urge incontinence episodes. 11/14 (78.5%) went on to permanent implantation, with 71.4% reporting greater than 50% improvement in symptoms [35]. Mean number of voids per day decreased from 25 (range 13–50, SD 11.7) to 10.2 (range 7–15, SD 2.75), nocturia episodes decreased from 5.8 to 2.2, and daily pad use decreased from 7.3 to 1.6 pads daily. By final evaluation at a mean of 18 months (range 9–49 months), six patients were totally dry on a 3-day bladder diary. Repeat urodynamics showed improved maximum cystometric capacities, from 159 (range 80–230 mL) to 312 mL (range 160–500 mL). No patients developed urinary retention.

In a large group of women ($N = 106$) with refractory idiopathic OAB in China, long acupuncture needles were used to stimulate four sacrococcygeal points to perform electrical pudendal nerve stimulation (EPNS). 42.5% of women indicated complete OAB symptom resolution and 91 (85.8%) reported greater than 50% symptom improvement after a mean of 21.2 sessions. These findings were durable, with 62/91 who had >50% symptom improvement followed at a median of 98 months. Of these, 53/62 had either maintained or improved response [40]. The same group randomized 120 women with refractory idiopathic urge incontinence to EPNS or transvaginal electrical stimulation and showed significantly better improvement in women who underwent EPNS, with a complete resolution rate of urge UI of 42.5% and greater than 50% symptom improvement in 70.1% of patients receiving EPNS [41].

Pudendal After Failed Sacral Stimulation Trial

Although SNM has a high success rate, between 10 and 25% of patients fail to respond to first-stage implant [42, 43], with an additional percentage losing efficacy after that; management of this population can be challenging. Another third-line therapy, such as detrusor chemodenervation with onabotulinumtoxin-A or PTNS, can be offered. PNM is a particularly safe and effective therapy in patients who have failed SNM. One study of 84 patients with refractory OAB and IC/BPS symptoms, of whom 44 had failed SNM treatment, showed a 93% (41/44) response to PNM in this subset [37]. The study population of Groen et al. was notable for having a high failure rate of previous forms of neuromodulation, including 9/14 who failed test peripheral nerve evaluation (PNE), 2/14 who failed SNM, and 4/14 who failed percutaneous tibial nerve stimulation (PTNS) [39]. Similarly, Possover presented nine patients who previously failed SNM, of whom 93.2% responded to PNM [35].

As previously discussed, PNM can be offered at second-stage procedure if symptom response is inadequate after SNM as part of preoperative counseling, or as a salvage for patients who have undergone SNM with inadequate improvement in OAB symptoms.

Neurogenic OAB

One of the earliest studies looked at acute PNM in three people with neurogenic bladder and demonstrated detrusor inhibition and increased micturition thresholds in all subjects on cystometrogram; no chronic implant was used [32]. Fifteen neurogenic bladder patients had a dorsal transcutaneous placement of pudendal lead, with 12 undergoing chronic IPG implant [30]. Incontinence episodes per day decreased from 7 ± 3.3 to 2.6 ± 3.3 ($p = <0.02$). Urodynamic follow-up in six patients showed decreased detrusor pressures and increased maximum cystometric capacity.

Urinary Retention

Chronic non-obstructive urinary retention (UR) is an FDA-approved indication for sacral neuromodulation, but if unsuccessful, PNM is considered a viable alternative approach. In a small subset of 13 patients with UR, Peters et al. found no difference in catheterized volumes and number of catheterizations at 1-year follow-up; however, two of these patients (both of whom had failed multiple attempts at SNM) regained complete ability to void at 3 months post-implant [37]. While this may seem like a minor success, PNM should remain a tool in the armamentarium of the clinician treating UR due to underactive bladder. Further studies with longer follow-up are necessary to identify accurate outcomes of PNM for UR.

Pelvic Pain

Chronic pelvic pain due to pudendal neuralgia, a challenging condition to manage that can be debilitating. The Nantes criteria delineates pudendal neuralgia using the following criteria: (1) pain in the anatomical distribution of the pudendal nerve, (2) worse with sitting, (3) pain does not wake the patient at night, (4) no objective sensory loss on examination, and (5) positive anesthetic pudendal block. Not all criteria need to be met to diagnose pudendal neuralgia [44]. In our practice, we will perform one or more blocks, either in the office setting or under sedation, with or without ultrasound, fluoroscopic, and/or EMG guidance. If patients respond to these blocks, they can be considered for PNM, if in addition to pain they have refractory OAB, chronic retention, voiding dysfunction, or fecal incontinence (FI), as these are the FDA-approved indications for neuromodulation using InterStim®.

A cohort of 19 complex subjects with pudendal neuralgia, 18 of whom had undergone a total of 77 pudendal blocks, received a pudendal lead for neuromodulation [45]. Pain relief was "significant/remarkable," "almost complete," or "complete" in 10, 3, and 3 patients, respectively. While 5/19 had explantation at a mean of 3 years, only three were for loss of efficacy. A pilot study was conducted in 20 patients with chronic pelvic pain, using four different techniques. They report that the mean pain intensity decreased statistically significant from a baseline of 85 mm to 40 mm ($p = 0.018$) using the STAR and Bock technique [33]. Carmel et al. presented a report of three patients who had PNM via the Spinelli transgluteal approach for pelvic pain [46]. Pudendal nerve terminal motor latency (PTNML) was measured using multiple EMG needles. All three women reported almost complete pain relief at >2 years follow-up.

Fecal Incontinence

The relationship between the pudendal nerve and FI has been studied mainly in the context of pudendal neuropathy or injury. Anorectal function studies in people with pudendal neuropathy have shown that unconscious contraction of the external anal sphincter is not affected in those with pudendal neuropathy; however, conscious contraction of the anal sphincter is mediated by the PN [47]. Given these findings, the authors concluded that pudendal neuropathy results in fecal urge incontinence, and not complete FI.

Currently, the literature on neuromodulation for FI is limited to sacral nerve stimulation, with only a few series describing outcomes with PNM for this troublesome condition. As cited previously, Bock et al. reported on a feasibility study in two women using the technique described by Spinelli, with both patients having excellent outcomes in terms of bowel control at short-term follow-up [31]. Given the innervation of the external anal sphincter by the PN, and the outcomes seen thus far for OAB, one would expect that PNM should not be inferior to sacral stimulation, but larger studies focused on PNM for FI are required to corroborate this statement.

Conclusion

The ability to access the pudendal nerve offers the neuromodulation specialist an alternative approach to addressing refractory overactive bladder, but also has proven to benefit select patients with neuralgia, pelvic pain, and other complex pelvic floor and voiding disorders. The procedure to place the lead is an extension of the sacral lead placement, which is familiar to many clinicians who practice in this field, but requires some careful adjustments and the use of neurophysiologic guidance to insure proper positioning. Despite the enthusiasm for this procedure, it should be tempered by the lack of large, multicenter studies to prove its role beside sacral stimulation, as well as long-term outcomes.

References

1. Swanson LW. Neuroanatomical terminology: a lexicon of classical origins and historical foundations. Oxford: Oxford University Press; 2015.
2. Schmidt RA. Neural prostheses and bladder control. Eng Biol Med Mag. 1983;2:31.
3. Vodusek B, Keith Leigh J, Libby J. Detrusor inhibition induced by stimulation of pudendal afferents. Neurourol Urodyn. 1986;5:381–9.
4. Siegel SW. Management of voiding dysfunction with an implantable neuroprosthesis. Urol Clin North Am. 1992;19(1):163–70.
5. Shafik A, Doss SH. Pudendal canal: surgical anatomy and clinical implications. Am Surg. 1999;65(2):176–80.
6. Barber MD, Bremer RE, Thor KB, et al. Innervation of the female levator ani muscles. Am J Obstet Gynecol. 2002;187(1):64–71.
7. Maldonado PA, Chin K, Garcia AA, et al. Anatomic variations of pudendal nerve within pelvis and pudendal canal: clinical applications. Am J Obstet Gynecol. 2015;213:727.e1–6.
8. Xiao Z, Reese J, Schwen Z, et al. Role of spinal GABA-A receptors in pudendal inhibition of nociceptive and nonnociceptive bladder reflexes in cats. Am J Physiol Renal Physiol. 2014;306:F781–9.
9. Schwen Z, Matsuta Y, Shen B, et al. Involvement of 5-HT_3 receptors in pudendal inhibition of bladder overactivity in cats. Am J Physiol Renal Physiol. 2013;205:F663–71.
10. Matsuta Y, Schwen Z, et al. Effect of methysergide on pudendal inhibition of micturition reflex in cats. Exp Neurol. 2013;247:250–8.
11. Kadow BT, Lyon TD, et al. Sympathetic β-adrenergic mechanism in pudendal inhibition of nociceptive and non-nociceptive reflex bladder activity. Am J Physiol Renal Physiol. 2016;311(1):F78–84.
12. Lyon TD, Ferroni MC, Kadow BT, et al. Pudendal but not tibial nerve stimulation inhibits bladder contractions induced by stimulation of pontine micturition center in cats. Am J Physiol Regul Integr Comp Physiol. 2016;310(4):R366–74.
13. Tai C, Shen B, et al. Bladder inhibition by intermittent pudendal nerve stimulation in cat using transdermal amplitude-modulated signal (TAMS). Neurourol Urodyn. 2012;31:1181–4.
14. Uy J, Yu M, et al. Glutamatergic mechanisms involved in bladder overactivity and pudendal neuromodulation in cats. J Pharmacol Exp Ther. 2017;362(1):53–8.
15. Cheng CL, de Groat WC. Role of 5HT receptors in control of lower urinary tract function in anesthetized rats. Am J Physiol Renal Physiol. 2010;298(3).
16. Mally AD, Matsuta Y, Zhang F, et al. Role of opioid and metabotropic glutamate 5 receptors in pudendal inhibition of bladder overactivity in cats. J Urol. 2013;189(4):1574–9.
17. Zhang Z, Slater RC. Role of μ, κ, and δ opioid receptors in tibial inhibition of bladder overactivity in cats. J Pharmacol Exp Ther. 2015;355(2):228–34.
18. Jiang X, Yu M, et al. Role of cannabinoid receptor type 1 in tibial and pudendal neuromodulation of bladder overactivity in cats. Am J Physiol Renal Physiol. 2017;312:F482–8.
19. Bansal U, Fuller TW, et al. Lumbosacral spinal segmental contributions to tibial and pudendal neuromodulation of bladder overactivity in cats. Neurourol Urodyn. 2016;36(6):1496–502.
20. Boggs JW, Wenzel BJ, et al. Frequency-dependent selection of reflexes by pudendal afferents in cats. J Physiol. 2006;577(1):115–26.
21. Tai C, Wang J, Wang X, et al. Bladder inhibition or voiding induced by pudendal nerve stimulation in chronic spinal cord injured cats. Neurourol Urodyn. 2007;26:570–7.
22. Reese JN, Rogers MJ, Xiao Z, et al. Role of spinal metabotropic glutamate receptor 5 in pudendal inhibition of the nociceptive bladder reflex in cats. Am J Physiol Renal Physiol. 2015;308(8):F832–8.
23. Tian Y, Liao L, Wyndaele JJ. Inhibitory effect and possible mechanism of intraurethral stimulation on overactive bladder in female rats. Int Neurourol J. 2015;19(3):151–7.
24. Jen E, Tsung-Hsun H, et al. Effects of pulsed-radiofrequency neuromodulation on rats with overactive bladder. Neurourol Urodyn. 2016;36(7):1734–41.

25. Yoo PB, Woock JP, Grill WM. Bladder activation by selective stimulation of pudendal nerve afferents in cats. Exp Neurol. 2008;212(1):218–25.
26. Zempleni MZ, Michels L, Mehnert U, et al. Cortical substrate of bladder control in SCI and the effect of peripheral pudendal stimulation. NeuroImage. 2010;49(4):2983–94.
27. Huang JC, Deletes V, Vodusek DB, et al. Preservation of pudendal afferents in sacral rhizotomies. Neurosurgery. 1997;41(2):411–5.
28. Reitz A, Schmid DM, Curt A, et al. Afferent fibers of the pudendal nerve modulate sympathetic neurons controlling the bladder neck. Neurourol Urodyn. 2003;22(6):597–601.
29. Schmidt RA. Technique of pudendal nerve localization for block or stimulation. J Urol. 1989;142:1528–31.
30. Spinelli M, Malaguti S, Giardiello G, et al. A new minimally invasive procedure for pudendal nerve stimulation to treat neurogenic bladder: description of the method and preliminary data. Neurourol Urodyn. 2005;24:305–9.
31. Bock S, Folie P, Wolff K, et al. First experiences with pudendal nerve stimulation in fecal incontinence: a technical report. Tech Coloproctol. 2010;14:41–4.
32. Vodusek DB, Plevnik S, Vrtacnik P, et al. Detrusor inhibition on selective pudendal nerve stimulation in the perineum. Neurourol Urodyn. 1988;6:389–93.
33. Heinze K, Hoermann R, Fritsch H, et al. Comparative pilot study of implantation techniques for pudendal neuromodulation: technical and clinical outcome in first 20 patients with chronic pelvic pain. World J Urol. 2015;33:289–94.
34. Martens FMJ, Heesakkers JPFA, Rijkhoff NJM. Surgical access for electrical stimulation of the pudendal and dorsal genital nerves in the overactive bladder: a review. J Urol. 2011;186:798–804.
35. Possover M. A novel implantation technique for pudendal nerve stimulation for treatment of overactive bladder and urgency incontinence. J Minim Invasive Gynecol. 2014;21:888–92.
36. Konschake M, Brenner E, Moriggl B, et al. New laparoscopic approach to the pudendal nerve for neuromodulation based on an anatomic study. Neurourol Urodyn. 2017;36:1069–75.
37. Peters KM, Killinger KA, et al. Chronic pudendal neuromodulation: expanding available treatment options for refractory urologic symptoms. Neurourol Urodyn. 2010;29(7):1267–71.
38. Peters KM, Feber KM, Bennett RC. Sacral versus pudendal nerve stimulation for voiding dysfunction: a prospective, single-blinded, randomized, crossover trial. Neurourol Urodyn. 2005;24:643–7.
39. Groen J, Amiel C, Bosch JC. Chronic pudendal nerve neuromodulation in women with idiopathic refractory detrusor overactivity incontinence: results of a pilot study with a novel minimally invasive implantable mini stimulator. Neurourol Urodyn. 2005;24:226–30.
40. Wang S, Zhang S, Zhao L. Long-term efficacy of electrical pudendal nerve stimulation for urgency-frequency syndrome in women. Int Urogynecol J. 2014;25:397–402.
41. Wang S, Lv J, Feng X, et al. Efficacy of electrical pudendal nerve stimulation versus transvaginal electrical stimulation in treating female idiopathic urgency urinary incontinence. J Urol. 2017;197:1496–501.
42. Siegel S, Noblett K, et al. Three-year follow-up results of a prostpective, multicenter study in overactive bladder subjects treated with sacral neuromodulation. Urology. 2016;94:57–63.
43. Bartley J, Gilleran J, Peters K. Neuromodulation for overactive bladder. Nat Rev Urol. 2013;10:513–21.
44. Labat JJ, Riant T, et al. Diagnostic criteria for pudendal neuralgia by pudendal nerve entrapment (Nantes criteria). Neurourol Urodyn. 2008;27(4):306–10.
45. Peters KM, Killinger KA, Jaeger C, et al. Pilot study exploring chronic pudendal neuromodulation as a treatment option for pain associated with pudendal neuralgia. LUTS. 2015;7:138–42.
46. Carmel M, Lebel M, Tu LM. Pudendal nerve neuromodulation with neurophysiology guidance: a potential treatment option for refractory chronic pelvi-perineal pain. Int Urogynecol J. 2010;21:613–6.
47. van Meegdenburg MM, Heineman E, Broens PMA. Pudendal neuropathy alone results in urge incontinence and not total fecal incontinence. Dis Colon Rectum. 2015;58:1186–93.

Neuromodulation for Chronic Pelvic Pain

8

Jessica C. Lloyd and Courtenay K. Moore

Overview

The goal of this chapter is to provide an in-depth overview of the pathophysiology of chronic pelvic pain (CPP), more specifically interstitial cystitis/painful bladder syndrome (IC/PBS) as well as review the AUA IC/PBS treatment guidelines with an emphasis on neuromodulation.

Pathophysiology of Chronic Pelvic Pain

The pelvic floor plays a critical role in supporting the pelvic viscera, as well as permitting the storage and evacuation of urine and feces, sexual function and, in women, parturition. Given these complex functions, it follows that the pelvic viscera and musculature would be at risk for chronic pain states. The nature of pelvic innervation further complicates the matter, as the sympathetic, parasympathetic, and somatic nervous systems all play a role, sometimes acting in consort and at other instances, singularly. The pelvic structural configuration and complex neuroanatomy make identifying noxious stimuli in this area troublesome. Indeed, delays in diagnosis can lead to a delayed treatment, which may risk conversion of an acute, unpleasant stimulus into a state of CPP [1].

CPP is a complex condition defined as "non-malignant pain perceived in the pelvis in either men or women.In the case of documented nociceptive pain that becomes chronic, the pain must have been chronic or continuous for at least 6 months" [2]. This disease can be debilitating, with negative cognitive, behavioral, sexual, and emotional consequences that have a major impact on quality of life. CPP is seen more commonly in the female population, and was estimated in 2010 to affect over nine million American women [3]. The direct costs of CPP have been estimated at over $2.8 billion [4].

The etiology of CPP is likely multifactorial and variable between patients, but development of this pain syndrome is more common in women who have a history of endometriosis, sexual abuse [5, 6], vulvar vestibulitis, fibromyalgia [7], and irritable bowel syndrome [8]. In men, the most commonly suspected inciting factor is prostate pain, arising from either infectious or aseptic inflammatory etiologies [9, 10]. There is, however, no gold standard for diagnostic algorithm of chronic pelvic pain, and it remains a diagnosis of exclusion.

Although unclear, the pathophysiology of CPP seems to parallel many common centralized neuropathic and sympathetically driven pain models [1]. The prevailing hypothesis is

J. C. Lloyd · C. K. Moore (✉)
Glickman Urological Institute, Cleveland Clinic, Cleveland, OH, USA
e-mail: lloydj2@ccf.org; moorec6@ccf.org

J. P. Gilleran, S. A. Alpert (eds.), *Adult and Pediatric Neuromodulation*,
https://doi.org/10.1007/978-3-319-73266-4_8

that an insult or injury damages a specific structure or organ, leading to either: (1) somatic pain from skin, muscles, or soft tissues transmitted via sensory afferent nerves, or (2) visceral pain originating from a viscous structure transmitted through autonomic or sympathetic fibers (or both), which over time develops into neuropathic pain characterized by unpleasant paresthesias, allodynia, and hyperalgesia [11]. Just as patients with complex regional pain syndrome suffer hyperesthesia and allodynia in the affected extremity, patients with CPP often experience similar painful sensations with routine pelvic functions, such as urination, sexual intercourse, or ovulation. Indeed, in 2003, Janicki and colleagues postulated that CPP was a variant of complex regional pain syndrome, secondary to an inciting insult and subsequent "wind-up" phenomenon that subsequently hypersensitized local pelvic neurons, leading to the perception of pain with non-noxious stimuli [12].

In a pelvic medicine practice, one condition commonly associated with chronic pelvic pain is IC/BPS. IC/BPS is characterized by urinary frequency, urgency, dyspareunia, nocturia, and pelvic pain [13]. In 2009, the Rand Interstitial Cystitis Epidemiology study detailed a prevalence of 3–6% in the general population, affecting approximately 3.4 million US women [14].

The exact causal cascade of IC/BPS remains elusive though many experts agree that a defect in the urothelial glycosaminoglycan layer is the most likely primary underlying factor [3]. When the urothelium is exposed to urine due to inadequate GAG covering, mast cell activation occurs within the bladder wall, generating an influx of potassium ions that upregulates the afferent nerves, which in turn activate more mast cells, creating a positive feedback loop that leads to increased sensory nerve fiber activity in the bladder, chronic inflammation, and ultimately neuropathic pain, which can be manifested through visceral allodynia and hyperalgesia of the bladder and adjacent pelvic organs [15].

AUA Guidelines for Treatment of Interstitial Cystitis/Bladder Pain Syndrome

In an effort to clarify and standardize care for patients with IC/BPS, the American Urological Association published guidelines in 2014 [16]. With regard to diagnosis, the authors recommend that basic assessment should include "a careful history, physical examination, and laboratory examination to rule symptoms that characterize IC/BPS and rule out other confusable disorders." Moreover, they encourage that baseline voiding symptoms and pain scores be captured, in order to measure subsequent treatment effects. Per the diagnostic guidelines, cystoscopy and urodynamics are not necessary for the diagnosis of IC/BPS, but may be considered in complex presentations.

Treatments that may be offered are divided into first- through sixth-line groups based on the potential benefits to the patient, potential severity of the side effects, and reversibility of the treatment.

First-Line Treatments: Patient Education and Lifestyle Modification

First-line treatments should include patient education regarding normal bladder function and what is known and not known about IC/BPS. The multimodal approach to therapy should be explained to patients, as well as the rationale for a stepwise approach to therapy. Behavioral modification strategies include manipulating urine concentration and/or volume, application of local heat or cold to the suprapubic region, avoidance of foods known to irritate the bladder, meditation, guided imagery, pelvic floor muscle relaxation, and bladder training to suppress urinary urgency [17–20]. These interventions are recommended based on an NIDDK multicenter trial focused on treatment naïve IC/BPS patients. After undergoing a standardized education and behavioral modification program, including increased understanding of bladder and voiding physiology, stress management strategies, and avoidance of symptom triggers, 45% of patients reported markedly or moderately improved symptoms on the Global Response Assessment [18]. In addition to global management of psychological stress, the guidelines also emphasize that clinicians may want to include multidisciplinary assistance when appropriate for management of factors that may exacerbate IC/BPS, such as irritable bowel syndrome symptoms, endometriosis, recurrent vaginitis/vestibulitis, menstrual pain, panic attacks, depressive episodes, and the like.

Second-Line Treatments: Physical Therapy, Pain Management, Medications, and Intravesical Instillations

Second-line treatments are numerous. They include manual physical therapy techniques, multimodal pain management, provision of certain medications (i.e., amitriptyline, cimetidine, hydroxyzine, or pentosan polysulfate), and instillation of intravesical therapies, such as DMSO, heparin, lidocaine, or a combination thereof.

Patients with IC/BPS often exhibit tenderness and/or banding of the pelvic floor musculature [21, 22]. It is unclear if these musculoskeletal findings represent primary pain generators or are themselves secondary phenomena elicited by the primary bladder pain of IC/BPS. Regardless of etiology, literature supports that manual physical therapy can provide symptom relief by treating these soft tissue abnormalities [23–25]. Preferred physical therapy techniques include myofascial and trigger point release. These targeted interventions fared better than global therapeutic massage in a 2012 randomized controlled trial, with 59% of patients undergoing myofascial release reporting moderate or marked improvement, versus only 26% of those receiving massage therapy [25]. Pelvic floor strengthening interventions, such as Kegel exercises, may exacerbate symptoms and should be avoided.

Multimodal pain management is encouraged in the AUA IC/BPS guideline. The goal of pharmacotherapy is to find a medication regimen that will provide significant pain relief with minimal side effects; tools include urinary analgesics, NSAIDs, narcotics, and a variety of non-opioid medications now being used for treatment of chronic pain, such as antidepressants, antiepileptics, and the like. The panel's clinical experience reflected diverse approaches to effective pain management, ranging from primary management by the urologist to use a multidisciplinary team incorporating an anesthesiologist or pain specialist provider. Complementary therapies, including physical therapy, psychological counseling, and stress management, are also recommended. Ultimately, the panel concluded that "the decision regarding how to approach [pain management] depends on the judgment and experience of the involved clinician, the severity of the patient's symptoms, and the availability of expertise and resources."

Also included in second-line therapies are a variety of oral medications directed specifically at the underlying mechanisms of IC/BPS, including (in alphabetical order) amitriptyline, cimetidine, hydroxyzine, and pentosan polysulfate. Amitriptyline has central and peripheral anticholinergic actions, it blocks the active transport system in the presynaptic nerve ending that is responsible for the reuptake of serotonin and noradrenaline, and it is a sedative with action that is presumably centrally based but is perhaps also related to antihistaminic properties [18]. This may explain the potential benefits in patients with IC/BPS. One randomized, controlled trial reported efficacy of oral amitriptyline (25 mg daily titrated over several weeks to 100 mg daily if tolerated) to be superior to placebo at 4 months, with 63% of the treatment group clinically improved compared to 4% of the placebo group [26]. However, side effects, including drowsiness, sedation, and nausea, were very common and were the major reason for withdrawal from the study.

The antihistamine cimetidine is proposed to benefit IC/BPS patients by competitive antagonism of the H_2 histamine receptor [27]. In their randomized controlled trial, Thilagarajah and colleagues reported efficacy of oral cimetidine (400 mg twice daily) to be statistically significantly superior to placebo in terms of total symptoms, pain, and nocturia after 3 months of treatment [27]. Two observational studies reported that oral cimetidine (300 mg twice daily or 200 mg three times daily) resulted in 44–57% of patients reporting clinically significant improvement in symptoms at follow-up intervals of one and more than 2 years [28, 29]. No adverse events (AEs) were reported in these studies.

Hydroxyzine is a long-standing oral pharmacotherapeutic agent used for IC/BPS patients, on the principle that it prevents bladder mastocytosis via its antihistamine effects [30]. There is one randomized, controlled trial that, though underpowered, failed to show a statistically significant difference in symptom control relative to placebo with hydroxyzine therapy [31]. In contrast, an observational study reported 92% of patients experienced clinically significant improvement on hydroxyzine therapy, though this population all had systemic allergies, and may represent a subset of patients that is more likely to respond to hydroxyzine [32]. Adverse effects were common, but usually minor and self-limited, including short-lasting sedation and subjective weakness.

Pentosan polysulfate is hypothesized to improve IC symptoms by adhering to the bladder wall, buffering against cell permeability and penetration by irritating solutes. It is by far the most-studied oral medication for use in IC/BPS. Indeed, the AUA panel was able to consider seven randomized trials reporting on more than 500 patients including five trials that compared PPS to placebo, one trial that examined PPS dose–response effects, and one that compared PPS to cyclosporine A. Ultimately, after consideration of the data, the panel concluded that there was a statistically significant but clinically weak improvement in IC/BPS symptoms with use of pentosan polysulfate [16]. Adverse events were rare and generally not serious. The panel did specify that pentosan polysulfate appears to have lower efficacy in patients with Hunner's lesions.

Finally, intravesical therapies are also included in the second-line category, including (listed in alphabetical order) dimethyl sulfoxide (DMSO), heparin, and lidocaine instillations. DMSO is an organosulfur compound that is believed to reduce inflammation, relax the detrusor muscle, and act locally as an analgesic [33]. It may also cause temporary urothelial injury that allows for better penetration of other agents. If DMSO is to be used, the panel recommended limiting dwell time to 15–20 min, as DMSO is rapidly absorbed into the bladder wall and longer dwell periods are paradoxically associated with worsening pain. Additionally, the panel noted that if DMSO is administered in conjunction with other agents, such as heparin, sodium bicarbonate, steroid, or lidocaine, it potentially enhances absorption of these other substances, which could yield toxicity, particularly from local anesthetics such as lidocaine. No clinical studies have addressed the safety or potential for increased efficacy of these "cocktail" regimens relative to DMSO alone

Heparin is a highly sulfonated glycosaminoglycan (GAG) best known for its use in anticoagulation. However, when instilled intravesically, it can act as an exogenous GAG to decrease urothelial penetrability in IC patients [33]. Side effects with heparin instillation are infrequent and appear minor. Placebo-controlled trials are lacking.

Intravesical lidocaine functions as a topical anesthetic. Notably, alkalinization increases urothelial penetration of lidocaine and therefore is believed to increase efficacy; however, this can increase systemic absorption and potential toxicity. Relief is generally short term and limited to 2 weeks or less. Researchers are attempting to remedy this problem with an implantable lidocaine-eluting device, but this technology is not yet available to patients [34].

Third-Line Treatments: Hydrodistension and Fulguration of Hunner's Lesions

As third-line treatment, cystoscopy under anesthesia with hydrodistension can be performed. This intervention should be at low pressure (60–80 cm H2O) and for short duration (<10 min). This intervention is intended to serve three purposes: first, prior to distension, to inspect the bladder for other potential sources of symptoms (bladder stones, tumors, etc.) and for Hunner's lesions; second, the distension itself may offer therapeutic benefit, and finally distension allows for disease "staging" by determining the anatomic as opposed to functional bladder capacity, thus identifying the subset of patients with substantially reduced capacity due to fibrosis. Three observational studies reported that one or two exposures to low-pressure, short-duration hydrodistention resulted in clinically significant relief of symptoms for a subset of patients. However, these benefits did decline over time: at 1-month efficacy ranged from 30 to 54%; at 2–3 months, from 18 to 56%; at 5–6 months, from 0 to 7% [35–37]. No adverse events were reported. The panel warns that potential benefits must be balanced against the possibility of a flare in symptoms following instrumentation.

During cystoscopy, if Hunner's lesions are visualized, the panel recommends fulguration with laser or electrocautery and/or injection of triamcinolone. Patients with Hunner's lesions who experience relief after fulguration or injection should be counseled that periodic retreatment is often required to maintain symptom control. Adverse events for these interventions are rare in the literature though the panel does recommend that patients undergoing laser fulguration be warned of the risk for forward energy scatter and resultant delayed bowel perforation.

Fourth-Line Treatments: Intradetrusor Botulinum Toxin and Trial of Sacral Nerve Stimulation (SNS)

Intradetrusor onabotulinum toxin-A (BTX-A) injection is a fourth-line off-label therapy for IC/BPS. It has more recently been combined with hydrodistension in the IC/BPS population, and clinicians are becoming more comfortable repeating dosing (typically 100 units, u) when symptoms return. A single RCT has been performed, by Kuo and Chancellor in 2009 [38]. Three groups were compared: Botox 200u with hydrodistension 2 weeks after injection, Botox 100u with hydrodistension at the time of initial injection, and Botox 100u with hydrodistension at the time of initial injection and 2 weeks afterward. Side effects, including elevated post-void residual and dysuria were markedly higher in the 200u group, such that randomization to this group was stopped prior to completion of the study. Patients were followed for 2 years, and success ranged from 80% at 3 months to 47% at 24 months in the BTX-A 200+ hydrodistension group, 72% at 3 months to 21% at 24 months in the BTX-A 100 + hydrodistension group, and 48% at 3 months to 17% at 24 months in the hydrodistension only group.

Pinto injected 100u into the trigone with retreatment at symptom return and followed patients for up to 3 years [39]. All patients reported subjective improvement at 1- and 3 months follow-up. Pain, daytime and nighttime voiding frequency and quality of life (QoL) improved significantly. Treatment remained effective in greater than 50% of the patients at 9-month follow-up. Retreatment was also effective in all patients with return of symptoms (62% of patients), with similar duration. Nearly one-third of patients had UTIs post-treatment 2 (but not after the other treatments); there was no urinary retention or clean intermittent catheterization required in this study. In the absence of placebo-controlled studies, the true effect of Botox injection for IC/BPS remains unclear. However, the existing studies suggest that a subset of patients will experience symptom relief for several months after treatment. Given the frequency and potential seriousness of side effects with the 200u dose, the AUA guideline panel recommends injection of the 100u dose as a fourth-line intervention for IC/BPS.

The guidelines also state that a trial of SNS may be offered to patients with refractory IC/BPS symptoms. Nonetheless, it is important to note that SNS is currently not FDA approved for the treatment of CPP or IC/BPS. However, many patients meet the urgency/frequency indication, for which SNS is FDA approved. While there are no prospective randomized trials a variety of observational studies were considered by the panel [40–43]. Follow-up ranged from 60 to 86 months across the studies, with success rates ranging from 72 to 80%. Significant improvements in urgency, frequency, nocturia, voided volumes, and pain scores were noted amongst the studies. Device explantation for lack of efficacy or intractable side effects occurred in 0–28% of patients, and revision procedures for battery replacement, lead revision, or site change ranged from 21 to 50%. Mean battery life was approximately 93 months. Notably, Powell and Kreder note that patients are significantly less likely to proceed with stage 2 SNS implantation after PNE, relative to a stage 1 SNS trial [43]. Given the paucity of high-quality evidence and the moderately invasive nature of SNS, this remains a fourth-line treatment option per guidelines.

Fifth-Line Treatments: Cyclosporine A Therapy

Cyclosporine A (CyA) immunomodulatory therapy has been designated as a fifth-line intervention for refractory IC/BPS. One randomized trial compared CyA versus PPS, and demonstrated 75% improvement in the patients taking CyA versus only 19% in those on PPS after 6 months of treatment [44]. One recent retrospective study in the USA reported on 44 patients followed for a mean of 15 months, and reveals 59% reporting a meaningful clinical response with CyA therapy [45]. Notably, success rates were much higher in patients with Hunner's lesions (85% vs. 30% in those without). AE rates were high, with half of patients reporting at least one. These included rising serum creatinine, hypertension, alopecia, cutaneous lymphoma, mouth ulcers, and gout flares. Amongst the Hunner's lesion group, attrition due to AEs decreased the intention-to-treat effectiveness to 68%. Ultimately, these data suggest substantial efficacy of CyA, particularly in patients with Hunner's lesions; however, the lack of long-term data and the potential for serious adverse events is not trivial. The AUA guidelines panel encourages clinicians unfamiliar with CyA administration to seek guidance from experts regarding dosing and monitoring.

Sixth-Line Treatments: Major Surgical Intervention

Per AUA guidelines, major surgical interventions, such as substitution cystoplasty and urinary diversion with or without cystectomy, may be undertaken in carefully selected patients for whom all other therapies have proven ineffective with regard to symptom control or quality of life. The panel cautions that "major surgery should be reserved for the small proportion of patients with severe, unresponsive disease, who are motivated to undergo the risks and lifelong changes associated with irreversible major surgery." The panel emphasizes that pain relief is not guaranteed, even with this aggressive intervention, as pain can persist even after cystectomy, especially in non-ulcer IC/BPS [46].

The AUA guidelines committee also comments on inappropriate therapies. Neither long-term oral antibiotic therapy nor long-term systemic steroid treatment should be offered. Similarly, intravesical Bacillus Calmette–Guérin (BCG) vaccine should not be administered. In terms of surgical interventions, the panel specifies that high-pressure, long-duration hydrodistension is potentially harmful and should not be offered. The panel concludes by emphasizing that the IC/BPS population constitutes an underserved group in need of adequate medical management, and encourages future efforts both at the basic science and clinical levels to develop better, safer treatment modalities for this complex condition. In particular, there is emerging interest in determination of an IC/BPS biomarker, both for diagnosis and outcomes measurement.

SNS for the Treatment of CPP and IC/PBS

An understanding of pelvic neuroanatomy is critical prior to consideration of sacral neuromodulation for CPP. The pelvic viscera are parasympathetically innervated by the S2–S4 nerve roots, and sympathetically innervated by the T12-L2 nerve roots. The parasympathetic outflow is transmitted via the pelvic splanchnic nerves (S2–S4), which converge into the preganglionic pelvic splanchnic nerves. Sympathetic input to the pelvis arises from the thoracolumbar cord by way of the superior hypogastric plexus. The somatic afferents and efferents to the pelvis originate from the S2–S4 cord via the pudendal nerve, with S3 offering the primary supply to the anterior perineal musculature [1].

The first reported use of pelvic nerve electrostimulation occurred in 1878, when Saxtroph described his treatment of patients with urinary retention due to an a contractile bladder [47]. Over time, this modality evolved into modern day sacral neuromodulation when, in 1971, Nashold et al. described the first successful implantation of an SNS system to initiate voiding in a patient with spinal cord injury [48]. In 1981, Tanagho and Schmidt subsequently demonstrated that stimulation of the S3 nerve root could be applied to a variety of urologic pathologies, including incontinence and refractory urgency/frequency, by modulating detrusor and urinary sphincter function [49]. This research ultimately led to FDA approval of SNS for urinary urgency, frequency, and urgency incontinence in 1997. Later, in 1999, the SNS system was approved for idiopathic urinary retention and in 2011 for fecal incontinence. To date IC/PBS is not an FDA-approved indication for SNS.

The exact mechanism by which SNS modulates micturition remains unclear. It may activate or reset the somatic afferents involved with sensory processing and the micturition reflex pathways in the spinal cord [49]. Additional theories propose that SNS may interfere with the sympathetic signals to the bladder involved in the guarding and the vesicosympathetic reflexes, which control continence and filling, respectively [50]. On PET study, SNS has also been correlated with increased activity of the paraventricular gray area of the brain, which is involved in activation or inhibition of the micturition reflex [51].

Given that the etiology and pathophysiology of chronic pelvic pain can be hard to delineate and may vary between patients, if follows that the mechanism by which SNS may improve CPP symptoms is also unknown. However, most researchers agree that dysregulated central nervous system responses to non-noxious stimuli are the major underlying feature [52, 53]. Therefore, reason suggests that effective therapies work to modulate the nervous system. A possible mechanism for neuromodulation as therapy for CPP is based on the gate control theory, which states that pain perception depends on a pattern of peripheral nervous input. It is believed that a gate control mechanism is present at the spinal segment level that regulates the interaction between afferent nerve signals and pain sensation [54]. Interneurons of the spinal cord dorsal horn create gating components, and inhibition or facilitation of afferent fibers modulates pain signal input to the spinal transmission neurons. Impulses from the dorsal horn are controlled by a descending system containing fibers from the brainstem, thalamus, and limbic lobes [55]. Neuromodulation is believed to restore control at the spinal segmental gate as well as at the supraspinal sites such as the brainstem and limbic system nuclei, thereby "gating" peripheral stimuli and preventing the CNS signaling that leads to hyperalgesia. In essence, SNS restores the balance between excitatory and inhibitory impulses to and from the pelvic organs at the sacral and suprasacral levels.

Another possible mechanism of action lies in the treatment of underlying pelvic floor dysfunction. Hypertonia of the pelvic floor is commonly associated with CPP. SNS may inhibit inappropriate excitation of the pelvic floor musculature, thereby facilitating voiding and other pelvic floor functions [56].

SNS has shown consistent efficacy in the treatment of refractory overactive bladder, idiopathic urinary retention, and fecal incontinence. However, while studies suggest that SNS can relieve the concomitant voiding symptoms seen in IC/BPS, pain relief has proven more difficult to achieve [57]. One evolution of the therapy to address this deficit includes bilateral, rather than unilateral, lead placement, since pain is seldom unilateral [52]. Subsequent small-scale studies have suggested reductions in pain and narcotic use with this more aggressive approach to SNS. Indeed, Maher reported reduction in pain of

27% with SNS in a cohort of 15 patients [58], and Siegel described 60% improvement in pain with ten patients followed for a median of 19 months [59]. In addition to IC/BPS, SNS has proven effective for treatment of other pathologies, such as coccydynia, vulvodynia, anorectal pain, and pain from pelvic floor muscle dysfunction in small-scale studies [1]. Nonetheless, the extent of pain control varies greatly amongst patients and from one study to the next, and research has failed to consistently demonstrate an overall improvement in quality of life for CPP patients following SNS [60].

Everaert and colleagues performed one of the initial studies suggesting improvement in pelvic pain with SNS in a cohort of 26 patients with CPP refractory to conservative management [61]. S3 stimulation was effective in 16 of 26 patients, 11 of whom underwent implantation. At a mean follow-up of 36 months, all had improvement in pain, achieving pain scores <3/10 and reporting >50% pain relief relative to baseline.

Comiter prospectively studied a group of 25 patients with refractory IC/BPS undergoing trial of SNS [13]. Of these, 17 had at least 50% improvement in their voiding and pain symptoms and went on to permanent implantation. Average reported pain decreased from 5.8 to 1.6 on a 0–10 visual analog scale (VAS). Ultimately, 94% of patients who underwent implantation reported sustained improvement in all pain and voiding parameters at their last postoperative visits, with a mean follow-up of 14 months.

Whitmore et al. conducted a prospective multicenter clinical trial in 2003, for women with refractory IC/BPS [62]. They enrolled 33 patients with intractable IC/BPS who failed alternative therapies. Analysis of voiding diaries showed statistically significant decreases in urinary frequency, bladder pain, average volume voided, and maximum volume voided following SNS.

Siegel and colleagues used SNM to treat ten patients with refractory CPP, inserting leads into S3 for eight patients and S4 in two patients [59]. At follow-up of 19 months, 9 of the 10 patients reported decreased pain, with mean hours of pain per day decreasing from 13.1 to 6.9 following SNS implantation. The severity of pain decreased from 9.7 to 4.4 on a 0–10 pain scale.

Maher and colleagues prospectively evaluated 15 women undergoing SNS with IC/BPS using pain scores, voiding diaries, and validated quality of life surveys [58]. Mean bladder pain decreased from 8.9 to 2.4 points on a 0–10 pain scale. Quality of life parameters related to social functioning, bodily pain, and general health significantly improved during the stimulation period. Of the subjects, 73% requested to proceed to complete device implantation.

Peters and Konstandt retrospectively assessed the efficacy of long-term SNS in treating chronic pelvic pain associated with IC/BPS in a cohort of 21 patients [63]. Of these, 20 reported moderate or marked improvement in pain following SNS implantation. In those using chronic opioids, the mean dose decreased by 36% and 4 of 18 patients stopped all narcotics after SNS implantation.

Several studies have assessed the long-term efficacy of SNM for IC/BPS. Rackley and colleagues followed 22 patients with refractory IC/BPS who underwent implantation of SNS [64]. Over a 2-year period, five devices were explanted; two devices were removed because of infection and three because of failure to maintain efficacy. Amongst those whose devices remained in situ, 13 expressed continued benefit and 4 complained of loss of efficacy. The overall success rate at 2 years was 48%, suggesting that the device may lose some degree of success over time.

In 30 patients who underwent SNS, Marinkovic et al. report a 64% reduction in pain at an average of 86 months follow-up [42]. Similarly, Powell and Kreder report 78% ongoing efficacy in their cohort of nine patients followed for 5 years [43]. In their retrospective review, Gajewksi and Al-Zahrani reported on their cohort of 46 patients who underwent SNS implantation for CPP; these patients were then followed for an average of 62 months, and 13 of the 46 (28%) underwent removal, most commonly for poor outcome or painful stimulation [40]. In a follow-up study of 21 female patients with SNS for bladder pain syndrome, they had an implant rate of 52% after

PNE, with durable long-term improvements in reported visual analog pain scale scores at 5 years of follow-up [41].

Given the inconclusive data regarding long-term efficacy of SNS, management of patient expectations at the time of trial stimulation and device implantation is essential. Patients must be told that SNS is not FDA approved for the treatment of chronic pelvic pain and counseled that the long-term durability of SNS for management of chronic pelvic pain remains unclear.

Technical Considerations and Lead Placement

Despite interest in SNS for treatment of chronic pelvic pain, conflict remains regarding the correct lead position for optimal benefit. Targeting of non S3 nerve roots or multiple unilateral nerve roots, as well as bilateral stimulation, has been proposed. Indeed, some authors even postulate that a spinal cord stimulator, rather than a sacral nerve stimulator, offers the greatest potential for benefit [1]. With neuropathic pelvic pain, the sacral portion of the cord theoretically appears to be the most ideal target for neuromodulation. However, even though the pelvis receives both somatic and visceral innervation from the sacral cord, the unpredictable course of the sympathetic nervous system fibers means that some innervation could escape neuromodulation directed at the sacral cord, diminishing pain relief. Thus, coming to consensus regarding optimal lead placement proves difficult.

For FDA-approved indications, SNS targets the S3 nerve root. However, some authors have inquired as to whether targeting other nerve roots may offer greater benefit for CPP patients. In their 2008 study, Zabihi and colleagues evaluated the efficacy of bilateral caudal epidural sacral neuromodulation for the treatment of refractory pelvic pain in the setting of IC/BPS [52]. This was accomplished by deploying a quadripolar lead in a retrograde fashion under fluoroscopy over the S2–S4 nerve roots. In their study, 30 consecutive female patients underwent bilateral S2–S4 sacral neuromodulation via the retrograde approach. Of these patients, 77% had good responses and underwent permanent implantation. At last follow-up (mean 15 months, minimum 6 months), quality of life measures were significantly improved relative to pre-implantation, with mean 40% improvement in pain scores by VAS. Thus, the authors conclude that in patients with refractory CPP, bilateral caudal epidural sacral neuromodulation is another possible mode of treatment.

Since CPP is likely mediated by more than one sacral root, either unilaterally or bilaterally, the stimulation of only one nerve root may not be sufficient for symptom control. To date, no trial has compared unilateral versus bilateral stimulation although several studies suggest efficacy of the bilateral approach. Steinberg and colleagues retrospectively reviewed 15 patients who underwent bilateral S3 stimulators for refractory IC/BPS symptoms, including pain [65]. At a mean follow-up of 14 months, the mean decrease in frequency and nocturia was 10.4 voids and 2.6 voids, respectively. Pain scores were not captured independently, but patient satisfaction did improve as measured by the urinary distress inventory short form, which queries pain levels.

Future Directions for Treatment of CPP Using Neuromodulation

In addition to SNS, other neuromodulatory approaches have been suggested for the treatment of CPP, including posterior tibial nerve stimulation (PTNS), pudendal nerve stimulation (PNS), and caudal epidural S2–S4 SNS placement. Kim et al. evaluated the effect of PTNS in 15 patients (10 women and 5 men) with CPP in an open prospective clinical trial [66]. After 12 weeks of PTNS, 60% of patients had an improvement of more than 50% on a visual analog pain scale, and 40% achieved a mean VAS less than 3. Van Balken et al. evaluated PTNS in 33 patients with CPP as their primary complaint in a prospective multicenter trial [67]. In 21% of patients, mean VAS decreased more than 50%, and after 12 weeks of treatment, 7 patients (21%) had a mean VAS less than 3. In aggregate, PTNS boasts modest overall success rates for chronic pelvic pain, and randomized, placebo-controlled trials with longer term follow-up are warranted.

The pudendal nerve originates from the S2, S3, and S4 nerve roots, such that PNS provides broader stimulation compared to targeting S3 alone. In a retrospective study by Peters et al., 84 patients underwent PNS for IC/BPS and overactive bladder [68]. A positive pudendal response, defined as greater than 50% improvement in symptoms following pudendal lead placement, was achieved in 71% of subjects. Notably, almost all (93%) with a history of failed sacral neuromodulation responded to the pudendal lead. This may be due to the unique ability of the pudendal approach to offer increased afferent stimulation through the S2–S4 nerve roots. However, accurate placement of the tined lead in the pudendal location can prove challenging and time consuming for the surgeon. To combat this pitfall, Heinze and colleagues devised the STAR (ischial Spine, ischial Tuberosity, acetabulum, and anal Rim) technique using fixed anatomic landmarks to improve PNS placement in their 2014 pilot study using this technique in 20 patients with refractory chronic pelvic pain [69]. In the ten patients who underwent placement by the STAR technique, they noted a mean operative time of 85 min for bilateral PNS lead placement, versus a mean of 105 min for unilateral PNM lead placement using techniques previously described in the literature. In the patients who underwent STAR PNS placement, there was a statistically significant decrease in pain at the conclusion of the 4-week trial, with 90% proceeding to generator implantation.

In a follow-up study in 2007, Peters and colleagues compared sacral neuromodulation versus PNS for refractory IC/BPS symptoms [70]. In their study, 22 patients with refractory IC/BPS underwent placement of a tined lead at S3 and another lead at the pudendal nerve. Each was tested in a blinded manner for 7 days. The authors found that the time required to place a pudendal lead was about 30% less than that required for a sacral lead. Of the 22 patients, 77% responded and had a permanent implant placed. PNS was chosen as the better lead in 77% and SNS in 24%. The order in which the lead was stimulated had no effect on the final lead implanted, and there was no measurable "carry-over" effect. The overall reduction in symptoms was 59% for PNS and 44% for SNS, leading the authors to conclude that PNS may offer advantages beyond traditional SNS in some patients with refractory IC/BPS.

Caudal epidural SNS also provides stimulation of the S2–S4 nerve roots. This procedure involves deploying a quadripolar lead over the S2–S4 sacral nerve roots. While literature regarding this technique is scarce, Zabihi et al. did evaluate the efficacy of bilateral caudal epidural SNS for the treatment of refractory chronic pelvic pain and IC/BPS in a 2008 study [52]. In his trial of 30 patients, 77% had a successful trial stimulation and underwent permanent implantation. At mean follow-up of 15 months, median pain scores were improved by 40% relative to baseline. Similar improvements were seen on validated patient symptom questionnaires. On average, patients reported a 42% improvement in symptoms. However, four patients eventually underwent explantation due to treatment failure. Subsequent studies are still needed.

Before SNS is widely adopted for the treatment of chronic pelvic pain, further investigation is warranted. Indeed, large-scale, multicenter randomized controlled trials with long-term follow-up data, comparing SNS with other non-neuromodulatory modalities, as well as non-sacral neuromodulation, for treating CPP would help clinicians counsel patients and offer appropriate interventions. Moreover, such studies could offer insight into predictors of SNS treatment response. Given that this intervention is moderately invasive, it is important to avoid it in patients who are unlikely to benefit and rather target it toward likely responders, and we currently do not have high-quality evidence regarding how to make this distinction.

Summary

SNS has been shown to be an effective treatment for refractory non-obstructive urinary retention, urgency/frequency, urgency urinary incontinence, and fecal incontinence. However, SNS currently has no FDA approval for the treatment of chronic pelvic pain. Since many patients with CPP experience insufficient results with conservative treatment, minimally invasive intervention such as SNS could offer a promising middle ground that avoids a major surgery, such as bladder augmentation or urinary diversion. The currently published results suggest that SNS may be a valuable alternative treatment option for CPP patients. However, the majority of published studies were small, retrospective, and lacking in long-term follow-up. Inclusion and exclusion criteria varied between studies and outcomes were not uniform. In particular, not all studies clarified improvements in voiding outcomes versus pain outcomes. These features make the current body of literature regarding SNS for CPP difficult to generalize. Large-scale randomized trials with long-term follow-up and clearly stated, strict inclusion criteria are needed in order to more thoroughly evaluate SNS as a treatment for CPP.

References

1. Hunter C, Dave N, Diwan S, Deer T. Neuromodulation of pelvic visceral pain: review of the literature and case series of potential novel targets for treatment. Pain Pract. 2013;13(1):3–17.
2. Kothari S. Neuromodulatory approaches to chronic pelvic pain and coccygodynia. Acta Neurochir Suppl. 2007;97(Pt 1):365–71.
3. Fariello JY, Whitmore K. Sacral neuromodulation stimulation for IC/PBS, chronic pelvic pain, and sexual dysfunction. Int Urogynecol J. 2010;21(12):1553–8.
4. Mathias SD, Kuppermann M, Liberman RF, Lipschutz RC, Steege JF. Chronic pelvic pain: prevalence, health-related quality of life, and economic correlates. Obstet Gynecol. 1996;87(3):321–7.
5. Lampe A, Solder E, Ennemoser A, Schubert C, Rumpold G, Sollner W. Chronic pelvic pain and previous sexual abuse. Obstet Gynecol. 2000;96(6):929–33.
6. Heim C, Ehlert U, Hanker JP, Hellhammer DH. Abuse-related posttraumatic stress disorder and alterations of the hypothalamic-pituitary-adrenal axis in women with chronic pelvic pain. Psychosom Med. 1998;60(3):309–18.
7. Martinez-Lavin M. Is fibromyalgia a generalized reflex sympathetic dystrophy? Clin Exp Rheumatol. 2001;19(1):1–3.
8. Longstreth GF. Irritable bowel syndrome and chronic pelvic pain. Obstet Gynecol Surv. 1994;49(7):505–7.
9. de la Rosette JJ, Hubregtse MR, Meuleman EJ, Stolk-Engelaar MV, Debruyne FM. Diagnosis and treatment of 409 patients with prostatitis syndromes. Urology. 1993;41(4):301–7.
10. Krieger JN, Nyberg L Jr, Nickel JC. NIH consensus definition and classification of prostatitis. JAMA. 1999;282(3):236–7.
11. Raj P. Practical management of pain. St. Louis, MO: Mosby Inc.; 2000.
12. Janicki TI. Chronic pelvic pain as a form of complex regional pain syndrome. Clin Obstet Gynecol. 2003;46(4):797–803.
13. Comiter CV. Sacral neuromodulation for the symptomatic treatment of refractory interstitial cystitis: a prospective study. J Urol. 2003;169(4):1369–73.
14. Prevalence of interstitial cystitis/painful bladder syndrome in the United States: The RAND Interstitial Cystitis Epidemiology study. Annual Meeting of the American Urological Association; 2009.
15. Nazif O, Teichman JM, Gebhart GF. Neural upregulation in interstitial cystitis. Urology. 2007;69(4 Suppl):24–33.
16. Hanno P, Burks D, Clemens J, Dmochowski R, Erickson D, et al. Diagnosis and Treatment of Interstitial Cystitis/Bladder Pain Syndrome. 2014. https://www.auanet.org/common/pdf/education/clinical-guidance/IC-Bladder-Pain-Syndrome-Revised.pdf. Accessed 11 Nov 2016.
17. Carrico DJ, Peters KM, Diokno AC. Guided imagery for women with interstitial cystitis: results of a prospective, randomized controlled pilot study. J Altern Complement Med. 2008;14(1):53–60.
18. Foster HE Jr, Hanno PM, Nickel JC, Payne CK, Mayer RD, Burks DA, et al. Effect of amitriptyline on symptoms in treatment naive patients with interstitial cystitis/painful bladder syndrome. J Urol. 2010;183(5):1853–8.
19. Hsieh TF, KJ Y, Lin SY. Possible application of Raman microspectroscopy to verify the interstitial cystitis diagnosis after potassium sensitivity test: phenylalanine or tryptophan as a biomarker. Dis Markers. 2007;23(3):147–52.
20. Herati AS, Shorter B, Srinivasan AK, Tai J, Seideman C, Lesser M, et al. Effects of foods and beverages on the symptoms of chronic prostatitis/chronic pelvic pain syndrome. Urology. 2013;82(6):1376–80.
21. Peters KM, Carrico DJ, Kalinowski SE, Ibrahim IA, Diokno AC. Prevalence of pelvic floor dysfunction in patients with interstitial cystitis. Urology. 2007;70(1):16–8.
22. Weiss JM. Pelvic floor myofascial trigger points: manual therapy for interstitial cystitis and the urgency-frequency syndrome. J Urol. 2001;166(6):2226–31.
23. Anderson RU, Wise D, Sawyer T, Chan C. Integration of myofascial trigger point release and paradoxical relaxation training treatment of chronic pelvic pain in men. J Urol. 2005;174(1):155–60.
24. FitzGerald MP, Anderson RU, Potts J, Payne CK, Peters KM, Clemens JQ, et al. Randomized multicenter feasibility trial of myofascial physical therapy for the treatment of urological chronic pelvic pain syndromes. J Urol. 2009;182(2):570–80.

25. FitzGerald MP, Payne CK, Lukacz ES, Yang CC, Peters KM, Chai TC, et al. Randomized multicenter clinical trial of myofascial physical therapy in women with interstitial cystitis/painful bladder syndrome and pelvic floor tenderness. J Urol. 2012;187(6):2113–8.
26. van Ophoven A, Pokupic S, Heinecke A, Hertle L. A prospective, randomized, placebo controlled, double-blind study of amitriptyline for the treatment of interstitial cystitis. J Urol. 2004;172(2):533–6.
27. Thilagarajah R, Witherow RO, Walker MM. Oral cimetidine gives effective symptom relief in painful bladder disease: a prospective, randomized, double-blind placebo-controlled trial. BJU Int. 2001;87(3):207–12.
28. Dasgupta P, Sharma SD, Womack C, Blackford HN, Dennis P. Cimetidine in painful bladder syndrome: a histopathological study. BJU Int. 2001;88(3):183–6.
29. Seshadri P, Emerson L, Morales A. Cimetidine in the treatment of interstitial cystitis. Urology. 1994;44(4):614–6.
30. Theoharides TC, Sant GR. Hydroxyzine therapy for interstitial cystitis. Urology. 1997;49(5A Suppl):108–10.
31. Sant GR, Propert KJ, Hanno PM, Burks D, Culkin D, Diokno AC, et al. A pilot clinical trial of oral pentosan polysulfate and oral hydroxyzine in patients with interstitial cystitis. J Urol. 2003;170(3):810–5.
32. Theoharides TC. Hydroxyzine in the treatment of interstitial cystitis. Urol Clin North Am. 1994;21(1):113–9.
33. Colaco MA, Evans RJ. Current recommendations for bladder instillation therapy in the treatment of interstitial cystitis/bladder pain syndrome. Curr Urol Rep. 2013;14(5):442–7.
34. Nickel JC, Jain P, Shore N, Anderson J, Giesing D, Lee H, et al. Continuous intravesical lidocaine treatment for interstitial cystitis/bladder pain syndrome: safety and efficacy of a new drug delivery device. Sci Transl Med. 2012;4(143):143ra100.
35. Cole EE, Scarpero HM, Dmochowski RR. Are patient symptoms predictive of the diagnostic and/or therapeutic value of hydrodistention? Neurourol Urodyn. 2005;24(7):638–42.
36. Erickson DR, Kunselman AR, Bentley CM, Peters KM, Rovner ES, Demers LM, et al. Changes in urine markers and symptoms after bladder distention for interstitial cystitis. J Urol. 2007;177(2):556–60.
37. Ottem DP, Teichman JM. What is the value of cystoscopy with hydrodistension for interstitial cystitis? Urology. 2005;66(3):494–9.
38. Kuo HC, Chancellor MB. Comparison of intravesical botulinum toxin type A injections plus hydrodistention with hydrodistention alone for the treatment of refractory interstitial cystitis/painful bladder syndrome. BJU Int. 2009;104(5):657–61.
39. Pinto R, Lopes T, Frias B, Silva A, Silva JA, Silva CM, et al. Trigonal injection of botulinum toxin A in patients with refractory bladder pain syndrome/interstitial cystitis. Eur Urol. 2010;58(3):360–5.
40. Gajewski JB, Al-Zahrani AA. The long-term efficacy of sacral neuromodulation in the management of intractable cases of bladder pain syndrome: 14 years of experience in one centre. BJU Int. 2011;107(8):1258–64.
41. Ghazwani YQ, Elkelini MS, Hassouna MM. Efficacy of sacral neuromodulation in treatment of bladder pain syndrome: long-term follow-up. Neurourol Urodyn. 2011;30(7):1271–5.
42. Marinkovic SP, Gillen LM, Marinkovic CM. Minimum 6-year outcomes for interstitial cystitis treated with sacral neuromodulation. Int Urogynecol J. 2011;22(4):407–12.
43. Powell CR, Kreder KJ. Long-term outcomes of urgency-frequency syndrome due to painful bladder syndrome treated with sacral neuromodulation and analysis of failures. J Urol. 2010;183(1):173–6.
44. Sairanen J, Tammela TL, Leppilahti M, Multanen M, Paananen I, Lehtoranta K, et al. Cyclosporine A and pentosan polysulfate sodium for the treatment of interstitial cystitis: a randomized comparative study. J Urol. 2005;174(6):2235–8.
45. Forrest JB, Payne CK, Erickson DR. Cyclosporine A for refractory interstitial cystitis/bladder pain syndrome: experience of 3 tertiary centers. J Urol. 2012;188(4):1186–91.
46. Rossberger J, Fall M, Jonsson O, Peeker R. Long-term results of reconstructive surgery in patients with bladder pain syndrome/interstitial cystitis: subtyping is imperative. Urology. 2007;70(4):638–42.
47. Madersbacher H. Conservative therapy of neurogenic disorders of micturition. Urologe A. 1999;38(1):24–9.
48. Nashold BS Jr, Friedman H, Boyarsky S. Electrical activation of micturition by spinal cord stimulation. J Surg Res. 1971;11(3):144–7.
49. Van Kerrebroeck PE. Advances in the role of sacral nerve neuromodulation in lower urinary tract symptoms. Int Urogynecol J. 2010;21(Suppl 2):S467–74.
50. Mayer R, Howard F. Sacral nerve stimultation: neuromodulation for voiding dysfunction and pain. Neurotherapeutics. 2008;5:107–13.
51. Dasgupta R, Critchley HD, Dolan RJ, Fowler CJ. Changes in brain activity following sacral neuromodulation for urinary retention. J Urol. 2005;174(6):2268–72.
52. Zabihi N, Mourtzinos A, Maher MG, Raz S, Rodriguez LV. Short-term results of bilateral S2-S4 sacral neuromodulation for the treatment of refractory interstitial cystitis, painful bladder syndrome, and chronic pelvic pain. Int Urogynecol J Pelvic Floor Dysfunct. 2008;19(4):553–7.
53. Fall M, Baranowski AP, Elneil S, Engeler D, Hughes J, Messelink EJ, et al. EAU guidelines on chronic pelvic pain. Eur Urol. 2010;57(1):35–48.
54. Melzack R, Wall P. Pain mechanisms: a new theory. Science. 1965;150:971.
55. van der Pal F, Heesakkers JP, Bemelmans BL. Current opinion on the working mechanisms of neuromodulation in the treatment of lower urinary tract dysfunction. Curr Opin Urol. 2006;16(4):261–7.

56. Marcelissen T, Jacobs R, van Kerrebroeck P, de Wachter S. Sacral neuromodulation as a treatment for chronic pelvic pain. J Urol. 2011;186(2):387–93.
57. Hohenfellner M, Dahms SE, Matzel K, Thuroff JW. Sacral neuromodulation for treatment of lower urinary tract dysfunction. BJU Int. 2000;85(Suppl 3):10–9; discussion 22–3.
58. Maher CF, Carey MP, Dwyer PL, Schluter PL. Percutaneous sacral nerve root neuromodulation for intractable interstitial cystitis. J Urol. 2001;165(3):884–6.
59. Siegel S, Paszkiewicz E, Kirkpatrick C, Hinkel B, Oleson K. Sacral nerve stimulation in patients with chronic intractable pelvic pain. J Urol. 2001;166(5):1742–5.
60. Brookoff D, Bennett D. Neuromodulation in intractable interstitial cystitis and related pain syndromes. Pain Med. 2006;7(suppl 1):S166–84.
61. Everaert K, Plancke H, Lefevere F, Oosterlinck W. The urodynamic evaluation of neuromodulation in patients with voiding dysfunction. Br J Urol. 1997;79(5):702–7.
62. Whitmore KE, Payne CK, Diokno AC, Lukban JC. Sacral neuromodulation in patients with interstitial cystitis: a multicenter clinical trial. Int Urogynecol J Pelvic Floor Dysfunct. 2003;14(5):305–8; discussion 308–9.
63. Peters KM, Konstandt D. Sacral neuromodulation decreases narcotic requirements in refractory interstitial cystitis. BJU Int. 2004;93(6):777–9.
64. Rackley R, Vasavada S, Daneshgari F. Neuromodulation for interstitial cystitis. Cleveland Clinic Glickman Urologic Institute. 2005. https://my.clevelandclinic.org/ccf/media/files/Urology/AUA%20Abstracts%202005.pdf.
65. Steinberg AC, Oyama IA, Whitmore KE. Bilateral S3 stimulator in patients with interstitial cystitis. Urology. 2007;69(3):441–3.
66. Kim SW, Paick JS, Ku JH. Percutaneous posterior tibial nerve stimulation in patients with chronic pelvic pain: a preliminary study. Urol Int. 2007;78(1):58–62.
67. van Balken MR, Vandoninck V, Messelink BJ, Vergunst H, Heesakkers JP, Debruyne FM, et al. Percutaneous tibial nerve stimulation as neuromodulative treatment of chronic pelvic pain. Eur Urol. 2003;43(2):158–63; discussion 163.
68. Peters KM, Killinger KA, Boguslawski BM, Boura JA. Chronic pudendal neuromodulation: expanding available treatment options for refractory urologic symptoms. Neurourol Urodyn. 2010;29(7):1267–71.
69. Heinze K, Hoermann R, Fritsch H, Dermietzel R, van Ophoven A. Comparative pilot study of implantation techniques for pudendal neuromodulation: technical and clinical outcome in first 20 patients with chronic pelvic pain. World J Urol. 2015;33(2):289–94.
70. Peters KM, Feber KM, Bennett RC. A prospective, single-blind, randomized crossover trial of sacral vs pudendal nerve stimulation for interstitial cystitis. BJU Int. 2007;100(4):835–9.

9 Sacral Neuromodulation for Fecal Incontinence

Dadrie Baptiste and Jason Shellnut

Introduction

Fecal incontinence refers to the involuntary passage of gas or liquid stool (minor incontinence) or the involuntary passage of solid stool (major incontinence). The condition is common, and affects an estimated 8.3% of all noninstitutionalized adults in the United States [1]. The prevalence of fecal incontinence in institutionalized adults is thought to be higher. The prevalence of fecal incontinence is likely underestimated as many patients affected by it are reluctant to report or discuss it. Greater than 70% of patients who suffer from fecal incontinence do not seek treatment, for a variety of reasons ranging from limited health care access to self-blame [2] (Fig. 9.1).

In a meta-analysis performed on fecal incontinence in the community with face to face or phone interviews, the prevalence was established at 8.4%. In patients who submitted mail-in surveys, the prevalence of fecal incontinence was 12.4% [3]. This study demonstrates that patients with fecal incontinence may underreport their symptoms when they have to disclose them to another individual. Fecal incontinence can have a devastating impact on the quality of life of those affected as it can lead to issues with self-esteem and even social isolation. While sacral neuromodulation has been performed for disorders of the urinary system since 1999, it was not FDA approved for the indication of fecal incontinence until March 2011.

Background

One of the challenges of treating fecal incontinence is that continence is an incompletely understood phenomenon. In terms of the factors contributing to fecal incontinence, there are four general categories: sphincteric, neurologic, stool characteristics, and the rectum. The internal sphincter muscle is tonically contracted. This, along with the natural hemorrhoidal tissue, creates a water and air tight ring of closure of the anal canal. Sphincteric injury often leads to fecal incontinence; common causes being obstetric injuries and iatrogenic injuries secondary to anorectal surgery. The pelvic floor muscles, when contracted, help to maintain continence. During the process of defecation, these muscles conversely will relax and assist in opening the anus. Intact rectal and anal sensations are also important in maintaining continence mechanism as the

D. Baptiste
Department of Colorectal Surgery, Beaumont Health, Royal Oak, MI, USA
e-mail: dadrie@gmail.com

J. Shellnut (✉)
Colon and Rectal Surgery, William Beaumont Hospital, Royal Oak, MI, USA
e-mail: Jason.shellnut@beaumont.org

J. P. Gilleran, S. A. Alpert (eds.), *Adult and Pediatric Neuromodulation*,
https://doi.org/10.1007/978-3-319-73266-4_9

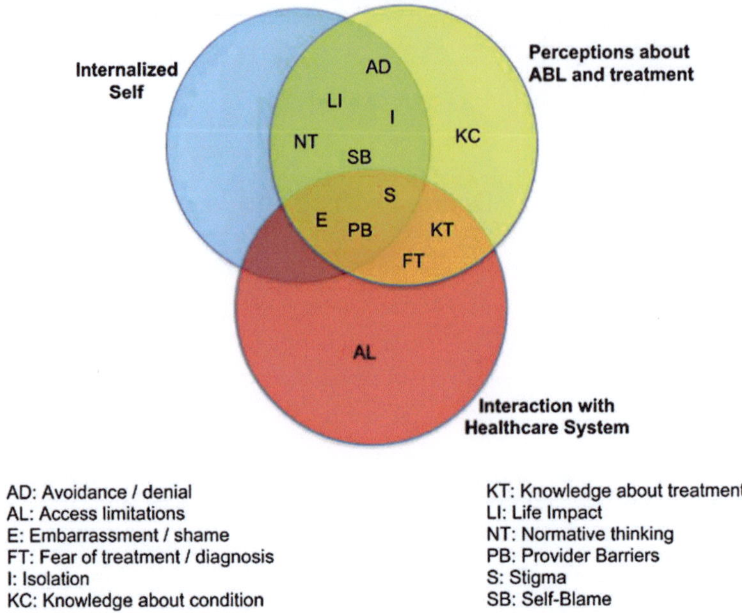

Fig. 9.1 Themes across barriers to care-seeking for accidental bowel leakage. From Brown HW, et al. [2]. Reprinted with permission from Springer

sensation of stool within the distal rectum generates contraction of the external sphincter, which assists the internal sphincter. Neurologic pathology which can cause fecal incontinence includes diabetic neuropathy and injury to the internal pudendal nerve. Rectal compliance is an important factor in achieving continence of stool as the rectum is responsible for relaxing when a bolus of stool enters it. This relaxation decreases the intrarectal pressure and assists both the sphincter muscles and pelvic floor in retaining stool until the individual opts to defecate. A rectum which is not capable of distending can cause patients to experience frequency, urgency, and potential incontinence if a bathroom is not immediately available. Diseases which decrease rectal compliance and place the patient at risk for fecal incontinence include ulcerative colitis and radiation proctitis. Finally, stool consistency is an important factor in fecal continence, as liquid stool is more difficult to retain than solid stool. Stool consistency can be altered in a variety of medical conditions and an increased liquid component can overwhelm the continence mechanisms, listed previously, leading to incontinence. Given the number of factors which contribute to fecal continence, all of which have incompletely understood mechanisms of action, there are many potential causes for the development of incontinence.

Evaluation

History

A thorough history of the patient presenting with fecal incontinence is paramount. Symptoms should be documented in terms of severity, onset, duration, and the degree of incontinence from fecal seepage to overflow incontinence. Any associated pathology including rectal or vaginal prolapse, and urinary incontinence should be documented. A detailed obstetrical and surgical history should be obtained as well as coexisting previous treatments, medical conditions, and current medications.

Physical Examination

A thorough abdominal exam should be performed with any scars from previous operations noted. The perianal region should then be examined in the prone or lateral Sim's position. The presence of feculent material on the perianal skin or irritation of the perianal skin may indicate the patient is experiencing fecal incontinence. Scars on the perianal skin should also be noted and may be an indication of previous anorectal surgery or if located anteriorly may represent a previous obstetric injury. On digital rectal exam, a patulous anus can be an indication of rectal prolapse, but can also occur in the setting of a patient who frequently engages in ano-receptive intercourse. The resting tone of the internal anal sphincter can be noted during digital rectal exam. Decreased tone may be caused by previous anorectal surgery, obstetric injuries, rectal prolapse, and frequent ano-receptive intercourse. The function of the external sphincter can be established by assessing squeeze pressure on the examiner's finger. The rectum should be examined for the presence of a rectocele and the vagina should also be examined for evidence of an enterocele, cystocele, rectocele, and/or vaginal prolapse. Assessment of the perineal body can be performed by simultaneously placing the examiner's index finger in the rectum and thumb in the vagina. A short or absent perineal body may indicate an obstetric injury to the sphincter complex.

Assessment of Severity and Impact on Quality of Life

Grading of the severity of fecal incontinence and the subjective effect on the patient's quality of life are important as well. Establishing an objective measure of the severity, in which a patient is experiencing fecal incontinence prior to treatment, allows for a more accurate evaluation of the success of the patient's treatment regimen. Several severity scales have been developed and one of the most commonly used is the Wexner (Cleveland Clinic) fecal incontinence score, which utilizes five parameters scored on a scale from zero (absent) to four (daily). These parameters include frequency of incontinence to gas, liquid stool, and solid stool; in addition to the need to wear a pad, and lifestyle changes. Another commonly used system is the fecal incontinence severity index (FISI), based on four types of leakage (gas, mucus, liquid stool, solid stool) and five frequencies (once to three times per month, once per week, twice per week, once per day, and twice or more per day) (Fig. 9.2). While other scoring systems exist, in general, the more detailed summary scales such as the Wexner and FISI are thought to have greater validity and can be utilized to quantify improvements in continence scores after treatment [4–7].

Diagnostics

As part of the workup for incontinence, careful consideration to other etiologies of fecal leakage should be considered. There are many patients who are considered to be incontinent, yet on further examination are diagnosed with diarrhea of various etiologies. This illustrates the importance of a carefully documented history and sequential workup. If there is concern for concomitant or solitary diarrhea resulting in "incontinence," it is important to perform endoscopic evaluation with modalities such as flexible sigmoidoscopy or colonoscopy to rule out etiologies such as mucosal inflammation, masses, or strictures. Other etiologies of diarrhea such as infections and metabolic derangements need to be ruled out as well by performing stool studies and testing for thyroid dysfunction, diabetes, and food intolerances. The studies ordered to evaluate for infection include stool culture, ova and parasites, fecal leukocytes, and *Clostridium difficile* toxin [8].

Anal Manometry

The primary utility of anal manometry in evaluation of a patient with fecal incontinence is to rule out impaired function of the sphincter muscles. Typically, the resting pressure, squeeze pressure, rectoanal inhibitory reflex (RAIR), rectal compliance, and rectal distensibility are measured. The resting pressure is a function of the internal anal sphincter, whereas the squeeze pressure is a function of the external anal sphincter. Resting and squeeze pressures are typically lower in patients with fecal incontinence. These pressures do not typically correspond with the degree of fecal

a

	2 or More Times a Day	Once a Day	2 or More Times a Week	Once a Week	1 to 3 Times A Month
Gas					
Mucus					
Liquid					
Solid					

b

	2 or More Times a Day	Once a Day	2 or More Times a Week	Once a Week	1 to 3 Times A Month	Never
a. Gas	☐	☐	☐	☐	☐	☐
b. Mucus	☐	☐	☐	☐	☐	☐
c. Liquid Stool	☐	☐	☐	☐	☐	☐
d. Solid Stool	☐	☐	☐	☐	☐	☐

Fig. 9.2 Fecal incontinence severity index (Each event is weighted from "0" as never to the highest score "4/5" as 2 or more times a day). From Rockwood TH, et al. [4]. Reprinted with permission from Wolters Kluwer Health

incontinence. Even those patients who experience fecal soilage typically have decreased resting pressures and normal squeeze pressures. Men typically have higher resting and squeeze pressures than women which may be related to prior obstetric injuries to the sphincter complex.

Pudendal Nerve Motor Latency

Pudendal nerve terminal motor latency (PNTML) testing has proven to be a useful diagnostic tool in fecal incontinence. It has also been used as a predictive factor in sphincteroplasty repairs. Patients who demonstrate a bilateral pudendal nerve neuropathy on PNTML testing generally do not have good outcomes with a sphincteroplasty. The procedure is performed by placing an electrode mounted on a glove within the rectum on the internal pudendal nerve. Electrical stimulation of the nerve is then performed, and the time until a motor response from the sphincter complex and muscles of the pelvic floor is determined. A value of greater than 2 ms is considered abnormal and consistent with a pudendal nerve neuropathy. In a study reviewing over 1000 patients being evaluated for fecal incontinence, a subcohort of 83 patients who had intact anal sphincters, and no evidence of prolapse on imaging were evaluated with PNTML. Twenty eight percent of patients had prolonged latency unilaterally and 12% bilaterally when using a 2.2-ms threshold. When comparing fecal incontinence scores, patients who had bilateral prolonged PNTML testing were noted to have normal mean squeeze pressure, decreased mean resting pressure, and increased fecal incontinence scores. Those with unilateral prolonged PNTML had no association with changes in pressures or fecal incontinence scores [9].

Imaging

Endoanal Ultrasound

Endoanal ultrasound and anal manometry are complementary studies. This study is utilized to evaluate the sphincter muscles and is considered the gold standard of sphincter evaluation. Sensitivity has been reported as high as 100% for detection of sphincter defects, though the technique is heavily operator dependent. Defects indicate a tear; internal anal sphincter tears are hyperechoic while external anal sphincter tears are typically hypoechoic. Scarring is noted on visualization of loss of normal texture and low reflectiveness. Measurement of the perineal body is thought to be important in the technique of determining a sphincter defect on endoanal ultrasound such that a perineal body measuring 12 mm or greater is not likely to have a sphincter defect unless some surgical augmentation has occurred in the past. To appropriately document sphincter defects, both the location(s) and extent of the defect(s) should be noted. The extent of the defect is reported by the estimated number of degrees of the tear based on a circle having 360° [10–13]. It is also important to document any sphincter atrophy as this is associated with poor outcomes in those patients who subsequently undergo sphincteroplasty.

Magnetic Resonance Imaging

MRI allows for enhanced and precise visualization of the pelvic structures. The addition of an endo-coil allows for an improved evaluation of the anal sphincters. While endoanal ultrasound is considered the gold standard for imaging of the anal sphincters in general, endoanal MRI is considered more specific for identifying external anal sphincter defects with specificity ranging 90–95%, in some reports. MRI is not operator dependent like endoanal ultrasound; however, it does have its drawbacks. In comparison to ultrasound, it is significantly more expensive, is not readily available at many institutions, and cannot be performed in some patients who have metallic implants [14].

Defecating Proctography

This study involves the fluoroscopic evaluation of the process of defecation. It provides an interactive evaluation of the patient's defecation by recording the expulsion of rectal barium, which is thought to simulate the consistency of feces. The study serves to evaluate the sequential phases of defecation. In the evaluation of a patient with fecal incontinence, a defecating proctogram mainly serves to evaluate for the presence of external rectal prolapse or an outlet obstruction caused by internal rectal intussusception. Obstructed defecation secondary to internal rectal prolapse can lead to overflow incontinence in patients with the condition. In addition to rectal barium, the patient ingests oral barium for evaluation of enteroceles and the vagina is coated with a diatrizoic acid containing gel. Patients are then imaged in a lateral position at rest, during pelvic floor contracture, and during evacuation of the rectum, which in turn estimates completeness of defecation and measurement of pelvic floor descent. Morphological abnormalities are also discernible during this part of procedure [15].

Treatment of Fecal Incontinence

Treatment algorithms can be divided into nonsurgical medical and surgical interventions.

Medical Management

Dietary Modification

Dietary modification involves such interventions as increasing the patient's daily fiber intake and consuming the BRAT diet. The BRAT diet (Bananas, Rice, Applesauce, and dry Toast) is usually prescribed for diarrhea treatment in children; however, it typically works in adults as well. It serves to decrease the liquid component of stool. It should be noted that this diet should not be adhered to in sole fashion as a long-term solution given its lack of protein and other necessary dietary supplements as prescribed by the Center for Nutrition Policy and Promotion. Foods which tend to promote leakage of feces should also be avoided. The most common dietary culprits are caffeine products (coffee, soda, and tea), alcohol, spicy foods, and chocolate. In patients with only mild leakage issues, cotton balls placed against the anus or perineal pads may provide sufficient treatment. If dietary modification is unsuccessful in bulking the stool, then antidiarrheal medications including loperamide (Imodium), diphenoxylate (Lomotil), and tincture of opium should be considered.

Biofeedback Therapy

The purpose of biofeedback is to use sensory information including visual, auditory, and touch to improve the patient's sensation of rectal distension and reinforce appropriate sphincter contraction. Balloon training using a Miller–Abbott balloon as a sensor attached to a polygraph to improve the quality of Kegel exercises can be incorporated into pelvic floor physical therapy. By increasing the volume of water within a rectally placed balloon over time rectal sensation can be improved. Published studies typically demonstrate over 70% improvement in continence for both adults and children. Described methods are highly variable and studies indicate no one regimen is superior to the next. Patients with decreased rectal compliance generally do not respond well to biofeedback therapy [16].

Surgical Management

Dynamic and Adynamic Gracilis Flap

This surgical procedure involves mobilizing the gracilis muscle while preserving its neurovascular bundle so that the muscle can be wrapped around the anal canal. The gracilis muscle is not tonically contracted as the anal sphincter muscles are, and it is widely believed that optimal results with this procedure require an Implantable Pulse Generator (IPG) in order to stimulate the muscle. Patients who undergo an Adynamic Graciloplasty (no IPG) typically experience improvement in their fecal incontinence; however, those who undergo a Dynamic Graciloplasty (DGP, with an IPG) often experience superior results. The addition of an IPG to the procedure increases the complication rates of the procedure which mainly involve infection or malfunction of the device. The IPG for this procedure is currently not approved by the FDA, and therefore dynamic graciloplasty is only available outside of the United States. A meta-analysis which reported on dynamic graciloplasty found an overall success rate of 49.3%. The rates of surgical revisions and explantations were 46.2% and 32.5%, respectively. The overall complication rate for DGP in the study was 82.8% [17].

Overlapping Sphincteroplasty

The initial technique was described by Parks and McPartlin in 1971 [18] and slightly modified to the currently utilized technique by Slade in 1977. This technique is largely indicated for patients with fecal incontinence related to a sphincter defect usually caused by an obstetric or iatrogenic anterior injury. Sphincteroplasty for posterior or lateral injuries is typically less successful. The procedure is performed under general anesthesia with the patient in the prone jackknife position. The sphincter is repaired via a curvilinear incision made transversely between the anus and the vagina parallel to the outer edge of the external sphincter separating the scar from the vagina and the rectum. Mobilization of the sphincters is performed generously to avoid tension on the repair. Once mobilized circumferentially, the two ends of the sphincter are overlapped and secured typically with absorbable suture. The skin is closed loosely over the repair to allow for drainage. Some surgeons will also perform a levatorplasty at the time of the repair. Initial success rates of the procedure are generally reported in the 70–90% range; however, many patients experience a decline in results over time, with only 40% of patients reporting good control of their bowel movements at a median of 10 years after the operation [19]. In one retrospective study [20] which reviewed 31 patients followed for 36 months postoperatively, 15 patients had complete continence or incontinence to gas only while five had incontinence to liquid or solid stool. Incontinence to anything but gas was considered a failure. Bravo-Gutierrez reviewed 130 patients followed for a median of 10 years post sphincteroplasty. In this study, complete continence was reported in only 6% of patients while 58% of patients reported incontinence to solid stool [19]. The issue of when to perform definitive repair of injured sphincter muscles is often debated. No study has ascertained whether immediate primary repair versus delayed secondary repair months to years later is best [21]. Several studies have looked at the success rates of primary repair. In one such study [22], 34 women undergoing primary (end to end) repair after enduring a third degree tear during delivering were followed for an extended period ranging from 42 to 651 days. In follow-up, a persistent defect was found on endoanal ultrasound in 85% of the patients, 41% had incontinence to flatus or flatus and liquid stool, and 26% had fecal urgency. Other studies have revealed similar results, thus indicating that for more extensive obstetrical injuries (i.e., third or fourth degree tears) there is a high incidence of persistent sphincter defects and symptomatic incontinence following primary repair and perhaps these should be referred for delayed repair with a colorectal surgeon [23].

Artificial Bowel Sphincter

The typical approach is through the perineum or alternatively through the vagina. The device consists of three components, including a fluid-filled silicone cuff which encircles the anus, a fluid-filled pressure regulating balloon which is placed in the peritoneal cavity, and a control pump which connects the previous two components and is placed either in the scrotum or the labia majora. The silicone cuff and control pump are connected by tubing which allows for manual pumping of fluid into and out of the cuff. When the cuff is inflated, the anus is closed preventing defecation. When the patient wishes to defecate, the pump can be used to transfer the fluid into the balloon which desufflates the cuff and opens the anus. A meta-analysis which reviewed the literature on the artificial bowel sphincter procedure found an overall 42.6% success rate of the procedure. Surgical revisions and explantations were commonly required and occurred in 45.5% and 33% of patients, respectively [17]. In this study, the total complication rate was 168% for the ABS procedure due to a large number of patients suffering multiple complications. The success rate for this procedure is high in the subset of patients who have a functioning device without complication; however, the total complication rates are high enough that the procedure is not widely accepted and is performed at a limited number of specialized centers worldwide.

Injectables

Urologists have utilized injectable bulking agents to treat urinary incontinence for more than a decade, which has been extrapolated into the treatment of fecal incontinence [24]. The proposed mechanism of action is augmentation by mechanical bulking of proximal portion of the internal anal sphincter. This was first implemented in 1992 [25]. There are several different methods of injection and injectable bulking agents [26]. Perhaps one of the most studied injectable is Solesta® also known as dextranomer in stabilized sodium hyaluronate (dextranomer/hyaluronic acid). This substance is injected into the submucosa of the anal canal just proximal to the dentate line. In a study by Danielson [27], 34 patients were injected with Solesta® and observed for a 50% reduction in fecal incontinence episodes post injection. Patients were followed out to 12 months. Pre-treatment, the median number of incontinent episodes was 22, and reduced to 9 at 6 months, and 10 at 12 months post injection. Forty-four percent of patients were responders at 6 months and 56% at 12 months. No long-term side effects were noted in this study. While encouraging, until 2011 a randomized trial had not been conducted. Graf conducted a randomized, double-blind, sham-controlled, multinational study and a non-comparative, multinational study in 2011. The primary endpoint was greater than 50% reduction in incontinent episodes at 6 months and greater than 25% reduction at 12 months. Subjects undergoing Solesta® injections achieved the primary endpoints at a statistically significantly higher rate than the sham group. The treatment group also experienced an improvement in quality of life scores in comparison to the sham group. Adverse events were typically mild in nature and limited to transient injection site bleeding or pain. Two abscesses were encountered with one being a prostatic abscess and the other a rectal abscess requiring operative drainage [28].

SECCA®: Radiofrequency Ablation

The SECCA® procedure involves the administration of temperature-controlled radiofrequency energy to the anal canal. The procedure is targeted to the muscle and collagen component of the anal sphincter to improve sphincter function and sensitivity of the anal canal, and it requires adequate muscle availability. It was first approved by the FDA in 2002 for use in the USA for fecal incontinence though it was piloted in Mexico in 1999. The proposed mechanism of action is thought to be locally induced fibrosis, which may in turn help with improved continence. The procedure is performed on an outpatient basis, typically with only a local anesthetic block. Patient positioning is prone jackknife, with a clear anoscopic handle with four nickel-titanium electrodes. These electrodes are deployed into the internal sphincter muscle through the mucosa of the anal canal. The ablation is secured via these electrodes. During the ablation, while the deeper tissue is ablated, chilled water is perfused through the anoscope to keep the anoderm cool. Several clinical studies, though small in terms of patient numbers, have shown positive results with the use of SECCA® with patients reporting improvements in quality of life scores. These improvements have been shown to be durable to at least 6 months with some suggestion of benefit out to 5 years [29, 30]. In one such study, the SECCA® procedure was performed in 24 patients of whom 16 were followed for 12 months. There was a noted improvement in the fecal incontinence quality of life scores in all areas except for depression. Most patients continued to have moderate fecal incontinence on reporting but still indicated quality of life improvements [31]. In another study, similar positive results were reported in 15 patients followed out to 12 months, with the mean Wexner incontinence score decreasing from 14.07 at baseline to 12.33 at 1 year ($P = 0.02$). The mean fecal incontinence quality of life score had only improved in the domain of depression [32].

Diverting Colostomy

While not a particularly desirable option for many patients, diverting colostomy is an effective treatment for fecal incontinence and should remain in the physician's armamentarium, though it is reasonable to consider this as a last resort when faced with other treatment failures. The sigmoid colon is most commonly used and is brought up to the abdominal wall via either an open or laparoscopic approach. Physicians often avoid discussing this option as it is perceived that the quality of life with fecal incontinence is better than with a stoma. Recent investigations on this subject have demonstrated the opposite [33, 34]. In a direct comparison of patients who were treated with or without a colostomy, those with a colostomy reported a higher level of social function, coping, less embarrassment, depression, and improved lifestyle scores in comparison to those with ongoing fecal incontinence. Patients who had received a stoma reported over 80% satisfaction with the stoma and little to no restriction on their quality of life. It is important that the decision to proceed with a diverting stoma not be rushed, allowing the patient to come to terms with the upcoming changes. Involvement of enterostomal nurses is key in the preoperative discussion and planning and the postoperative follow-up for these patients. Patients should be counseled preoperatively on the continued intermittent loss of small amounts of fluid or mucous from the anus, as the bowel distal to the colostomy will continue to generate mucous. In unprepared patients, this can be a source of angst.

Neuromodulation

Fecal incontinence refractory to dietary modification, biofeedback, and antidiarrheal medications often warrants more aggressive management. Other surgical procedures briefly outlined above have been shown to lack durability and are fraught with high complication rates. While overlapping sphincteroplasty addresses the underlying mechanical defect, it has not shown long-term durability. Artificial bowel sphincter and dynamic graciloplasty are complex procedures with high complication rates. Given the anecdotal reports in improvement in fecal incontinence in patients who underwent placement of a sacral nerve stimulator for the indication of urinary incontinence, investigation into the efficacy in stand-alone fecal incontinence was undertaken. The results were positive with an overall 80% success rate in patients with a neurologically intact sacral plexus and an anatomically intact anal sphincter and rectum. Unfortunately, until the early 2000s there were no randomized trials to substantiate the efficacy of sacral neuromodulation for fecal incontinence. In 2005, Le Roi et al. published the first double-blind multicenter European trial examining the effectiveness of sacral nerve stimulation in fecally incontinent patients. Thirty-four patients underwent sacral nerve stimulation for fecal incontinence. After implantation, 27 of 34 patients were randomized in a double-blind crossover design to stimulation ON or OFF for 1-month periods. While still blinded, the patients chose the period of stimulation that they had preferred. The mode of stimulation corresponding to the selected period was continued for 3 months. Results indicated a statistically significant improvement in the reduction of episodes of fecal incontinence when the patient's device was set to ON. The ability to postpone defecation, anal sphincter function, the score for symptom severity, and quality of life were improved. The authors concluded that given the improvements in the crossover period these results were not related to placebo effect [35]. Following the approval of sacral nerve stimulation for fecal incontinence in Europe, investigations into the morbidity and quality of life during long-term stimulation were undertaken. Hetzer et al. conducted a prospective trial aimed at this between 2001 and 2005. Forty-four patients were assessed with the main outcome measures being morbidity, improvements in the stool diary, Wexner Score for fecal incontinence, Hanley Score for urinary incontinence, and quality of life questionnaires. A permanent stimulator was implanted in 37 patients (84%). Eight patients (22%) experienced complications with reimplantation successful in five of those patients. Wexner Scores decreased from a median of 16 points preoperatively (range, 6–20), to a median of five points postoperatively (range, 0–13; $P < 0.001$). The median number of involuntary stool losses and urge defecations also decreased significantly. Significant improvement in quality of life was found in both generic and incontinence-specific questionnaires ($P < 0.05$). The success rate of the sacral nerve stimulator (SNS) in this study overall was 77 and 92% in patients with permanent implantation. Patients who underwent a placement of a SNS reported significant improvement in quality of life from both a physical and psychological standpoint with low overall morbidity [35]. Despite these encouraging results, the SNS (*InterStim®* device) remained unapproved by the FDA for fecal incontinence until 2011, following publication of a landmark study performed by Mellgren et al. investigating the safety and efficacy of sacral nerve stimulation using an FDA-approved protocol in a multicenter prospective nonrandomized trial. The patient cohort included 129 patients from 16 centers in North America and Australia between 2002 and 2008. A temporary electrode was placed in the S2, S3, or S4 foramen. Patients experiencing a reduction of ≥50% in the number of incontinent episodes or days per week in the 2-week test period underwent implantation of a permanent neurostimulation device. Patients completed a bowel diary at baseline, during the test period at 3, 6, 12 months, and annually. Of the 129 who underwent the 2-week test stimulation, 120 demonstrated therapeutic success and underwent permanent implantation. Therapeutic success was seen in 83% at 12 months, 85% at 2 years, and 87% at 3 years. Perfect continence was achieved in 40% of the patients. Weekly frequency of incontinent episodes decreased from 9.4 at baseline to 1.9 at 12 months, 2.7 at 2 years, and 1.4 at 3 years. Logistic regression analysis demonstrated that internal anal sphincter defects decreased the success rate (65% vs. 87%, p 0.025). Patients had improvement in all four quality of life domains. Adverse effects occurred in 26 patients, and were primarily listed as implant site pain or infection which led to device explant in 4% of patients [36].

More recently sacral nerve stimulation has emerged as the surgical procedure of choice for patients experiencing fecal incontinence. This is the case even in patients with a sphincter defect. A retrospective study comparing a 26-patient cohort matched for age, gender, body mass index, and duration of follow-up with the main outcome measure of the change in the Cleveland Clinic Florida Fecal Incontinence Score (CCF-FIS). The analysis demonstrated a statistically significant reduction in this score among the 13 patients who received the SNS, but not amongst the 13 who underwent a sphincteroplasty. There were no differences observed in parity, the rate of concurrent urinary incontinence of early postoperative complications. The differences observed in CCF-FIS were not observed in side by side comparisons of the groups [37].

Method of Neurostimulator Implantation

Sacral neuromodulation is delivered via the InterStim® system manufactured by Medtronic. The device consists of a stimulating electrode attached to an implanted pulse generator. This system sends electrical pulses to an area near the sacral nerve root to modulate the neural activity between the brain, the pelvic floor, lower urinary tract, urinary and anal sphincters, and colon. The precise mechanism of action remains largely unknown and is under investigation. Once the decision to perform sacral nerve stimulator implantation has occurred, the procedure is typically performed in a two-stage process. Both stages are performed in the prone position under general anesthesia without paralysis or which short acting paralytics for intubation purposes. Some studies have described the procedure performed under local anesthetic with intravenous sedation. For the Stage I procedure, a 22-gauge insulated needle is inserted into the S3 foramen and the location confirmed with fluoroscopy and monitoring of functional response. The functional response evaluated may include plantar flexion of the great toe, bellowing of the buttocks, or tightening of the levator muscles. In those patients undergoing implantation under local sedation, sensations such as tightening or vibration in the rectum, vagina, and scrotum are often described. Once response is confirmed, a quadripolar stimulating electrode is attached to a modified connecting lead and tunneled subcutaneously where it is attached to an external neurostimulator [38]. The patient is then discharged with instructions to keep a bowel diary for a 2-week period of time. For those patients experiencing a 50% reduction in episodes of incontinence, the neurostimulator is deemed successful and the patient returns for stage II of the implantation. During this stage, a permanent implantable pulse generator is placed in a subcutaneous pocket in the upper buttock, attached to the lead, and secured in twist-lock fashion. This generator can be manipulated by adjusting the stimulation amplitude for improved symptom management.

Complications of Sacral Nerve Stimulation

Serious complications involving sacral nerve stimulation are infrequent. Several studies have reported on these with the most common related to lead migration (12%), pain (3%) though other studies report up to 34%, infection (10%), and re-operation (15%) [39, 40]. Re-operation generally is undertaken for decreased response, infection, lead migration, and less frequently for pain [39]. Infection can be severe resulting in immediate explantation, or mild requiring subcutaneous debridement and antibiotic management with interim salvage of the stimulator. In terms of pain, initially the site of generator placement was thought to play a role, but comparison of placement in the flank, sacral, and abdominal regions did not yield a difference. Pain has been reported to improve with physiotherapy. Lead migration can be managed with reprogramming and does not typically require insertion of a new lead. Electrical circuitry responses have been reported in up to 11% of patients. Poor response to stimulation is thought to be due to issues of impedance, thus patients with poor or a sudden decrease in response should undergo impedance testing. High impedance measurements are indicative of an open circuit caused by a fractured lead, loose wires, or loose connections. In these circumstances, patients will generally feel no stimulation. When the impedance measurements are low, patients typically experience stimulation distant to the desired site. This happens in instances where the wires are crushed and crossed or bodily fluids have leaked into the connectors. Ultimately if unable to troubleshoot and repair with reprogramming in these situations, contralateral lead insertion or explantation with re-insertion may be required [41, 42]. Most of these electrical complications provide only minor forms of irritation or decrease in stimulation which requires only reassurance to the patients while the troubleshooting is ongoing.

Conclusions

Fecal incontinence remains a significant medical concern which can be socially and emotionally devastating for those carrying the diagnosis. The algorithm for surgical management of fecal incontinence has changed significantly in the past several years due to the addition of sacral neuromodulation. Patients presenting with fecal incontinence should initially be treated medically achieving a significant quality of life improvement in many through augmentation of stool consistency and improvement in pelvic floor tone. For those patients in whom medical management fails, though long-term data on efficacy and complication rates are absent for the specific indication of fecal incontinence, sacral neuromodulation is currently the most effective surgical option available with a low morbidity rate as compared to other surgical options. This remains the case even for those patients with anatomical sphincter defects. For patients in whom neuromodulation fails to improve quality of life, there remains a variety of surgical options with varying degrees of success, and the selection of a specific procedure will generally need to be tailored to the individual patient.

References

1. Whitehead WE, Borrud L, Goode PS, Meikle S, Mueller ER, Tuteja A, Weidner A, Weinstein M, Ye W, Pelvic Floor Disorders Network. Fecal incontinence in US adults: epidemiology and risk factors. Gastroenterology. 2009;137(2):512–7.
2. Brown HW, Rogers RG, Wise ME. Barriers to seeking care for accidental bowel leakage: a qualitative study. Int Urogynecol J. 2016;28:1–9.
3. Sharma A, Yuan L, Marshall RJ, Merrie AE, Bissett IP. Systematic review of the prevalence of faecal incontinence. Br J Surg. 2016;103(12):1589–97.
4. Rockwood TH, Church JM, Fleshman JW, Kane RL, Mavrantonis C, Thorson AG, Wexner SD, Bliss D, Lowry AC. Patient and surgeon ranking of the severity of symptoms associated with fecal incontinence. Dis Colon Rectum. 1999;42(12):1525–31.
5. Rockwood TH, Church JM, Fleshman JW, Kane RL, Mavrantonis C, Thorson AG, Wexner SD, Bliss D, Lowry AC. Fecal incontinence quality of life scale. Dis Colon Rectum. 2000;43(1):9–16.
6. Boreham MK, Richter HE, Kenton KS, Nager CW, Gregory WT, Aronson MP, Vogt VY, McIntire DD, Schaffer JI. Anal incontinence in women presenting for gynecologic care: prevalence, risk factors, and impact upon quality of life. Am J Obstet Gynecol. 2005;192(5):1637–42.
7. Rothbarth J, Bemelman WA, Meijerink WJ, Stiggelbout AM, Zwinderman AH, Buyze-Westerweel ME, Delemarre JB. What is the impact of fecal incontinence on quality of life? Dis Colon Rectum. 2001;44(1):67–71.
8. Rao SS. Diagnosis and management of fecal incontinence. Am J Gastroenterol. 2004;99(8):1585.
9. Ricciardi R, Mellgren AF, Madoff RD, Baxter NN, Karulf RE, Parker SC. The utility of pudendal nerve terminal motor latencies in idiopathic incontinence. Dis Colon Rectum. 2006;49(6):852–7.
10. Albuquerque A. Endoanal ultrasonography in fecal incontinence: current and future perspectives. World J Gastrointest Endosc. 2015;7(6):575.
11. Tjandra JJ, Dykes SL, Kumar RR, Ellis CN, Gregorcyk SG, Hyman NH, Buie WD. Standards Practice Task Force of the American Society of Colon and Rectal Surgeons. Practice parameters for the treatment of fecal incontinence. Dis Colon Rectum. 2007;50(10):1497–507.
12. Law PJ, Kamm MA, Bartram CI. A comparison between electromyography and anal endosonography in mapping external anal sphincter defects. Dis Colon Rectum. 1990;33(5):370–3.
13. Law PJ, Kamm MA, Bartram CI. Anal endosonography in the investigation of faecal incontinence. Br J Surg. 1991;78(3):312–4.

14. Maier A, Fuchsjäger M, Funovics M. Endoanal magnetic resonance tomography in fecal incontinence. Radiologe. 2000;40(5):465–8.
15. Wiersma TG, Mulder CJ, Reeders JW. Dynamic rectal examination: its significant clinical value. Endoscopy. 1997;29(06):462–71.
16. Heymen S, Jones KR, Ringel Y, Scarlett Y, Whitehead WE. Biofeedback treatment of fecal incontinence. Dis Colon Rectum. 2001;44(5):728–36.
17. Belyaev O, Müller C, Uhl W. Neosphincter surgery for fecal incontinence: a critical and unbiased review of the relevant literature. Surg Today. 2006;36(4):295–303.
18. Parks AG, McPartlin JF. Late repair of injuries of the anal sphincter. Proc R Soc Med. 1971;64(12):1187–9.
19. Gutierrez AB, Madoff RD, Lowry AC, Parker SC, Buie WD, Baxter NN. Long-term results of anterior sphincteroplasty. Dis Colon Rectum. 2004;47(5):727–32.
20. Sitzler PJ, Thomson JP. Overlap repair of damaged anal sphincter. Dis Colon Rectum. 1996;39(12):1356–60.
21. Engel AF, Kamm MA, Sultan AH, Bartram CI, Nicholls RJ. Anterior anal sphincter repair in patients with obstetric trauma. Br J Surg. 1994;81(8):1231–4.
22. Goetz LH, Lowry AC. Overlapping sphincteroplasty: is it the standard of care? Clin Colon Rectal Surg. 2005;18(01):22–31.
23. Vaizey CJ, Kamm MA. Injectable bulking agents for treating faecal incontinence. Br J Surg. 2005;92(5):521–7.
24. Shafik A. Polytetrafluoroethylene injection for the treatment of partial fecal incontinence. Int Surg. 1992;78(2):159–61.
25. Luo C, Samaranayake CB, Plank LD, Bissett IP. Systematic review on the efficacy and safety of injectable bulking agents for passive faecal incontinence. Color Dis. 2010;12(4):296–303.
26. Danielson J, Karlbom U, Sonesson AC, Wester T, Graf W. Submucosal injection of stabilized nonanimal hyaluronic acid with dextranomer: a new treatment option for fecal incontinence. Dis Colon Rectum. 2009;52(6):1101–6.
27. Graf W, Mellgren A, Matzel KE, Hull T, Johansson C, Bernstein M, NASHA Dx Study Group. Efficacy of dextranomer in stabilised hyaluronic acid for treatment of faecal incontinence: a randomised, sham-controlled trial. Lancet. 2011;377(9770):997–1003.
28. Frascio M, Mandolfino F, Imperatore M, Stabilini C, Fornaro R, Gianetta E, Wexner SD. The SECCA procedure for faecal incontinence: a review. Color Dis. 2014;16(3):167–72.
29. Parisien CJ, Corman ML. The Secca® procedure for the treatment of fecal incontinence: definitive therapy or short-term solution. Clin Colon Rectal Surg. 2005;18(01):42–5.
30. Ruiz D, Pinto RA, Hull TL, Efron JE, Wexner SD. Does the radiofrequency procedure for fecal incontinence improve quality of life and incontinence at 1-year follow-up? Dis Colon Rectum. 2010;53(7):1041–6.
31. Lefebure B, Tuech JJ, Bridoux V, Gallas S, Leroi AM, Denis P, Michot F. Temperature-controlled radio frequency energy delivery (Secca® procedure) for the treatment of fecal incontinence: results of a prospective study. Int J Color Dis. 2008;23(10):993–7.
32. Norton C, Burch J, Kamm MA. Patients' views of a colostomy for fecal incontinence. Dis Colon Rectum. 2005;48(5):1062–9.
33. Colquhoun P, Kaiser R, Efron J, Weiss EG, Nogueras JJ, Vernava AM, Wexner SD. Is the quality of life better in patients with colostomy than patients with fecal incontience? World J Surg. 2006;30(10):1925–8.
34. Leroi AM, Parc Y, Lehur PA, Mion F, Barth X, Rullier E, Bresler L, Portier G, Michot F. Efficacy of sacral nerve stimulation for fecal incontinence: results of a multicenter double-blind crossover study. Ann Surg. 2005;242(5):662–9.
35. Hetzer FH, Hahnloser D, Clavien PA, Demartines N. Quality of life and morbidity after permanent sacral nerve stimulation for fecal incontinence. Arch Surg. 2007;142(1):8–13.
36. Mellgren A, Wexner SD, Coller JA, Devroede G, Lerew DR, Madoff RD, Hull T, SNS Study Group. Long-term efficacy and safety of sacral nerve stimulation for fecal incontinence. Dis Colon Rectum. 2011;54(9):1065–75.
37. Rodrigues FG, Chadi SA, Cracco AJ, Sands DR, Zutshi M, Gurland B, Da Silva G, Wexner SD. Faecal incontinence in patients with a sphincter defect: comparison of sphincteroplasty and sacral nerve stimulation. Color Dis. 2017;19(5):456–61.
38. Brazzelli M, Murray A, Fraser C. Efficacy and safety of sacral nerve stimulation for urinary urge incontinence: a systematic review. J Urol. 2006;175(3):835–41.
39. Peeren F, Hoebeke P, Everaert K. Sacral nerve stimulation: Interstim® therapy. Expert Rev Med Devices. 2005;2(3):253–8.
40. Zbar AP. Sacral neuromodulation and peripheral nerve stimulation in patients with anal incontinence: an overview of techniques, complications and troubleshooting. Gastroenterol Rep. 2014;2(2):112–20.
41. Hijaz A, Vasavada S. Complications and troubleshooting of sacral neuromodulation therapy. Urol Clin N Am. 2005;32(1):65–9.
42. Hijaz A, Vasavada SP, Daneshgari F, Frinjari H, Goldman H, Rackley R. Complications and troubleshooting of two-stage sacral neuromodulation therapy: a single-institution experience. Urology. 2006;68(3):533–7.

Check for updates

Posterior Tibial Nerve Stimulation

10

Gillian Frances Wolff and Ryan M. Krlin

Introduction

Percutaneous Tibial Nerve Stimulation (PTNS) is a lower urinary tract neuromodulation technique involving the intermittent, weekly stimulation of the tibial nerve at the ankle. PTNS is a minimally invasive technique that requires no permanent lead or implanted stimulator. It is currently approved by the United States Food and Drug Administration (FDA) for the treatment of overactive bladder (OAB) and its associated frequency, urgency, and urgency urinary incontinence, but its uses in other clinical contexts are still under investigation.

History and Mechanism of Action

The history and development of electrical stimulation therapy has been covered in depth in previous chapters. In this section, we will do a brief review with a focus on posterior tibial nerve stimulation. In the 1870s, researchers began experimenting with electrical stimulation to target organs and began developing methods to direct stimulation to select peripheral and sacral nerves [1]. In the 1980s, while Tanagho and Schmidt were developing the concepts of sacral nerve stimulation [2], McGuire was laying the groundwork for the development of PTNS. He used traditional Chinese acupuncture techniques and found that electrical stimulation of the tibial nerve inhibited bladder overactivity [3]. PTNS was approved by the FDA for non-neurogenic bladder overactivity in the late 1990s and its application to other symptoms has been expanding.

The mechanism of action of PTNS is not fully understood, but it is postulated to act upon existing innervation pathways to the lower urinary tract. The posterior tibial nerve is a mixed sensory-motor nerve arising from the L4-S3 spinal roots and then proceeds down the leg (Fig. 10.1). The peripheral nerves involved in sensory and motor control of the bladder and pelvic floor similarly arise from L4-S3, and it is thought that PTNS modulates the lower urinary tract via these shared spinal tracts.

In the normal micturition reflex, bladder afferent fibers signal fullness to bladder efferent fibers through spinal interneurons. These spinal interneurons are influenced by either negative inhibition of voiding or positive initiation of voiding through supraspinal feedback (Fig. 10.2). One theory is that PTNS remodels reflex loops such as the detrusor inhibition reflex, by stimulating afferent nerve fibers of the posterior tibial nerve

G. F. Wolff
Division of Urology, Albany Medical Center, Albany, NY, USA
e-mail: wolffg@amc.edu

R. M. Krlin (✉)
Department of Urology, Lousiana State University Health Sciences Center, New Orleans, LA, USA
e-mail: rkrli1@lsuhsc.edu

J. P. Gilleran, S. A. Alpert (eds.), *Adult and Pediatric Neuromodulation*,
https://doi.org/10.1007/978-3-319-73266-4_10

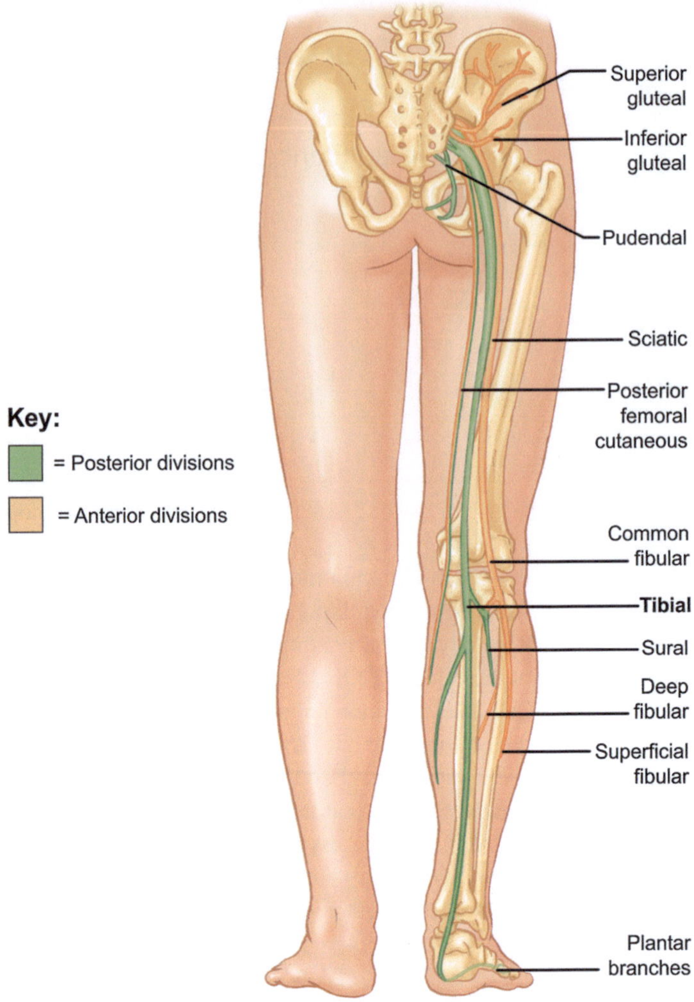

Fig. 10.1 The peripheral tibial nerve stimulation pathway to the sacral plexus.

that influence these reflex loops via the spinal cord [4]. It has also been proposed that neuromodulation may act centrally. Tai et al. [5] demonstrated in a cat model that stimulation of the posterior tibial nerve induces a persistent bladder inhibitory effect and increases bladder capacity. It was postulated that this effect resulted from direct modulation of the pontine micturition center (PMC) gating circuits of the suppression afferent input to the PMC.

Patient Evaluation

PTNS is most often utilized after behavioral and medical management has failed. As mentioned above, it is a noninvasive neuromodulation technique that can be performed in the outpatient setting and requires no local or general anesthesia. No permanent hardware is left in place such as leads or generators. Thus, PTNS may be an attractive option for patients who are either unable or unwilling to undergo a surgery, or who do not wish to have an implant such as those who may need magnetic resonance imaging (MRI) in the future. Absolute contraindications for PTNS include patients with pacemakers, implantable defibrillators, coagulopathies, or who are pregnant. However, PTNS can be performed safely even on most anticoagulants within therapeutic range.

The evaluation of patients for PTNS is no different from that of any patient unresponsive or refractory to first- and second-line therapies. Evaluations should begin with a directed history and physical exam. The history should reveal the nature and course of the patient's symptoms

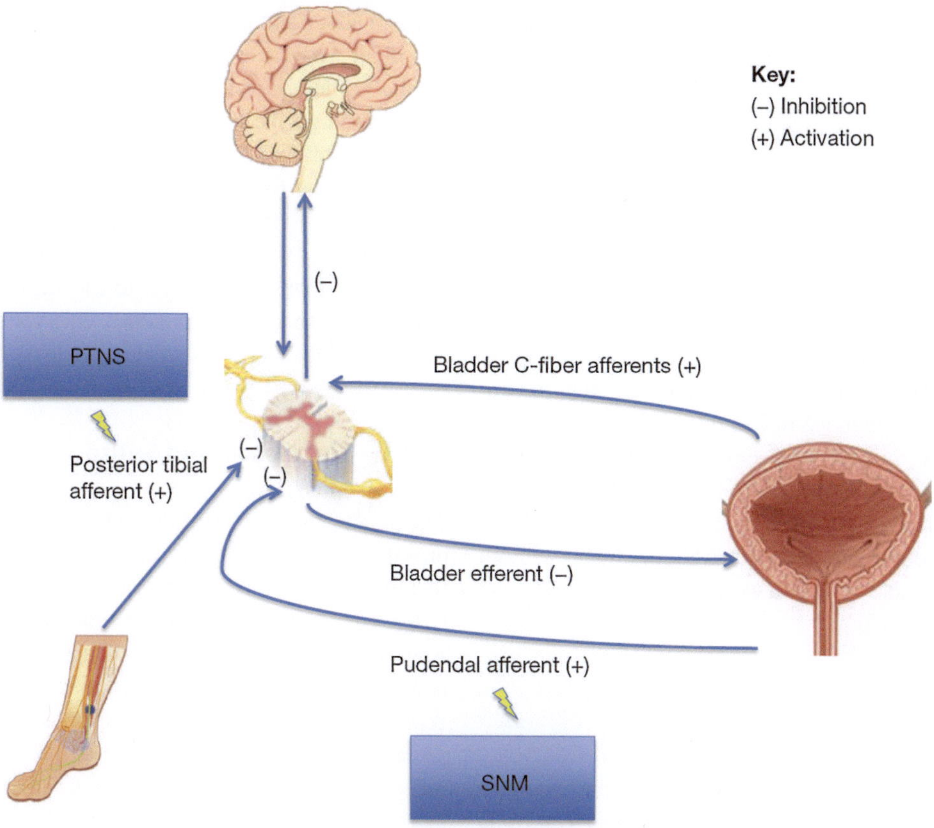

Fig. 10.2 In the normal micturition reflex, bladder C-fiber afferents signal bladder fullness. These signals affect bladder efferent fibers through spinal interneurons. These interneurons are themselves influenced by supraspinal feedback, both negative and positive. One theory of overactive bladder postulates that there is a derangement of supraspinal feedback regulation. PTNS is theorized to work by activating a peripheral afferent nerve, the posterior tibial nerve. This activation in turn inhibits signals from bladder afferents at the level of the spinal cord and disrupts aberrant micturition reflexes. From: Sanford MT, Suskind AM. Neuromodulation in neurogenic bladder. Transl Androl Urol 2016;5(1):117–126. Open Access

including chronicity, exacerbating factors, previous treatments, pelvic surgeries, comorbidities, and associated symptoms. Symptoms should be objectively measured and followed using bladder diaries and appropriate validated questionnaires. If present, incontinence should be evaluated including the presence of stress, urgency, or mixed incontinence. The number and type of pads should also be recorded.

A physical exam should note the patient's overall mobility and functional status and include a pelvic exam to evaluate for pelvic organ prolapse, urethral, uterine or vaginal pathology. The patient's neurological status may be assessed with a focused neurological exam, noting sensory and motor function of the S2-S4 distribution, and may include a cognitive assessment with a mini-mental status exam. Bladder emptying should also be evaluated with a post-void residual volume measured by either a bladder scanner or a catheterization.

As storage symptoms of urgency, frequency, and urgency incontinence may have other etiologies, persistent symptoms should be further evaluated. A urinalysis and urine culture should be performed to evaluate for hematuria and infection. One must also not ignore irritative storage symptoms in patients with risk factors such as tobacco use, environmental exposures, or family or personal history of urothelial carcinoma, as these should prompt a workup. This includes cystoscopy, upper tract studies such as a CT urogram, and urine cytology at the discretion of the clinician. Cystourethroscopy can also be performed to evaluate for foreign bodies, stigmata of interstitial cystitis, or any anatomic pathology.

Although not uniformly required, we often perform urodynamic studies (UDS) in patients who have failed behavioral and medical management. This includes uninstrumented uroflow, cystometrogram, and pressure-flow study with accompanying electromyogram (EMG) evaluation. UDS measure bladder capacity, compliance, sensation, and the presence of detrusor overactivity (DO) or incontinence. We utilize UDS to confirm our diagnosis and to rule out other etiologies of lower urinary tract symptoms such as dysfunctional voiding. Not all patients with overactive bladder have DO on urodynamic studies, however, one case series noted that patients without or with late onset DO were more likely to respond to PTNS [6].

Technique

To better understand PTNS needle placement, a brief review of the anatomy of the posterior tibial nerve will be reviewed (Fig. 10.3). The posterior tibial nerve is a mixed sensory-motor nerve that arises from L4-S3 nerve roots, and originates from the same spinal segments as the innervations to the bladder and pelvic floor [3, 7]. The posterior tibial nerve is a branch of the sciatic nerve, arising at the apex of the popliteal fossa. It then travels through the popliteal fossa and down the leg giving off motor branches to the leg. As it approaches the foot, the nerve passes posteriorly and inferiorly to the medial malleolus through the tarsal tunnel, where it gives rise to branches supplying cutaneous innervation to the heel it then terminates into sensory branches innervating the sole of the foot.

Needle Placement and Setup

The patient can be placed into a frog leg position or with the therapy leg elevated. It is imperative that they maintain a comfortable position, as they will need to stay there for the 30-min therapy session. The nerve is stimulated using a 34 gauge needle electrode. The needle is placed 4–5 cm cephalad to the medial malleolus and about 2 cm posterior to the tibia. The needle is inserted at a 60° angle to the skin and advanced 3–4 cm into the tissue (Figs. 10.4 and 10.5). A stick-on grounding pad is placed on the medial surface of the foot or leg or onto the sole of the foot. The stimulator is then attached to the needle and to the grounding pad.

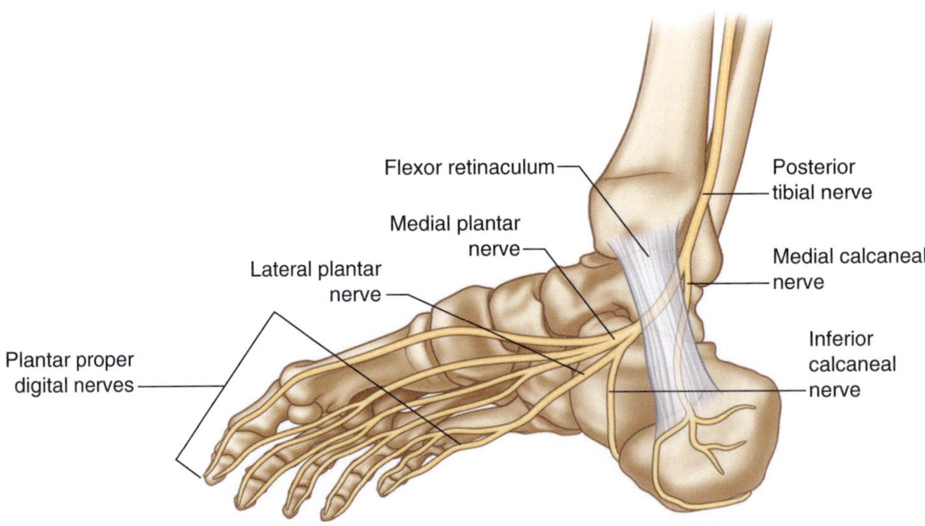

Fig. 10.3 The posterior tibial nerve passes into the foot running posterior to the medial malleolus. The nerve courses through the tibial tunnel prior to giving off its terminal branches, the medial and lateral plantar nerves. (Image courtesy of Springer)

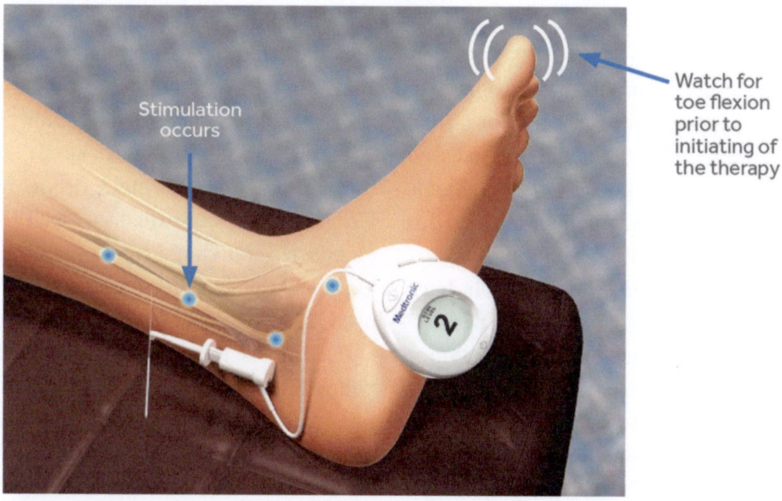

Fig. 10.4 Percutaneous access to the posterior tibial nerve is achieved by inserting the needle 4–5 cm cephalad to the medial malleolus and about 2 cm posterior to the tibia. In some patients, the correct placement spot can be palpated as a slightly hollow space between the flexor digitorum longus tendon and the flexor halluces longus tendon, where the nerve runs. Reprinted with the permission of Medtronic, Inc. ©

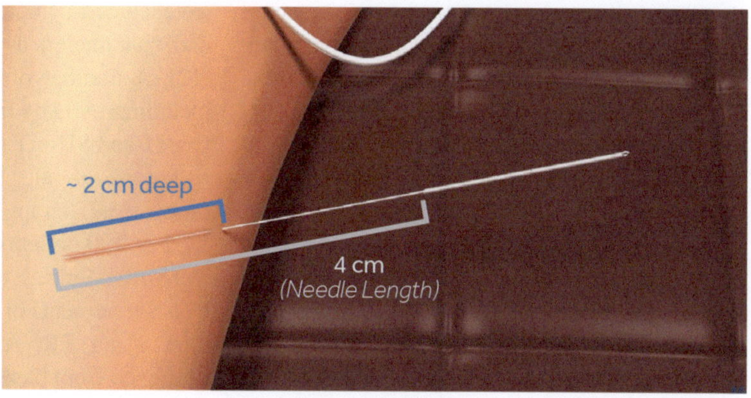

Fig. 10.5 The needle is inserted at a 60° angle to the skin and advanced 2–4 cm into the tissue (depending on tissue edema, etc.) Reprinted with the permission of Medtronic, Inc. ©

Current is then applied and slowly increased. The presence of motor responses, including flexion of the big toe, toe fanning, or extension of the entire foot, determines correct needle placement. Patients will describe sensory responses that accompany these reflexes as a tingling sensation that travels away from the insertion site to the arch, toes (ideally the first toe), or (rarely) up the leg. The electric current applied is a continuous, square waveform with a duration of 200 μs and a frequency of 20 Hz. Stimulation intensity is titrated based upon patient tolerance.

Troubleshooting

Lower extremity edema can prove a challenge to needle placement as the nerve is situated deeper than usual. In these circumstances, some alterations in technique may prove useful. In order to access deeper tissue, the needle may be placed at closer to a 90° angle than a 60° angle. Additionally, longer acupuncture needles can be helpful. Furthermore, the edema can be reduced prior to placing the needle by applying manual pressure to the limb.

Treatment Protocols

In most clinical trials, patients are assigned to undergo 30-min sessions once a week for a total of 12 weeks. Treatment effectiveness is assessed after the initial 12-week sessions. Patients responding to treatment are then monitored for the reappearance or worsening of symptoms.

Alternative PTNS scheduling protocols have also been evaluated. Finazzi Agro et al. [8] studied 35 patients undergoing 12 PTNS sessions either weekly or three-times per week. They found no significant difference in "success" (reduction >50% micturitions/24 h) between the two groups; 11/17 (63%) vs. 12/18 (67%) in the weekly vs. tri-weekly group, respectively. In both groups, subjective reports of initial improvement were reported after 6–8 sessions. From these data, the authors postulated that it is not the periodicity of stimulation, but rather the total number of sessions that impact success. They suggested that more frequent stimulation sessions could lead to earlier clinical improvement. Although there is no data regarding the durability of these treatments, patients wishing for sustained success would likely need to undergo maintenance therapy and require long-term periodic treatment regardless.

Yoong et al. [9] reported on an observational study of a shortened 6-week protocol with once a week PTNS sessions. Of the 43 women with OAB studied, there was a positive response rate of 69.7%, with reductions in daytime and nocturnal frequency, reductions in urge incontinence episodes, and improvements in reported quality of life (QOL.) Following the 6-week session, the median time to return of symptoms in the responders was 3 weeks.

Clinical Results

Idiopathic OAB

The International Urogynecological Association (IUGA) and International Continence Society (ICS) define OAB as a symptom complex of urinary urgency that may be associated with frequency and/or nocturia, with or without urinary urge incontinence (UUI), in the absence of urinary tract infection or other obvious pathology [10, 11]. OAB may cause significant bother, leading to a negative impact on a person's quality of life (QoL). American Urological Association (AUA)/Society for Urodynamics, Female Pelvic Medicine and Urogenital Reconstruction (SUFU) guidelines emphasize individual treatment plans to optimize QoL, and much of the research on PTNS and OAB use QoL measures as primary outcomes.

Diagnosis and treatment algorithms identify behavioral therapies, possibly combined with pharmacologic management, as first-line therapies for adult non-neurogenic OAB (Fig. 10.6). Medications likewise serve as the second-line therapy options. PTNS may be offered as third-line treatment in carefully selected patients with moderate to severe symptoms.

The evidence for PTNS in individuals with OAB includes randomized controlled trials (RCTs) and systematic reviews. Outcomes studied included symptoms, QoL measures, voiding diary parameters as well as urodynamic findings [12]. A number of RCTs have been published, including two key industry-sponsored RCTs, the OrBIT and SUmiT trials.

Peters et al. [13] conducted the OAB Innovative Therapy trial (OrBIT), a multicenter RCT of 100 patients with urinary frequency who were randomized to receive either 12 weekly PTNS treatments or to receive once daily tolterodine 4 mg ER. After 12 weeks both groups improved from baseline with 79.5% of the PTNS arm reporting cure or improvement compared to 54.8% in the tolterodine arm ($p < 0.01$). Between the two arms no statistically significant difference was found in objective measures such as frequency, UUI episodes, and improvements in voided volume, with both groups similarly improving from baseline. No serious adverse events or device malfunctions were reported although there was a higher frequency of constipation and dry mouth in the medication arm.

The validity of PTNS treatment response was further supported by the SUmiT Trial (Sham Effectiveness in Treatment of Overactive Bladder Symptoms) [14]. In this study, 220 adults with OAB were randomized to either 12 weekly PTNS treatments or to sham PTNS treatments.

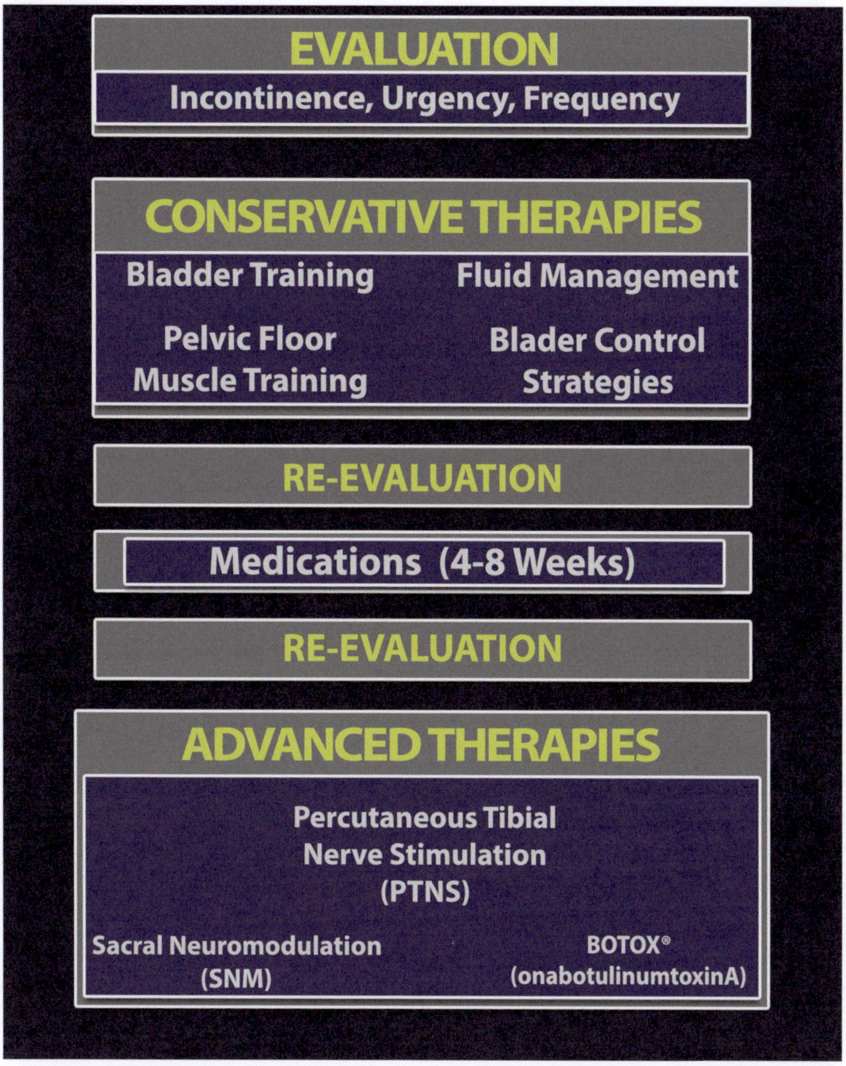

Fig. 10.6 The diagnosis and treatment algorithm: AUA/SUFU Guideline on non-neurogenic overactive bladder in adults. PTNS is considered as one possible third-line treatment for OAB in carefully selected and thoroughly counseled patients. From: American Urological Association. Diagnosis and Treatment of Non-Neurogenic Overactive Bladder (OAB) in Adults: AUA/SUFU Guideline. Published 2012; Amended 2014. Reprinted with permission. Available at: http://www.auanet.org/guidelines/overactive-bladder-(oab)-(aua/sufu-guideline-2012-amended-2014)

In order to blind the subjects, a sham Streitberger placebo needle was used in the control arm. The tip of the Streitberger needle, when applied to the skin, caused a slight prick but then retracted into the handle and never punctured the skin. A transcutaneous electrical nerve stimulation (TENS) unit was then applied to the foot in order to simulate the local sensation of stimulation; however, no PTNS ever occurred because no needle was placed percutaneously close to the nerve. The results of this study showed in the PTNS arm a statistically significant improvement in bladder symptoms from baseline (54.5%) compared to the sham arm (20.9%) ($p < 0.001$). Improvements were seen also in voiding diary parameters such as frequency, nighttime voids, urgency, and urge urinary incontinence episodes. Adverse reactions were uncommon and included discomfort or bleeding at the needle site and tingling of the leg.

Maintenance PTNS

Most studies report a decay in the effect of PTNS after the initial 12 weekly sessions. Van der Pal et al. [15] found that in 11 patients with medically refractory OAB who had previously responded to PTNS, 64% had worsening of symptoms 6 weeks after discontinuation of therapy. Repeated maintenance treatments, perhaps over a lifetime, are required for sustained PTNS efficacy, although the ideal maintenance schedule is not known.

The STEP (Sustained Therapeutic Effects of Percutaneous Tibial Nerve Stimulation) study was designed to assess the durability of PTNS effectiveness and to guide interval maintenance treatments [16]. This study was a 3-year extension of the 12-week SUmiT trial. As described above, the SUmiT trial provided level 1 evidence showing PTNS was superior to sham treatment for OAB. The STEP trial enrolled 50 patients who met the primary end point of moderately or markedly improved bladder symptoms after the initial 12 weekly treatments. These participants continued PTNS therapy under a fixed 14-week tapering process. The tapering protocol was designed to allow patients to recognize the return of their symptoms and to schedule appropriate intervals for further therapy. Following the tapering protocol each patient was individually assessed and personalized treatment plans were devised.

Of these 50 patients, about 75% had sustained symptom improvement though 3 years. Interval stimulations occurred at an average of 1 treatment per month. This sustained symptom improvement was documented subjectively and objectively through questionnaires and voiding diary parameters.

Similarly, a continuation of the OrBIT trial followed 33 PTNS responders for continued treatment for 1 year. Patients had a mean of 21 days between treatments and showed sustained improvement from 12 weeks to 6 and 12 months [17].

In summary, PTNS is FDA approved for idiopathic OAB and is recommended as a third-line therapy in the OAB pathway [11]. A number of RCTs have been published, including two key industry-sponsored RCTs, the OrBIT and SUmiT trials. Systematic reviews of the published trials have found short-term improvements with PTNS and have not identified long-term comparative studies. The largest, highest quality study was the double-blinded, sham-controlled SUmiT trial. It reported a statistically significant benefit of PTNS to sham at 12 weeks. The non-blinded OrBIT trial found that PTNS was non-inferior to medication treatment at 12 weeks. Unfortunately, longer term comparative data are not available after the initial 12-week treatment period. Up to 36 months of uncontrolled data are available, but only for patients who were enrolled in RCTs and responded to an initial course of treatment. However, these patients may not be representative of the patient population as a whole. Overall it appears that sustained efficacy from PTNS will require interval maintenance treatments. Further studies are underway evaluating home-based solutions.

Nonobstructive Urinary Retention

Unlike sacral nerve stimulation, PTNS is not FDA approved for nonobstructive urinary retention, and there is a paucity of robust data supporting its use in this clinical situation. A small number of published case series involving 12–39 patients show promising results for a number of outcomes including a reduction of total catheterized volume per 24 h and improvement in urodynamic voiding phase measures, including maximal flow and post-void residual urine [6].

Neurogenic Bladder

The neurogenic population was initially excluded from FDA approval of PTNS in the late 1990s as it was thought an intact nervous system was required for the procedure to be effective. More recently, however, there have been several small heterogeneous trials testing the use of PTNS in this population.

Multiple Sclerosis

Multiple sclerosis (MS) is a chronic demyelinating disease of the central and peripheral nervous system that can lead to a variety of symptomatic voiding dysfunctions including neurogenic detrusor overactivity, detrusor-sphincter dyssynergia, areflexia, or any combinations of these. Anticholinergic and antispasmodic medications, behavioral therapy, and clean intermittent catheterization (CIC) are all first-line therapies for MS-related voiding dysfunction. The cognitive symptoms of some MS patients may limit the use of anticholinergic medications, and limited hand dexterity may impede CIC. Intradetrusor injections of onabotulinumtoxinA and sacral neuromodulation (SNM) are both third-line therapies for management; SNM has been shown to have a high success rate in MS populations as well [18]. In patients unable to perform CIC and in those followed with MRI, PTNS may be an appropriate third-line option.

There are currently no randomized controlled trials evaluating the use of PTNS in MS patients. Unfortunately, the data available are limited by small sample sizes, heterogeneous patient populations, and lack of standardized treatment protocols.

Gobbi et al. [19] reported on a small study looking at 18 MS patients with LUTS treated with PTNS. At 3-month follow-up, 89% were subjectively pleased with the results as assessed by patient perception of bladder condition (PPBC) and a visual analog scale. Interestingly, no statistically significant decreases in urinary incontinence were observed. De Seze et al. [20] performed a multicenter prospective study of 70 ambulatory MS patients for a 3-month period. All patients were free of MS relapse for at least 3 months but had bothersome storage symptoms. Patients underwent daily 20-min PTNS sessions. The results were impressive with 82.6% of subjects reporting improved urgency, 51.3% urgency resolution, 66.7% improved frequency, 62% improved continence, and 44.9% resolution of incontinence.

Parkinson's Disease, Stroke, and Spinal Cord Injury

There is limited published data on the efficacy of PTNS in other neurogenic populations such as Parkinson's disease, stroke, and spinal cord injury. Two case series of 6 and 29 Parkinson's patients found improvements in subjective measures based on standardized patient questionnaires in 83–89% subjects [21, 22]. One randomized clinical trial is available examining the use of PTNS in patients with neurogenic OAB due to ischemic stroke. Twenty-four men were randomized to receive either PTNS twice weekly for 6 weeks or "general advice and stretching sessions" for 6 weeks. While not statistically better than controls, the PTNS arm did show a decrease in urgency, urgency urinary incontinence, nocturia, and nocturnal enuresis [23]. Chen et al. [24] randomized 100 patients with spinal cord injuries to either PTNS or solifenacin. At 2 weeks, both arms showed improvement in volumes per catheterization, leakage per day, and quality of life from baseline. The treatment results were similar in both arms with no significant differences observed between PTNS and solifenacin. The PTNS arm did appear to be more tolerable with fewer side effects. Five percent of patients in the solifenacin arm reported bothersome side effects, and as is often seen in practice, two patients discontinued the trial due to the intolerability of the medication.

Fecal Incontinence

The use of neuromodulation, specifically sacral nerve modulation, for the treatment of fecal incontinence (FI) is well established. SNM is considered first-line surgical treatment for FI after conservative management strategies such as diet, bowel training, and medications have failed. Because of shared sacral segmental innervation, PTNS has been proposed in the treatment algorithm for FI. The data supporting the use of PTNS for treatment of FI is less robust than that of SNM [25]. The Clinical Practice Guidelines Committee of the American Society of Colon and Rectal Surgeons notes a weak recommendation based upon low or very low quality evidence for the use of PTNS in FI, stating there are only limited case series showing improvements from baseline in several clinical parameters such as bowel diaries, symptom scores, and QOL improvements [26]. Despite these promising results, these findings did not bear out in a large multicenter clinical trial comparing PTNS to sham. The CONFIDeNT trial randomized 227 patients with FI who had failed medical management. Patients were included if their FI was sufficiently severe to warrant intervention as recommended by the principle investigator at each site. Patients underwent weekly sessions of either PTNS or sham electrical stimulation for 12 weeks. At the conclusion of the trial, PTNS did not show significant improvement over sham in the primary outcome of 50% or greater reduction in weekly FI episodes (38% of the PTNS vs. 31% of the sham). Similarly, no significant improvements were observed for summative symptom scores, disease-specific, or generic quality of life measures. The study group had heterogeneous cases of FI, including both passive and urge FI, and some efficacy was shown specifically in the reduction of urge FI [27]. At this time, PTNS is still considered investigational and is not approved by the FDA for FI.

Chronic Pelvic Pain

Neuromodulation has been used as treatment for many chronic pain conditions such as migraine headache, facial pain, back pain, and neuropathic pain [28]. The evidence supporting the use of PTNS for chronic pelvic pain (CPP) is limited. Several small, heterogeneous case series have examined the use of PTNS for CPP with mixed results. Zhao et al. examined 14 patients with interstitial cystitis (IC) undergoing 10 weekly sessions. After 0, 4, and 10 weeks, they found no difference in voiding frequency or volume, pain scores, IC-specific questionnaires, or general QOL scores [29]. Ragab et al. evaluated 12 weekly PTNS sessions in 20 women with IC and again found no significant improvement in pain scores, IC or general QOL questionnaires. Seventeen patients (85%) reported PTNS had no effect, one patient (5%) reported worsening pain, and two patients (10%) reported only having a "mildly good response" [30]. Kabay et al. [31] reported a trial on 89 men with medically refractory CPP who were randomized to either 12 weekly PTNS treatments or sham treatments. They found that compared to sham the PTNS group had improvements in pain scores with a good response in 18 (40%), and a partial response in 27 (60%). Further follow-up after these 12 weeks was not reported. While promising, further larger trials are needed.

Conclusion

Posterior tibial nerve stimulation remains a valid and FDA approved third-line option for overactive bladder. Multiple randomized controlled trials support short-term efficacy for treatment of OAB. PTNS may be an attractive option for patients either unwilling or unable to undergo more invasive therapies or who are unable to tolerate standard medical therapy. Multiple therapy sessions, as well as continued maintenance therapy, may pose a hurdle for some patients. The efficacy of PTNS for other conditions such as neurogenic bladder, nonobstructive urinary retention, and pain is still under investigation.

References

1. Sanford MT, Suskind AM. Neuromodulation in neurogenic bladder. Transl Androl Urol. 2016;5(1):117–26.
2. Gaziev G, Topazio L, Iacovelli V, Asimakopoulos A, Di Santo A, De Nunzio C, et al. Percutaneous Tibial Nerve Stimulation (PTNS) efficacy in the treatment of lower urinary tract dysfunctions: a systematic review. BMC Urol. 2013;13:61. https://doi.org/10.1186/1471-2490-13-61.
3. McGuire EJ, Zhang SC, Horwinski ER, Lytton B. Treatment of motor and sensory detrusor instability by electrical stimulation. J Urol. 1983;129(1):78–9.
4. Vodusek D, Light J, Libby J. Detrusor inhibition induced by stimulation of pudendal nerve afferents. Neurourol Urodyn. 1986;5:381–9.
5. Tai C, Shen B, Chen M, Wang J, Roppolo JR, de Groat WC. Prolonged poststimulation inhibition of bladder activity induced by tibial nerve stimulation in cats. Am J Physiol Renal Physiol. 2011;300(2):F385–92.
6. Vandoninck V, van Balken MR, Finazzi Agro E, Petta F, Micali F, Heesakkers JP, et al. Percutaneous tibial nerve stimulation in the treatment of overactive bladder: urodynamic data. Neurourol Urodyn. 2003;22(3):227–32.
7. Nguyen LN, Chowdhury ML, Gilleran JP. Outcomes for intermittent neuromodulation as a treatment for overactive bladder. Curr Bladder Dysfunct Rep. 2017;12(1):66–73.
8. Finazzi Agro E, Campagna A, Sciobica F, Petta F, Germani S, Zuccala A, et al. Posterior tibial nerve stimulation: is the once-a-week protocol the best option? Minerva Urol Nefrol. 2005;57(2):119–23.

9. Yoong W, Ridout AE, Damodaram M, Dadswell R. Neuromodulative treatment with percutaneous tibial nerve stimulation for intractable detrusor instability: outcomes following a shortened 6-week protocol. BJU Int. 2010;106(11):1673–6.
10. Haylen BT, de Ridder D, Freeman RM, Swift SE, Berghmans B, Lee J, et al. An International Urogynecological Association (IUGA)/International Continence Society (ICS) joint report on the terminology for female pelvic floor dysfunction. Neurourol Urodyn. 2010;29(1):4–20.
11. Gormley EA, Lightner DJ, Faraday M, Vasavada SP. American Urological Association, Society of Urodynamics, Female Pelvic Medicine. Diagnosis and treatment of overactive bladder (non-neurogenic) in adults: AUA/SUFU guideline amendment. J Urol. 2015;193(5):1572–80.
12. Klingler HC, Pycha A, Schmidbauer J, Marberger M. Use of peripheral neuromodulation of the S3 region for treatment of detrusor overactivity: a urodynamic-based study. Urology. 2000;56(5):766–71.
13. Peters KM, Macdiarmid SA, Wooldridge LS, Leong FC, Shobeiri SA, Rovner ES, et al. Randomized trial of percutaneous tibial nerve stimulation versus extended-release tolterodine: results from the overactive bladder innovative therapy trial. J Urol. 2009;182(3):1055–61.
14. Peters KM, Carrico DJ, Perez-Marrero RA, Khan AU, Wooldridge LS, Davis GL, et al. Randomized trial of percutaneous tibial nerve stimulation versus Sham efficacy in the treatment of overactive bladder syndrome: results from the SUmiT trial. J Urol. 2010;183(4):1438–43.
15. van der Pal F, van Balken MR, Heesakkers JP, Debruyne FM, Bemelmans BL. Percutaneous tibial nerve stimulation in the treatment of refractory overactive bladder syndrome: is maintenance treatment necessary? BJU Int. 2006;97(3):547–50.
16. Peters KM, Carrico DJ, Wooldridge LS, Miller CJ, MacDiarmid SA. Percutaneous tibial nerve stimulation for the long-term treatment of overactive bladder: 3-year results of the STEP study. J Urol. 2013;189(6):2194–201.
17. MacDiarmid SA, Peters KM, Shobeiri SA, Wooldridge LS, Rovner ES, Leong FC, et al. Long-term durability of percutaneous tibial nerve stimulation for the treatment of overactive bladder. J Urol. 2010;183(1):234–40.
18. Kessler TM, La Framboise D, Trelle S, Fowler CJ, Kiss G, Pannek J, et al. Sacral neuromodulation for neurogenic lower urinary tract dysfunction: systematic review and meta-analysis. Eur Urol. 2010;58(6):865–74.
19. Gobbi C, Digesu GA, Khullar V, El Neil S, Caccia G, Zecca C. Percutaneous posterior tibial nerve stimulation as an effective treatment of refractory lower urinary tract symptoms in patients with multiple sclerosis: preliminary data from a multicentre, prospective, open label trial. Mult Scler. 2011;17(12):1514–9.
20. de Seze M, Raibaut P, Gallien P, Even-Schneider A, Denys P, Bonniaud V, et al. Transcutaneous posterior tibial nerve stimulation for treatment of the overactive bladder syndrome in multiple sclerosis: results of a multicenter prospective study. Neurourol Urodyn. 2011;30(3):306–11.
21. Ohannessian A, Kabore FA, Agostini A, Lenne Aurier K, Witjas T, Azulay JP, et al. Transcutaneous tibial nerve stimulation in the overactive bladder syndrome in patients with Parkinson's syndromes. Prog Urol. 2013;23(11):936–9.
22. Krivoborodov GG, Gekht AB, Korshunova ES. Tibial neuromodulation in the treatment of neurogenic detrusor hyperactivity in patients with Parkinson's disease. Urologiia. 2006;(4):3–6.
23. Monteiro ES, de Carvalho LB, Fukujima MM, Lora MI, do Prado GF. Electrical stimulation of the posterior tibialis nerve improves symptoms of poststroke neurogenic overactive bladder in men: a randomized controlled trial. Urology. 2014;84(3):509–14.
24. Chen G, Liao L, Li Y. The possible role of percutaneous tibial nerve stimulation using adhesive skin surface electrodes in patients with neurogenic detrusor overactivity secondary to spinal cord injury. Int Urol Nephrol. 2015;47(3):451–5.
25. Paquette IM, Varma MG, Kaiser AM, Steele SR, Rafferty JF. The American Society of Colon and Rectal Surgeons' clinical practice guideline for the treatment of fecal incontinence. Dis Colon Rectum. 2015;58(7):623–36.
26. Horrocks EJ, Thin N, Thaha MA, Taylor SJ, Norton C, Knowles CH. Systematic review of tibial nerve stimulation to treat faecal incontinence. Br J Surg. 2014;101(5):457–68.
27. Knowles CH, Horrocks EJ, Bremner SA, Stevens N, Norton C, O'Connell PR, et al. Percutaneous tibial nerve stimulation versus sham electrical stimulation for the treatment of faecal incontinence in adults (CONFIDeNT): a double-blind, multicentre, pragmatic, parallel-group, randomised controlled trial. Lancet. 2015;386(10004):1640–8.
28. Rushton DN. Electrical stimulation in the treatment of pain. Disabil Rehabil. 2002;24(8):407–15.
29. Zhao J, Nordling J. Posterior tibial nerve stimulation in patients with intractable interstitial cystitis. BJU Int. 2004;94(1):101–4.
30. Ragab MM, Tawfik AM, Abo El-enen M, Elnady M, El-Gamal OM, El-Kordy M, et al. Evaluation of percutaneous tibial nerve stimulation for treatment of refractory painful bladder syndrome. Urology. 2015;86(4):707–11.
31. Kabay S, Kabay SC, Yucel M, Ozden H. Efficiency of posterior tibial nerve stimulation in category IIIB chronic prostatitis/chronic pelvic pain: a Sham-Controlled Comparative Study. Urol Int. 2009;83(1):33–8.

Management of Complications and Revisions of Sacral Neuromodulation

11

Ragheed M. Saoud and Adonis Hijaz

Introduction

Lower urinary tract symptoms (LUTS) may present in several forms, including chronic urinary retention (UR), overactive bladder (OAB), urinary urgency/urgency incontinence (UUI), etc. Such symptoms may vary from mild to debilitating and hence may jeopardize the patient's quality of life. The treatment of chronic urinary symptoms is of prime importance and varies based on symptom severity.

The treatment of LUTS has evolved. Historically, conservative therapy was the mainstay, ranging from bladder retraining to pelvic floor musculature (Kegel's) exercises and biofeedback [1]. Such regimens may provide relief in patients with mild LUTS; however, patients complaining of severe symptoms require additional pharmacological therapy like antimuscarinics or β-3 agonists, which have proven to be beneficial for overactive bladder and urgency/frequency symptoms [2, 3]. Despite this, roughly 40% of patients treated with medication will still complain of refractory symptoms and will require more invasive treatment [1]. Surgical interventions including urinary diversion and bladder augmentation have been proposed as radical solutions for chronic refractory LUTS, but those are invasive and are not free of associated morbidity. In 1979, Schmidt and colleagues proposed the idea of using electrical current to stimulate the sacral plexus, in an attempt to control bladder function. Currently known as sacral neuromodulation (SNM), this minimally invasive procedure has been approved by the United States Food & Drug Administration for the treatment of refractory UR, UUI, and OAB [4]. This chapter will briefly describe the surgical technique and further focus on its complications and how to troubleshoot in case of adverse events.

Surgical Technique

Sacral neuromodulation comprises two major phases—the initial screening phase and the permanent evaluation phase. The screening phase has undergone changes in technique since its initial description in 1979. Two different screening methods exist, the percutaneous nerve evaluation (PNE) test and the staged test [5]. The PNE test starts by inserting a test needle into the third sacral foramen to stimulate the sacral nerve root. Motor and sensory responses are then detected upon

R. M. Saoud
Division of Urology, Department of Surgery, American University of Beirut Medical Center, Beirut, Lebanon
e-mail: rs144@aub.edu.lb

A. Hijaz (✉)
Center of Female Pelvic Medicine and Surgery, University Hospitals Cleveland Medical Center, Urology Institute, Cleveland, OH, USA
e-mail: adonis.hijaz@uhhospitals.org

J. P. Gilleran, S. A. Alpert (eds.), *Adult and Pediatric Neuromodulation*, https://doi.org/10.1007/978-3-319-73266-4_11

stimulation. A bellows reflex of the pelvic floor musculature or plantar flexion of the great toe and genital/rectal/perineal paresthesias are indicative of S3 nerve stimulation. Patients with a positive response will carry a temporary electrode for few days to monitor the effect of PNE on their chronic urinary symptoms. Patients who report more than 50% improvement will be considered responsive and will undergo second stage permanent generator and lead placement for SNS therapy.

An alternative approach for screening is the two-stage tined lead implantation devised by Spinelli and colleagues in 1999. It is less invasive as it can be performed in an outpatient setting under sedation. The tined lead is self-anchoring and does not require a large incision for eventual implantation of the permanent lead. While the patient is in a prone position, local anesthetic is applied posterior to the sacrum around the area where the definitive lead will be eventually implanted. A foramen needle is inserted to the S3 foramen, followed by a guidewire, which will allow insertion of an 8-F dilator to accommodate placement of the definitive lead [6]. The procedure is guided by fluoroscopy to ensure the lead is implanted in the correct anatomical position. Moreover, electrical stimulation is applied to induce a motor and/or sensory response and confirm correct positioning of the electrode. Patients are then followed up with voiding diaries to monitor symptomatic improvement. Those who report more than 50% improvement are considered successful and will undergo permanent generator (IPG) insertion. The key to successful SNS treatment is patient selection. False positives during the testing phase are common. In a prospective study of 85 patients with UUI who underwent PNE testing with a temporary electrode, 40% of those who benefited from the PNE test ultimately failed neurostimulator treatment on the long term [7]. The advantage of the tined lead in such a situation is that it allows for a longer testing phase and hence true positive responders who would eventually benefit from IPG placement can be more accurately selected.

In a prospective randomized study by Borawski et al. of 30 patients with UUI, 17 underwent traditional PNE placement while 13 underwent two-stage tined lead placement. Subjects assigned to the tined lead (88%) were significantly more likely to undergo IPG placement than the PNE group (46%). When compared based on symptomatic improvement, both groups were not significantly different, indicating that the two-stage tined lead technique can better predict true responders to SNS therapy [8, 9].

Complications

With the increasing popularity of sacral neuromodulation as a minimally invasive means to treat chronic LUTS, it is important to discuss the complications of this procedure, especially that it has undergone technical changes over the past two decades. The complications of SNS therapy vary and can be categorized into device-related (mechanical), response-related, and patient-related complications. Depending on the type of complication encountered, the treating physician will revise the implant, explant it, or simply treat the presenting symptom.

Device-Related Complications

Traditionally, a one-stage approach was devised for testing response and lead implantation. The reoperation rate after such procedures was estimated to be 40% with an explantation rate of 11%. Currently, a shift has been towards a two-stage technique for implantation of the quadripolar lead and testing it. In a study of 60 implants using the staged technique performed by a single surgeon, Peters and colleagues showed that 83% of patients who were tested for symptom improvement eventually proceeded towards implantation. In addition, the percentage of patients who underwent revision was 15% while only 1.7% required explantation due to IPG infection [10]. Different leads may result in variable outcomes especially when comparing the old fascial anchoring lead to the newer tined lead. In a retrospective review of 104 patients between 1994 and 2004, Sutherland et al. found that the rate of reoperation is three times higher (73% vs. 28%, $p < 0.01$) with a higher risk of complications when using the non-tined lead in comparison to the tined lead [11]. Moreover, the newer tined leads (e.g., Model 3893 and 3058) are at least 50% lighter and require a shorter incision for percutaneous placement, resulting in a decreased operative time [12]. They also connect directly to the lead, eliminating the need for an extension cable and can accommodate multiple lead sizes. Another comparative study by Al-Zahrani and colleagues showed that the revision rate decreased from 51 to 31% using the tined lead ($p = 0.1$) with an increased "median time to revision" (21 months vs. 15.7 months, $p = 0.4$) [4].

The most common reasons for revision after implantation are lead migration and pain. Such complaints vary depending on surgical technique and the type of lead utilized. In a prospective review of 12 centers worldwide, Siegel et al. followed up 581 patients who underwent temporary percutaneous SNS (stage 1). Only patients with a 50% reduction in target symptoms (UUI, U/F, UR) over at least 3 days progressed to surgical implantation of a permanent Medtronic InterStim® lead and neurostimulator (stage 2). Lead implantation was performed through an incision over the sacral area followed by insertion of a 4-electrode lead into the chosen foramen. Stimulation of the electrodes and a consequent motor response ensured proper lead placement. At 3 years follow-up, the most commonly encountered complication was lead migration (11.8%) during stage 1, while the risk of lead migration in patients who proceeded to stage 2 was lower (8.4%) [13]. Displacement of a lead depends on the anchoring system utilized to fix it. Multiple anchoring systems have been devised. In a study of 32 patients undergoing the percutaneous approach to SNS, 22 patients underwent final generator placement after the initial trial period. Among those, four lead displacements were encountered, two of which occurred when silicon anchoring was used and another two where the electrode was fixed without anchoring. The rest of the patients who were implanted using the twist-lock anchor did not experience lead displacement [14]. The introduction of the tined lead electrode allows for a longer testing period after its minimally invasive percutaneous placement using four sets of self-anchoring tines. It can be performed under local anesthesia through a miniature incision. Its major advantage however is the decreased rate of reoperation to adjust its location and decreased rate of lead migration. In a European study of 127 patients undergoing tined lead placement, 77% achieved more than 50% improvement in chronic voiding symptoms at 30 days follow-up, and hence all of them underwent pulse generator placement as second stage. In another review of 167 patients who underwent SNM using the tined lead at the Cleveland Clinic Foundation, 27.8% of those patients had to be explanted during stage 1, but none of them were due to lead migration [15]. Similarly, 12.2% (22/180 implants) of the patients underwent revision during stage 1 either due to marginal response (13/22) or other causes; however, none of the revisions resulted from lead migration which further attests to the advantage of the self-anchoring lead in that regard. Deng and colleagues also report on their 3-year experience using the InterStim® tined lead. Among 235 patients who underwent implantation, only 1 suffered lead displacement during stage 1, and 4 others during stage 2, totaling 2.1% (5/235) [16]. Such complications can be managed easily without significant morbidity to the patient.

Pain is a frequently encountered complaint as well; however, patients commonly present because of pain after placement of the permanent generator. Among 219 patients who underwent permanent InterStim® implantation, 15.3% complained of pain at the neurostimulator site or new onset pain (9%), which was significantly higher than the pain complaints during stage 1 of the procedure (2.1%) [13]. Of the 219 patients who underwent stage 2 implantation, 73 (33%) needed surgical revision, and the most common reason for revision was pain at the subcutaneous pocket. This highlights the significance of pain as a potential complication of SNS therapy and the need to create solutions to avoid it. Different patients have variable pain thresholds, so the complaint itself can be subjective. However, pain may also vary depending on the site of implantation of the neurostimulator. In a multicenter European study conducted in 1999, 39 patients underwent buttock implantation of the IPG instead of traditional abdominal implantation. On follow-up, the former complained of less pain (10% vs. 35% for abdominal placement), and thus a decreased need for stimulator repositioning post-op [17]. Similarly, Van Kerrebroeck and colleagues reported on 152 patients who underwent InterStim® neurostimulator placement, 121 of which were implanted in the abdomen and 31 in the buttock. The most common indication necessitating revision was pain at the site of implantation (11.8%), namely the abdomen, as none of the buttock-implanted patients complained of pain [18].

Patient-Related Complications

Despite the utilization of pre-procedural antibiotics, infections at the implantation site or the connecting wires still constitute a major cause of morbidity after SNM. Even though the rate of lead site infection is reported in the range of 5–8% in the literature [9], several studies of the staged approach have reported higher rates. Among 76 patients who underwent staged SNM implantation, a total of 9 patients (12%) developed lead infection during stage 1 and 11% (5/45 patients) during stage 2. Multiple risk factors have been postulated, including steroid use (one patient) and psoriasis (one patient), but a few were proven to significantly cause post-procedural infections [19]. In the aforementioned cohort, the only significant difference identified between infected and noninfected patients was a longer mean operative time for stage 2 procedures (IPG placement) in patients with infection (68.8 min vs. 52.4 min). The most commonly isolated organism was *Staphylococcus aureus* [19]. A group in Germany studied the effect of prolonged testing with the permanent electrode on infection-associated explantation rates in 21 patients undergoing SNM. Despite the presence of bacterial colonization of the extension leads in 43% of patients, this did not affect outcomes and did not increase the risk of explantation of the chronic implant (94% success rate after stage 2) [20]; hence prolonged testing is essential to improve outcomes and bacterial colonization should not be a limiting factor in that regard. Other groups have also investigated risk factors for periprocedural infections like gender, existing comorbidities, history of urinary tract infections, location the procedure is performed (i.e., outpatient center vs. university hospital), and preoperative antibiotics [21]. Among 136 patients undergoing SNM implantation, Haraway and colleagues showed that the only significant risk factor for infection was the choice of antibiotic given before the procedure. Cefazolin was found to be the culprit as the majority of infections were *S. aureus* resistant to cephalosporins and the patients treated with a different class of antibiotics were seven times less likely to acquire a post-procedural infection. Of the 35 patients given cefazolin preoperatively, a total of 6 were explanted (17.1%) due to infection, while only 2% of those given vancomycin or vancomycin and gentamicin were explanted (2/101) [21]. None of the other variables proved to be a statistically significant contributor to the risk of implantation failure. There is currently no consensus on the best antibiotic regimen for perioperative coverage as long as the skin flora including methicillin-resistant *S. aureus* are covered. In cases of infection despite antibiotic therapy, explantation of the whole system is the optimal solution [15].

Response-Related Complications

The most common response-related cause of revision is failure of the permanent implant to generate an adequate response. However, the success of the implantable generator may vary depending on the testing technique utilized. In a review of 75 patients undergoing either first stage PNE testing (35/70) followed by second stage lead or initial permanent tined lead placement (35/70), Jenks and colleagues found that 30% (5/15) of the PNE patients failed to produce a complete response when converted to a permanent implant and thus required revision [22]. Two of the failed PNE patients were only salvaged with a second lead implantation. The tined lead patients, on the other hand, achieved significantly higher success rates upon permanent implantation further demonstrating the advantage of the latter over the staged PNE evaluation. Response failure can be witnessed at both stages. In stage 1, it is defined by a response lower than 50% reported by the patients, which requires revision prior to proceeding to stage 2. In the Cleveland Clinic review of SNM therapy, the most common reason for revision and explantation during stage 1 of the tined lead evaluation was response related [23]. Stage 1 revisions totaled 22 of the 180 operations (12.2%). Revisions were done for marginal response (13/22), frayed subcutaneous extension wire (6/22), lead infection (3/22), and improper localization of stimulus (1/22) [23]. Upon revision after stage 1, 38.5% of those achieved a satisfactory response eventually and proceeded to final implantation. Stage 2 revisions, on the other hand, occur in patients who show an adequate response after stage 1, but upon implantation of the permanent generator, the response and symptomatic improvement are mediocre. This may be due to an infection, failure at the generator-lead interface, or an intrinsic malfunctioning IPG issue. Otherwise, the device and its connectivity may be successful but the response failure is due to patient-related etiologies like scarring at the lead/neural interface, disease progression, and neural plasticity. Stage II complications may be solved either via explantation (generator and lead) or revision of the device. In the Cleveland Clinic cohort, explantation was performed in 16 of 130 (12.3%) patients, either due to infection (56.3%) or failure to maintain response (43.7%). Revisions were done for infection, mechanical (generator related), and response causes [23].

Impedance Measurements and Troubleshooting in Sacral Neuromodulation

The elements of SNM function as part of an electric circuit composed of the neurostimulator, extension wires, the connectors from the extension wires to the lead wires, the lead and its electrodes, and the patient's tissue surfaces. With the advent of the newer generation IPG-2, the lead now directly connects to the generator without the need for a connector. However, it is essential to understand the intricate details of the functionality of the circuit to be able to identify its shortcomings and manage them. Electrical current is the flow of electrons in the circuit, while impedance is the resistance to this flow induced by the components of the circuit. Impedance measurements are important as they play a role in identifying the problem and troubleshooting it. A high impedance circuit (>4000 Ω), otherwise known as an open circuit, is not functional due to inadequate electron flow. Multiple etiologies exist (e.g., nonfunctional generator, displaced lead, inadequate connectivity, fractured wires, etc.) that may lead to high impedance. A short circuit, on the other hand, is one where the impedance is so low (<50 Ω) that electrical current flows in excess and thus shortens the battery life of the generator until it dies out. This may be due to fluid intrusion into the connectors or crushed wires that are touching each other [23]. Patients with open circuits usually do not feel any stimulation, while those with a short circuit may feel stimulation in an area different from the generator site or may simply have a diminished response to stimulation.

When impedance testing is abnormal, one must first rule out malfunctioning extension wires and connectors. The first step in management is to disconnect the lead from its extensions, dry them well, and retest impedance. If still abnormal, the physician can then disconnect the generator from its extension wires, irrigate them with sterile water, dry them judiciously, and reconnect the generator. At this juncture, if impedance values are still abnormal, it is best that the lead is revised. In rare instances when the new lead does not resolve the problem, new extensions wires must also be installed. One must note however that this may be of historical value as the newer generation IPGs do not require extension wires to connect to the lead.

It is important to note that the utilization of the tined lead has led to a change in the frequency and type of encountered complications. In the past, lead migration and pain at the IPG site were the most frequent complications [13], but contemporary series have shown that with the tined lead, most complications were either impedance related or a failure of response after successful implantation [24].

Out of 161 implantations at the Cleveland Clinic, 12 patients had an aberrant clinical response; of

Table 11.1 Complications and management of InterStim® stage I

Complication	Management
Lead infection	Remove lead and treat with antibiotics
Injury to subcutaneous extension wire	If significant objective and subjective improvement reported, cut extension wire close to skin and proceed to stage II implantation If inadequate testing period, change subcutaneous extension and complete testing period
Equivocal response	Revise lead and add intraoperative sensory testing for lead positioning

From Carmel et al. [25]. Reprinted with permission from Springer

those, 11 suffered an equalization of impedance between the leads, despite the fact that the impedance value itself was within normal (400–1500 Ω) in the majority of them. In this situation, the physician must dry the connections between the leads and the extension cable and measure impedance values again. If they normalize, then the revision is concluded. Only the patients whose impedance values fail to normalize after reprogramming should undergo lead revision along with intraoperative sensory testing for lead positioning [15] (Table 11.1). Roughly 38% of the patients who undergo revision will succeed and eventually proceed to stage II implantation [24].

It is imperative that the physician measures impedances after IPG installation and before closure of the incision. This will allow reprogramming of the device and adjustment of the connection wires in case of aberrant measurement. If the patient response were not improved despite reprogramming, then surgical revision would be necessary [25].

Lack of Stimulation, Stimulation at a Wrong Area, and Intermittent Stimulation

Patients who present with recurrent symptoms after installation may perceive the stimulation at the wrong area, have no stimulation, or have intermittent stimulation. Patients who perceive the stimulation at a site different than the one just after first implantation will need reprogramming of the device. We recommend going back to each unipolar setting and mapping out where the patient feels the stimulation. That is performed by setting the device at "0-, case+" and asking the patient where (s)he feels the sensation; next we set the device at "1-, case+," "2-, case+," etc. If all combinations fail to identify the target area, then the physician must try bipolar combinations. If all reprogramming possibilities fail, then lead repositioning or relocation to the opposite side is recommended.

Patients who no longer report any stimulation may have a device that was inadvertently turned off, an IPG that has run out of battery life, a migrated lead, or simply device parameters that are not set high enough. One must first measure unipolar impedances because those will allow differentiation between intact lead wires and those that are not [15]. Programming of the device should then be performed, along with bipolar measurements to rule out short circuits. If a battery change or reprogramming does not solve the problem and resume function, then surgical revision would be necessary.

Intermittent stimulation may be due to positional sensitivity or loose connecting wires. The physician must measure impedance while the patient is experiencing intermittent stimulation. This will signify whether the problem is positional (normal impedance) or mechanical (high impedance). When a patient reports a change in sensitivity upon motion (e.g., when standing up or changing position), this points towards positional sensitivity, as the lead position would be shifting with motion. It is not always easy to troubleshoot such problems when they are encountered [15].

Conclusion

Sacral neuromodulation has become a popular treatment option for patients with refractory lower urinary tract symptoms refractory to pharmacological and intravesical therapy. With the increased utilization of this technology, urologists are faced with postimplantation complaints that require rapid identification and troubleshooting. The introduction of the tined lead has decreased the overall rate of complications and has made sacral neuromodulation a more reasonable treatment option for the patient and the physician. It is always important to follow the steps mentioned in this chapter to troubleshoot any challenges encountered after installation of the lead and its implantable generator.

References

1. Oerlemans D, van Kerrebroeck P. Sacral nerve stimulation for neuromodulation of the lower urinary tract. Neurourol Urodyn. 2008;27:28–33.
2. Kay GG, Abou-Donia MB, Messer WS Jr, et al. Antimuscarinic drugs for overactive bladder and their potential effects on cognitive function in older patients. J Am Geriatr Soc. 2005;53(12):2195–201.
3. Bridgeman MB, Friia NJ, Taft C, et al. Mirabegron: β3-adrenergic receptor agonist for the treatment of overactive bladder. Ann Pharmacother. 2013;47(7–8):1029–38.
4. Al-zahrani AA, Elzayat EA, Gajewski JB. Long-term outcome and surgical interventions after sacral neuromodulation implant for lower urinary tract symptoms: 14-year experience at 1 center. J Urol. 2011;185:981–6.
5. Banakhar M, Hassouna M. Percutaneous nerve evaluation test versus staged test trials for sacral neuromodulation: sensitivity, specificity, and predictive values of each technique. Int Neurourol J. 2016;20:250–4.
6. Spinelli M, Giardiello G, Gerber M, et al. New sacral neuromodulation lead for percutaneous implantation using local anesthesia: description and first experience. J Urol. 2003;70:1905–7.
7. Bosch R, Groen J. Sacral nerve neuromodulation in the treatment of patients with refractory motor urge incontinence: long-term results of a prospective longitudinal study. J Urol. 2000;163:1219–22.
8. Borawski KM, Foster RT, Webster GD. Predicting implantation with a neuromodulator using two different test stimulation techniques: a prospective randomized study in urge incontinent women. Neurourol Urodyn. 2007;26:14–8.
9. Janknegt RA, Weil EH, Eerdmans PH. Improving neuromodulation technique for refractory voiding dysfunctions: two-stage implant. Urology. 1997;49:358–62.
10. Peters K, Konstandt D. Complications of sacral neuromodulation. International Continence Society (abstract). https://www.ics.org/Abstracts/Publish/41/000174.pdf. Accessed 18 Sept 2017.
11. Sutherland SE, Lavers A, Carlson A, et al. Sacral nerve stimulation for voiding dysfunction: one institution's 11-year experience. Neurourol Urodyn. 2007;26:19.
12. Sievert KD, Matzel K, Ratto C, et al. Permanente sakrale Neuromodulation mittels InterStim1: Ergebnisseeiner Anwenderbefragung zu aktuellen technischen Entwicklungen. J Urol Urogynakol. 2007;14:14.
13. Siegel SW, Catanzaro F, Dijkema HE, et al. Long-term results of a multicenter study on sacral nerve stimulation for treatment of urinary urge incontinence, urgency-frequency, and retention. Urology. 2000;56:87.
14. Spinelli M, Giardiello G, Arduini A, et al. New percutaneous technique of sacral nerve stimulation has high initial success rate: preliminary results. Eur Urol. 2003;43:70–4.
15. Hijaz A, Vasavada S. Complications and troubleshooting of sacral neuromodulation therapy. Urol Clin North Am. 2005;32:65–9.
16. Deng DY, Gulati M, Rutman M, et al. Failure of sacral nerve stimulation due to migration of tined lead. J Urol. 2006;175(6):2182–5.
17. Scheepens WA, Weil EH, van Koeveringe GA, et al. Buttock placement of the implantable pulse generator: a new implantation technique for sacral neuromodulation—a multicenter study. Eur Urol. 2001;40:434.
18. Van Kerrebroeck P, Van Voskuilen A, Lycklama A, et al. Results of sacral neuromodulation therapy for urinary voiding dysfunction: outcomes of a prospective, worldwide clinical study. J Urol. 2007;178:2029–34.
19. Guralnick ML, Benouni S, O'Connor RC, et al. Characteristics of infections in patients undergoing staged implantation for sacral nerve stimulation. Urology. 2007;69(6):1073–6.
20. Amend B, Bedke J, Khalil M, et al. Prolonged percutaneous SNM testing does not cause infection-related explanation. BJU Int. 2013;111(3):485–91.
21. Haraway AM, Clemens JQ, He C, et al. Differences in sacral neuromodulation device infection rates based on preoperative antibiotic selection. Int Urogynecol J. 2013;24(12):2081–5.
22. Kass-Iliyya A, Jenks J, Hamid R, et al. Tined lead versus percutaneous nerve evaluation for sacral nerve stimulator assessment. J Clin Urol. 2015;8(1):46–51.
23. Vasavada SP, Rackley RR. Electrical stimulation and neuromodulation in storage and emptying failure. In: Wein AJ, Kavoussi LR, Partin AW, Peters CA, editors. eBook Campbell-Walsh urology. 11th ed. Philadelphia: Elsevier Health Sciences; 2015.
24. Hijaz A, Vasavada SP, Daneshgari F, et al. Complications and troubleshooting of two-stage sacral neuromodulation therapy: a single-institution experience. Urology. 2006;68(3):533–7.
25. Carmel M, Vasavada SP, Goldman HB. Troubleshooting sacral neuromodulation issues. Curr Urol Rep. 2012;13:363–9.

CNS Non-invasive Brain Stimulation

12

Mirret M. El-Hagrassy, Felipe Jones, Gleysson Rosa, and Felipe Fregni

Abbreviations

ADHD	Attention deficit hyperactivity disorder
AED	Antiepileptic drug
AMPA	α-amino-3-hydroxy-5-methyl-4-isoxazolepropionic acid
BCE	Before Common Era
BSD	Brain-scalp distance
CP	Cerebral palsy
CSWSS	Continuous spikes and waves during slow wave sleep
DLPFC	Dorsolateral prefrontal cortex
DTMS	Deep transcranial magnetic stimulation
ECT	Electroconvulsive therapy
EEG	Electroencephalography
EMCS	Epidural motor cortex stimulation
EPC	Epilepsia partialis continua
fMRI	Functional magnetic resonance imaging
GABA	Gamma-aminobutyric acid
HAMD	Hamilton Scale for Depression
HD-tDCS	High-Definition transcranial direct current stimulation
ICI	Intracortical inhibition
LDLPFC	Left dorsolateral prefrontal cortex
LTD	Long-term depression
LTP	Long-term potentiation
M1	Primary motor cortex
MADRS	Montgomery Åsberg Depression Rating Scale
MDD	Major depressive disorder
mGluRs	Metabotropic glutamate receptors
N	Number of subjects in study
NIBS	Non-invasive brain stimulation
NMDA	*N*-methyl-D-aspartate
NNT	Number needed to treat
NP	Neuropathic pain
PFC	Prefrontal cortex
ppTMS	Paired-pulse transcranial magnetic stimulation
RDLPFC	Right dorsolateral prefrontal cortex
RE	Rasmussen's encephalitis
rTMS	Repetitive transcranial magnetic stimulation
SI	Spike-index
SPECT	Single-photon emission computed tomography
spTMS	Single-pulse transcranial magnetic stimulation
SUDEP	Sudden unexpected death in epilepsy

M. M. El-Hagrassy (✉) · F. Jones · G. Rosa
F. Fregni
Spaulding Neuromodulation Center, Department of Physical Medicine & Rehabilitation, Spaulding Rehabilitation Hospital and Massachusetts General Hospital, Charlestown, MA, USA
e-mail: melhagrassy@neuromodulationlab.org; fjones@neuromodulationlab.org; grosa@neuromodulationlab.org; fregni.felipe@mgh.harvard.edu

J. P. Gilleran, S. A. Alpert (eds.), *Adult and Pediatric Neuromodulation*,
https://doi.org/10.1007/978-3-319-73266-4_12

tDCS	Transcranial direct current stimulation
TES	Transcranial electric stimulation
TMS	Transcranial magnetic stimulation
VGCC	Voltage-gated calcium channels

Introduction

The term non-invasive brain stimulation (NIBS) refers to the modulation of brain activity through specific techniques requiring no invasive maneuvers or instrumentation to the body. NIBS techniques generate electrical currents within neural networks, for example through the application of either a magnetic or direct electric field to the scalp. The two main types of NIBS are transcranial electric stimulation (TES) and transcranial magnetic stimulation (TMS).

Although TES and TMS have been considered relatively novel techniques, the application of electrical currents to the brain is not new. As far back as 43 BCE, Scribonius Largus, a court physician to the Roman Empire, described the use of electric torpedo fish to treat headaches and gouty arthritis [1]. Almost 1700 years later in the seventeenth century, the discovery of electricity and magnetism prompted the exploration of the body's electrical properties during the following centuries [2]. By around 1786 CE, Luis Galvani demonstrated that the application of electrical currents to the spinal nerves of frogs elicited muscle contractions in a series of experiments known as "animal electricity" [3, 4]. Galvani has thus been acknowledged for laying the foundations of modern neurophysiology. Following his discoveries, the eighteenth and nineteenth centuries witnessed the development of electrical stimulation as a therapeutic modality. It was used to treat a range of medical conditions, such as psychosis, melancholia, pain, and coma [2]. However, for reasons not well defined, NIBS techniques were almost completely overlooked by the scientific community for more than a century.

It was only in the second half of the twentieth century that NIBS techniques were reintroduced to the scientific community. From the 1960s towards the 1980s, experiments revealed that direct current delivery to the human scalp could influence cortical excitability [5–9]. A series of other studies showed that tDCS could modulate brain activity by promoting excitation or inhibition of neural signals [10–12]. These effects were shown to last longer than the stimulation itself, and to ultimately promote behavioral changes depending on the site, frequency, intensity, and duration of stimulation [11, 13].

Similarly, in 1985, Barker et al. presented the first TMS system, and subsequent studies showed that the application of a magnetic field to the scalp could alter cortical excitability and behavior depending on stimulation parameters (e.g., type of coil, frequency and intensity of stimulation, montage and duration of stimulation) [14–20].

These findings opened up a new pathway in using NIBS to better understand and treat neuropsychiatric disorders, and the knowledge and application of these techniques has been increasingly utilized in recent decades. TMS and tDCS have been shown to have varying degrees of efficacy and effectiveness in the treatment of depression, migraine, chronic pain, Parkinson's disease, stroke, epilepsy, and cerebral palsy, among other conditions.

This chapter aims to discuss the two most studied NIBS techniques: TMS and tDCS. We will explain the basic principles behind these two techniques, as well as the available data on their safety and effectiveness. We will provide some insight into two main clinical applications in the adult and pediatric populations for each technique in order to provide a deeper view of their effects as well as the unique challenges of research in this field.

Basic Principles

Transcranial Magnetic Stimulation (TMS)

Despite the name, transcranial magnetic stimulation (TMS) induces electrical fields in the brain. In the TMS device, a capacitor stores an electric charge, which is then discharged through a wire coil, resulting in a current pulse in this circuit. Within a TMS coil's wiring, there is rapid fluctuation of the electric current as the pulse peaks in strength then drops back to zero in less than 1 ms; this generates a magnetic field, within the coil's vicinity, that also rises to roughly 2.5 T and falls quickly. This time-varying magnetic field induces an electric field in the brain if the coil is held over a subject's head, unaffected by the subject's scalp or skull. This magnetic field is perpendicular to the plane of the coil, and the current induced in the brain is parallel to the plane of the coil, but in the opposite direction of the initial current; for example, if the initial current direction is anteroposterior, the induced current direction is posteroanterior.

The induced electric field leads to ion flow in the brain, with subsequent changes in the electric charges on both sides of cell membranes, which passive ion channels render permeable to the ions. These changes then lead to depolarization or hyperpolarization of neural elements. Greater membrane permeability and conductance leads to less change in electric field-induced membrane potential, as well as less time to leak the induced charge [21, 22].

The magnitude of the electric field induced by the magnetic field is directly proportional to the magnetic field's rate of change (Faraday's principle of electromagnetic induction [23]), so the higher the rate of magnetic field change, the greater the induced electric field, and vice versa. However, the interaction between the shape of the coil and that of the tissues can lead to significant variation in which neural elements are stimulated, and how strongly. Stimulation of neural elements should tend to occur where the induced electric field is most powerful, and also when this field is in a direction where a lower threshold is needed for stimulation, such as pointing towards where axons terminate (e.g., into synapses) or bend sharply, particularly longer axons with larger diameters.

When the coil is held in a tangential position, TMS-induced currents flow mainly parallel to the cortical surface of the brain, and the superficial layers (about 1.5–2 or 3 cm deep to the scalp) receive most of the TMS stimulation. This is because a magnetic field's power drops exponentially the further it is from the original current (inverse cube law), and thus, the current drops rapidly the further it is from the coil as well [24]. At intensities under 120% of the motor threshold (MT), stimulation cannot directly activate tissues deeper than 2 cm beneath the scalp (brain-scalp distance, or BSD).

The direction and depth of the current is affected by the type of TMS coil, with figure-of-eight coils leading to shallower, more focal stimulation, while double-cone coils stimulate deeper cortical areas but with less focality. Coils designed for deep brain tissue stimulation tend to be larger than conventional coils, and produce electric fields which have a slower rate of decay with distance, but they also have decreased focality. However, all TMS coils have maximum stimulation intensity at the brain surface, even if they can affect deeper tissues [25–27].

Stimulus waveforms and current directions also significantly affect stimulation thresholds. For example, to achieve stimulation using shorter stimulus duration, a larger pulse amplitude is needed. Meanwhile, over the motor cortex, monophasic pulses lead to lower thresholds when the induced current flows posteroanteriorly in the brain, and biphasic pulses lead to lower thresholds when the induced current flows posteroanteriorly in the *second* phase (in the opposite direction from the first phase), perhaps due to the membrane's capacitative response.

An important thing to note as well is that the types of neural elements (e.g., interneurons, cortical dendrites [28, 29]) involved in TMS stimulation may vary by location and between subjects, and that TMS effects on those elements will be influenced by their state of activity during stimulation. Additionally, on modeling healthy heads vs. those with pathologies such as stroke, atrophy, or tumor, significant changes were demonstrated in TMS-induced currents for stimulation proximal to each pathological area. In addition, there were changes in the magnitude and direction of current density distributions, which may have altered the neural element populations stimulated. This is largely due to the stimulation currents flowing along paths of altered resistance, which result from changes in brain tissue conductivity when these tissues are altered.

Early models of electromagnetic field distributions generated during TMS have been too simplified, and led to conjectures such as the absence of radial currents during TMS. This in turn influenced clinical trial interpretations and led to claims such as the preferential stimulation of interneurons, as they are tangential to cortical surfaces. However, when making calculations those clinical studies and their interpretations should be reassessed in light of more recent modeling work, accounting for variables such as tissue conductivities and subjects' actual head model geometries. It is known that head models and BSD vary by age, sex, and other factors. Realistic and individualized head models would be optimal, but even in the absence of such models, decades of TMS studies in diverse populations have shown this form of NIBS to be quite safe when guidelines are followed properly.

Transcranial Direct Current Stimulation (tDCS)

In tDCS, which is the most commonly used and simplest form of transcranial electrical stimulation (TES), a constant electric current flow of up to 2 mA is delivered via a current generator; this battery-operated device is connected to two sponge electrodes (saline- or water-soaked electrodes placed inside 20–35 cm^2 square or rectangular sponges), which deliver the direct current to the scalp. The sponges are held in their montage-specific positions on the scalp or forehead via nonconducting rubber bands.

Despite significant shunting of the current through the scalp, skull, and CSF, enough current reaches the brain to alter neuronal transmembrane potentials. The current does not induce action potentials directly; rather, the current modulates spontaneous neuronal activity by polarizing brain tissue. The direction of polarization is dependent on the orientation of the axons and dendrites within that electric field; overall, anodal stimulation generally increases the excitability of the underlying brain tissue (e.g., motor cortex, visual cortex) and cathodal stimulation generally decreases it.

The mechanisms of the neurophysiologic effects are not well understood. It is not clear whether tDCS increases or decreases a neuronal membrane's conductance of ions, or its likelihood of reaching a particular threshold. It is also not clear whether tDCS indirectly modulates spontaneous neuronal activity (e.g., by the induction of ionic shifts leading to the facilitation or inhibition of such activity), nor whether tDCS alters transmembrane proteins, or whether its long-term effects are NMDA-mediated [30](neuroplastic after-effects are considered NMDA-dependent, unlike acute effects [31, 32]).

Of major clinical importance, co-administering neuropharmacologics with tDCS can alter tDCS after-effects to the degree that they can be selectively prolonged, blocked, or even reversed. For example, carbamazepine (a voltage-gated sodium channel blocker) and flunarizine (a T-type voltage-gated calcium channel blocker) can suppress anodal after-effects [32]. On the other hand, 100 mg of l-dopa reverses anodal after-effects, making them inhibitory, but does not change cathodal inhibition; this addition of l-dopa to tDCS also leads to after-effects lasting 30 times longer than the addition of placebo to tDCS!

tDCS effects are considered specific to the site of stimulation (the area under the electrodes), but the effects extend to neural networks beyond this region. This has been demonstrated in a number of ways. For example, functional effects are often seen distant to the stimulation site, such as in the case of anodal stimulation of the primary motor cortex leading to ipsilateral excitatory effects but contralateral motor area inhibitory effects [33, 34]. Functional magnetic resonance imaging (fMRI) studies also show widespread and sustained effects in areas of the brain other than those stimulated, and electroencephalography (EEG) studies reveal that stimulation of a specific area can lead to synchronous oscillatory activity changes throughout the brain [35–38]. How these distant effects occur is not entirely clear, nor whether the clinical neuromodulatory effects occur due to after-effects in the area being directly stimulated, or whether they occur due to secondary effects (excitatory or inhibitory) on other cortical and/or subcortical areas. Indeed, it may be a combination of all the above factors, at least in some cases.

The outcomes of tDCS stimulation are dependent on the parameters used in the clinical montage, varying by current density (electric current intensity/electrode surface area), polarity, duration, frequency, and location of stimulation. The area under the anode tends to become more excitatory, while the area under the cathode tends to become more inhibitory. Longer durations of stimulation tend to have longer after-effects; for example, anodal stimulation of 5–13 min leads to after-effects lasting 1–2 h, respectively [10]. However, the excitatory after-effects of anodal stimulation have a limit (homeostatic plasticity ceiling effect), and have been shown to reverse to inhibition after 26 min of stimulation [39]. This may be avoided and the stimulation optimized by introducing intervals; for example, in Monte-Silva et al. [39], the after-effects lasted longer when stimulation was applied in 13 min intervals with 13–20 min breaks, compared to either 3 h intervals or continuous stimulation without intervals.

Cathodal stimulation is thought to have a longer duration of after-effects per time unit of stimulation [40]. Increasing the duration of stimulation does not appear to reverse excitatory after-effects; however, such as when it was applied continuously for 18 min in one study [41], the after-effects did not last as long as they did with more brief time increments. This finding may be related to calcium homeostasis [42].

Overall, repetitive tDCS stimulation over days tends to increase tDCS efficacy, which is particularly important for neurorehabilitation. The montage used, the positions and sizes of the electrodes play an important part in the clinical after-effects and thus their clinical utility (e.g., in stroke rehabilitation, pain management), as we discuss in the clinical applications section below.

In TES, an electric charge enters the scalp at the site of the electrodes, and low amplitude electric current flows through the skull to the brain. Because the skull has low conductivity, a large potential difference between the electrodes is applied to reach a current density (electric current intensity/electrode surface area) in the brain that is high enough to induce neuronal stimulation; this leads to a current density in the scalp that is even higher, and which may lead to pain. Note that TMS can stimulate neurons in the cortex without the pain that may accompany TES, simply because TMS does not lead to electric charges in the scalp.

It is important to note that the smaller the electrode size, the greater the focality of stimulation—and the greater the current density for the same applied intensity as well (current density = current intensity/electrode surface area), and thus the lower the tolerability of stimulation. Higher intensities are also less well tolerated, such that at 3 mA the current application to the scalp begins to get painful even with larger electrode sizes of 35 cm^2 [43].

Overall, tDCS is safe when properly applied, as we discuss below. Additionally, there is ongoing work on models intended to optimize electrode locations and sizes for more precise neuroanatomical targeting. Such models take into account the flow routes of different currents within the CSF of healthy volunteer brains vs. pathologies such as stroke, and some models integrate diffusion tensor-imaged MRI weighting to better account for conductivity along fiber tracts (rather than a perpendicular current flow) [44–46].

Safety

In this section we discuss the safety of the main NIBS techniques in current use, tDCS and TMS.

Almost all non-invasive or transcutaneously administered electrical stimulation devices have been considered Class II by the Food and Drug Administration (FDA). It is important to know that the FDA monitors reports of adverse events and other problems with medical devices, and that it alerts both health professionals and the public when needed to ensure proper use of devices as well as the health and safety of patients. According to the FDA, serious adverse events are the following: death, life-threatening adverse events (e.g., cardiorespiratory arrest, anaphylactic reactions), hospitalization, disability/permanent damage, congenital abnormalities (when applied to pregnant women), refractory seizures, etc.

tDCS

tDCS has been used in thousands of subjects, with some studies concentrating specifically on safety. It has been shown to provide clinical benefits without major side effects [47] when standardized current levels and experimental protocols are used.

The side effects associated with tDCS are mild and transient. In a systematic review, Brunoni et al. [48] found that the most commonly reported side effects are itching (39.3%), tingling (22.2%), headache (14.8%), burning sensation (8.7%), and discomfort (10.4%). Notably, the rates of common adverse effects did not differ between the active arms of the studies and the sham arms. Other less prevalent side effects include fatigue, nausea, and difficulty of concentration. Skin redness or erythema is frequently ignored as an adverse effect but it is more common in active groups compared to sham groups [49]. Presumably, the erythema is due to an increase in the blood flow of dermal vessels associated with the electrical current application.

To date, no serious adverse events were ascribed to tDCS, and unlike TMS, no seizures have been reported as a result of tDCS. Furthermore, studies have shown that tDCS has no significant changes on serum enolase [40], a protein associated with neuronal death. Studies have found no significant pathological changes in EEG activity [50], or in heart rate.

Although there have been limited tDCS studies in pediatric populations, as with adult studies, they have reported no significant side effects beyond itching or tingling at the site of stimulation [51].

In brief, tDCS presents minimal risk to adult and pediatric populations, although data on the latter is more limited. Typical adverse effects such as itching, tingling, and erythema are mild and short in duration. However, this is conditional on following previously validated guidelines for safety.

TMS

Safety guidelines for application of TMS and repetitive TMS (rTMS) have been established by the research and medical community. In general, TMS is safe and well tolerated [52]. Current safety precautions and practice recommendations are guided by the consensus conference held at the National Institutes of Health (NIH) in June 1996 and summarized in Clinical Neurophysiology [53]. A consensus conference that took place in Certosa di Pontignano, Siena (Italy) in 2008 updated the previous safety guidelines [21]. Safety of TMS has also been supported by meta-analyses [54].

The most noteworthy side effects and safety concerns associated with TMS are discussed below.

Hearing

When the TMS stimulating coil is energized, it produces a sound effect that may be greater than 140 dB of sound pressure level [55]. This exceeds recommended safety levels for the auditory system (OSHA).

A small fraction of adults has experienced transitory increments in auditory threshold [56, 57] but the majority of studies in which hearing protection was used report no change in hearing after TMS [26, 56, 58]. In a population of 18 children (a small sample size to assure safety in a pediatric population), Collado-Corona and colleagues [59] reported no change in hearing.

Hearing safety concerns can be addressed by using earplugs or ear muffs. Cochlear implants are an absolute contraindication to any form of TMS.

Seizures

The most serious adverse effect of repetitive TMS is a generalized tonic-clonic seizure [21]. However, the risk during a treatment course is probably less than 0.5% when safety guidelines regarding patient selection and stimulation parameters are followed [21].

A review on the safety of rTMS in epilepsy [60] pointed to a 1.4% per-subject risk to develop a seizure (4 out of 280 patients), and there were no cases of status epilepticus. The seizures reported were self-limited, required no medications and did not recur.

For safety precautions, it is very important that conditions that may increase the risk of inducing epileptic seizures—such as protocol of stimulation, patient's history of epilepsy, drugs that may potentially lower seizure threshold, sleep deprivation, and alcoholism—be considered in advance. Note that TMS has a potent neurophysiological effect on EEG and the after-effects can be demonstrated even in the absence of a behavioral effect [61–63].

Local Pain, Ephemeral Headache, and Burns from Scalp Electrodes

Local pain is the most common side effect (about 39%) induced by TMS, and its intensity varies. Short-lived headache is another common side effect (about 28% of cases). Discomfort due to the stimulus itself is described. These physical sensations are unpleasant but do not cause safety concerns [21]. Less than 2% of study participants discontinue TMS due to pain.

Burns from scalp electrodes have been reported occasionally with high-frequency rTMS only. Burns have not been reported with theta burst TMS, although it does have the potential to cause burns [21].

Cognitive and Neuropsychological Changes

TMS alters cognition [54], which may be improved or worsened, depending on the protocol and the circumstance in which it is applied. Some cognitive changes may be long-lasting. TMS is being studied as a therapy for different neurological and psychiatric diseases and despite its important effect in improving the symptoms of major depressive disorder, it can rarely cause cognitive deterioration, as evidenced by some studies [64].

Another safety concern is mood changes, including psychotic symptoms, anxiety, agitation, and suicidal ideation, as well as insomnia [65, 66]. However, the nocebo effect size on these findings is unclear. All these findings were transient and easily treatable.

Transitory acute hypomania induction has been rarely reported in low frequency [67]. It is a possible side effect following left prefrontal cortex stimulation using high-frequency rTMS; it has not been reported in other protocols [21].

Other Side Effects

Structural brain changes and histotoxicity have been inconsistently reported in low- and high-frequency rTMS studies.

Clinical Applications

TMS

Single-Pulse TMS

Clinically, single-pulse TMS (spTMS) has been used in the assessment and follow-up of various neurologic disorders, such as stroke, traumatic brain injury, neurodegenerative disorders (e.g., Parkinson's disease, Alzheimer's disease), epilepsy, as well as various psychiatric disorders, such as unipolar major depression, bipolar disorder, and schizophrenia. It is not used for induction of therapeutic effects, but as a diagnostic and prognostic tool ("Transcranial Magnetic Stimulation," n.d.).

For example, spTMS can be used to measure the motor threshold (MT) intensity needed to produce a motor response, the motor evoked potential (MEP), and the cortical silent period. These are important neurophysiological markers for monitoring the efficacy of pharmacological, behavioral, and electric/magnetic stimulation treatments. Moreover, spTMS can also be used with EEG or neuroimaging in order to study cortical excitability in specific areas [68].

In children, spTMS is used in disorders such as Tourette syndrome, autism, attention deficit hyperactivity disorder (ADHD), and periventricular leukomalacia [69–71], with evidence that spTMS protocols undergo maturational changes (e.g., resting MT (rMT) is difficult to identify in children younger than 6 years of age [72]).

Repetitive TMS

Repetitive TMS (rTMS) can be used as a diagnostic tool to investigate and measure cortical plasticity, sometimes using specialized rTMS protocols such as continuous and intermittent theta burst stimulation [73, 74]. Unlike single- and paired-pulse TMS whose effects last milliseconds, rTMS modulates cortical excitability over minutes to hours, and its clinical effects may last weeks to months. While rTMS has the dual advantages of spatiotemporal specificity and limited side effects, evidence of its therapeutic efficacy remains limited. However, it is used off-label as a therapeutic tool, and its effects depend on the protocol, including the number and frequency of rTMS sessions.

rTMS therapeutic protocols tend to fall under three categories according to Horvath et al. [75]: direct targeting (where a specific area is targeted for modulation), distance effect modulation (where a neural area that is functionally related to the dysfunctional area is targeted), and distributed modulation (which attempts to induce neurotransmitter release that is network-specific to normalize abnormal brain activity). Protocol selection requires being up to date with the literature as well as individualized tailoring to patients.

Off-label clinical applications of rTMS include protocols in depression, obsessive compulsive disorder, schizophrenia, post-traumatic stress disorder, chronic pain, tinnitus, and for motor function/dysfunction in Parkinson's disease and stroke respectively. rTMS is also sometimes used off-label in epilepsy.

Deep TMS will be discussed further as treatment for depression below. Other clinical applications of TMS including paired-pulse TMS and TMS-EEG are beyond the scope of this chapter.

While the overwhelming majority of NIBS techniques are used off-label, there is FDA approval for TMS depression protocol. Therefore, in this section, we will focus on TMS treatment of depression, and we will also present tDCS depression studies in comparison.

Depression

rTMS

The end goal of most rTMS depression protocols is to normalize abnormal activity via modulation of cortical excitability across targeted neural networks. Several meta-analyses are consistent with the utility of rTMS in alleviating many symptoms of medication-resistant depression: eight select meta-analyses listed in Horvath et al. [75] each included a range of 5–34 trials, and mean effect size ranged from 0.39 to 0.81 (active/high-frequency stimulation vs. sham, statistically significant differences) [76–82]. One meta-analysis of five trials showed a number needed to treat (NNT) of 2–3 [80], and one meta-analysis of 13 trials showed a standardized mean difference of −0.35 between high-frequency stimulation and sham following 2 weeks of treatment (but this was nonsignificant 2 weeks later at follow-up) [79].

The highest effect size was obtained from rTMS monotherapy (rather than add-on) studies [82], and low-frequency right dorsolateral prefrontal cortex (RDLPFC) stimulation (distance effect) showed a trend towards improved response compared to high-frequency left dorsolateral prefrontal cortex (LDLPFC) stimulation (most clinical rTMS protocols stimulate LDLPFC). Though the results of the studies overall were variable, they did suggest that rTMS is efficacious in the treatment of medication-resistant depression.

Major depressive disorder (MDD) is highly prevalent and disabling; an estimated 20–40% of patients do not improve sufficiently on the available interventions, including medications and psychotherapy [83]. Patients with clinical depression commonly have prefrontal cortex dysfunction; there is also evidence suggesting LDLPFC hypoactivity associated with the severity of symptoms in both primary and secondary depression. The research on TMS effects on depression falls under the three paradigms mentioned above, mostly direct targeting, although several researchers explored distance effect modulation and a couple of groups looked at the distributed modulation paradigm in humans with depression (compared to extensive animal research in the latter paradigm). See Table 12.1 for comparisons between the typical parameters of both [75, 84]. Note that the neurotransmitter affected in the distributed modulation paradigm was dopamine, and that the results were mixed.

Two highly influential multisite sham-controlled RCTs both showed that prefrontal rTMS applied daily led to an antidepressant effect in antidepressant-free resistant MDD patients that was clinically relevant and significantly greater than sham; those two studies were O'Reardon et al.'s industry-sponsored international study on 301 subjects (the study that led to FDA-approval K061053 of TMS depression protocol) [52], and George et al.'s NIH-sponsored US study on 109 patients [85]. Both studies applied 10 pulses/s (10 Hz) to the LDLPFC of antidepressant-free patients at 120% rMT with ON time 4 s and OFF time 26 s; 3000 magnetic pulses were delivered per treatment session over 37.5 min. In the first study, sessions were held five times/week over 4–6 weeks [52]; in the second study, after a 2-week lead-in no-treatment phase, they had a 3-week fixed-treatment phase, and then clinical improvers had a variable 3-week extension, while non-improvers were crossed over to open-label treatment, and continued for up to 3 more weeks if they improved sufficiently [85].

Reardon et al. [52] concluded that more than 2 weeks of rTMS were needed before a significant improvement was seen as compared to sham, and that 2 more weeks of rTMS beyond the initial 4 weeks can have an important impact clinically (e.g., remission rates doubled during that time period). At 6 weeks, active rTMS patients had remission at twice the rates—or more—of sham patients, with Montgomery Åsberg Depression Rating Scale (MADRS) 14.2% vs. 5.2%, Hamilton Rating Scale for Depression with 17 items (HAMD17) 15.5% vs. 7.1%, and HAMD24 (24 items) 17.4% vs. 8.2%.

George et al. [85] also found that the active rTMS had a significant effect on remission rates—14.1% vs. 5.1% in the active vs. sham group ($p = 0.02$) at 3–5 weeks (acute phase); there were 4.2 times greater odds of remission with active rTMS vs. sham (95% confidence interval, 1.32–13.24). They concluded that at least 3 weeks of treatment were necessary. Then about 30% remitted in the open-label period with similar proportions from previously active or sham groups. They also noted that although their sample overall had moderate treatment resistance in their lifetime and in the current episode, most remitters had lower degrees of treatment resistance. Both studies had effective blinding and low rates of serious adverse events.

There have been other open-label and sham-controlled RCTs investigating rTMS in depression as well. There is evidence that the antidepressant effects of conventional rTMS last beyond the acute stimulation without maintenance treatment. (Note also that in an open-label trial on post-traumatic stress disorder, there was improvement of comorbid depression symptoms on subthreshold LDLPFC stimulation for 600/10 sessions at 1 or 5 Hz—although post-traumatic stress disorder symptoms only had minimal improvement [86]; this was a distance effect paradigm.)

Table 12.1 Comparisons between the typical parameters for therapeutic rTMS protocols in depression in terms of location, frequency, intensity, and duration of stimulation

Therapeutic protocol in depression	Location	Frequency	Intensity	Duration
Direct targeting	LDLPFC	10–20 Hz (excitatory)	Suprathreshold	Variable
Distance effect modulation	RDLPFC	1 Hz (inhibitory)	Suprathreshold	Variable
Distributed modulation	LDLPFC	10 Hz (excitatory)	At threshold	750–3500 pulses

DTMS (Deep TMS, H-coil Deep Brain Stimulation)

RCT

In January 2013, the FDA also approved the Brainsway Deep TMS System for the treatment of depressive episodes in adults with major depressive disorder (MDD) who failed to improve sufficiently from previous antidepressants in the current episode [22, 84]. This was based on an international multicenter double-blind randomized sham-controlled trial studying 212 MDD (single or recurrent episode) outpatients who were not on antidepressants, had failed 1–4 antidepressant trials or who had not tolerated two or more antidepressant treatments in the current episode.

The study was sponsored by Brainsway and utilized their H-coil Deep TMS System. Levkovitz et al. [87] note that different DLPFC subregions stimulated by standard protocols vary in connectivity with medial prefrontal regions such as the subgenual cingulate gyrus (important in MDD) [88–90]. The H1-coil was designed to stimulate the prefrontal cortex, the fibers connecting the prefrontal cortex or the cingulate to the nucleus accumbens and ventral tegmental area (in order to modulate control of motivation, reward, and pleasure). In this way, without significantly increasing the electric field induced in superficial cortical layers [26, 91–93], more extensive neural networks, deeper cortical regions, and fibers targeting subcortical regions are affected.

After 1–2 weeks of washout/tapering of antidepressants, subjects randomly received 20 min of active DTMS (18 Hz over the LDLPFC, with 2 s pulse trains separated by 20 s inter-train intervals, 55 trains/session, MSO 120% of MT) or sham 5 days/week over 4 weeks (20 sessions); the maintenance phase then lasted 12 weeks, during which time subjects received active DTMS or sham twice a week (24 sessions).

Subjects' HDRS-21 total score (from baseline to Week 5, the primary endpoint) improved by 6.39 points on DTMS vs. 3.28 points in the sham group ($p = 0.008$, effect size 0.76). Additionally, response (drop of at least 50% in total HDRS-21 score during that period) and remission (total HDRS-21 score of under 10 at Week 5) were also better with DTMS vs. sham (response: 38.4% vs. 21.4%, remission: 32.6% vs. 14.6%, $p = 0.013$ and 0.005, respectively). The differences were stable over the 12-week maintenance phase, and the only serious adverse event in the trial was a seizure in the setting of protocol deviation. They concluded that DTMS was efficacious and safe in MDD patients not responding to antidepressants, and that its effect was stable over 3 months of maintenance treatment.

Open-Label Studies in Comparison

There have been multiple open-label trials and case studies on DTMS. Kezdior et al. [94] included nine open-label studies in a quantitative meta-analysis on H-coils in MDD, and added the RCT above [87] to the qualitative analysis for a total of 10 studies.

The stimulation parameters and patient characteristics were similar between the nine open-label studies and the RCT; however, only the RCT and 2/9 open-label studies in the analysis used DTMS as monotherapy. Also, 7/9 open-label studies and the RCT were conducted on unipolar patients, while 2/9 studies were on only or mostly bipolar patients.

They found that the magnitude of the antidepressant effect due to DTMS (as interpreted by HDRS improvements) was large, and they noted that antidepressant effects as well as response rates tended to increase, from 1.3 to 2.04 and from 43% to 60%, respectively, as studies were cumulatively added to the analysis, implying that the truth is likely closer to a higher value of improvement compared to a lower value. They also found improved antidepressant effect and response rate in studies where patients were on antidepressant medications compared to the studies in which they were not. The improved results on antidepressant *medications* are consistent with neuromodulation having an additive effect on neuroplasticity; neuromodulation tends to work best in combination with medications or other therapeutic measures, such as physical therapy.

Kezdior et al. [94] concluded that high-frequency DTMS was an efficacious and acceptable acute treatment for major depression, particularly unipolar depression. As the single RCT [87] showed a significantly greater effect in the active DTMS group compared to placebo, they noted that any added placebo effect presumed to contribute to the large effect sizes in the open-label studies may better reflect the antidepressant effects that would be seen in a clinical setting [95]; in fact, placebo effects tend to be lower in resistant depression [96, 97].

They also suggested that the higher effect sizes seen in the meta-analysis may reflect the effects of the H1-coil in stimulating a higher cortical volume, and/or penetration of stimulation more deeply [87, 93, 95], which may have led to improvements in other areas of cognitive functions. There is some limited evidence that DTMS may improve some cognitive function domains (e.g., working and visuospatial memory, cognitive planning, and sustained attention) [96–99], and it has also been shown to improve global, psychological, environmental, and social quality of life domain scores in treatment-resistant depression, with moderate to large effect sizes [95].

They added that the optimized stimulation parameters in the meta-analysis such as high-frequency (18–20 Hz) stimulation, high intensity, and stimulation daily for a month (20 sessions—in the acute phases) may have contributed to the consistently improved antidepressant effects in these heterogeneous populations [99]. The analysis suggested that while DTMS antidepressant effects may last up to 12 months after acute treatment without maintenance treatment, providing maintenance treatment might prolong and improve DTMS acute effects. Yet a second DTMS course in patients who had relapsed within a year of responding well to DTMS led to comparatively lower response rates [100].

To conclude, both rTMS and DTMS are potentially efficacious treatments for major depressive disorder. However, more well-designed sham-controlled RCTs are needed to optimize stimulation parameters, and to clarify other questions such as durability of acute clinical effects, what additional therapies might enhance TMS effects, and whether tolerance or resistance could occur when treatment is reintroduced.

tDCS

Palm et al. [101] performed a comprehensive review on tDCS in depression, from 2002 (as they believed this to be the first date seminal tDCS studies following good clinical practice standards were published) to mid-October 2015. They thus reported on 11 double-blind, placebo-controlled RCTs, 9 open-label studies, 8 case reports, and multiple meta-analyses. The clinical trials reported on tDCS treatment in heterogeneous patient samples (in terms of treatment resistance, co-medications, unipolar vs. bipolar depression) with variable aims (e.g., add-on or long-term therapy, comparison to pharmacotherapy or of different stimulation protocols) and mostly measured HAMD and MADRS. The case reports mainly reported on adverse effects, such as mania or hypomania.

The original articles had similar stimulation parameters, placing the anode over the LDLPFC (F3) and the cathode over the right supraorbital region or RDLPFC (F4), with the opposite modulation of both hemispheres/transcallosal effects aimed to improve efficacy. They used sponge electrodes typically 7 × 5 cm (35 cm^2), though some used smaller electrodes and a few used extra-cephalic 100 cm^2 electrodes. Initial studies used 1 mA, but later studies used 2 mA after it was shown to be safe by Boggio et al. [102]. Most stimulation sessions were at 20 min per day over 2–3 weeks, but in recent years, twice daily stimulation (20 min each) or prolonged stimulation duration (30 min) protocols were evaluated to enhance neuroplasticity.

Palm et al. [101] concluded that the meta-analyses suggested some tDCS efficacy with moderate effect size in treatment of acute depressive disorder, but low efficacy in treatment-resistant depression, and that its effects can be potentially decreased by other drugs (e.g., mood stabilizers, antiepileptic drugs, and benzodiazepines).

Rigonatti et al. [103] and Brunoni et al. [104] did head to head efficacy comparisons between antidepressants and tDCS. Rigonatti et al. [103] randomized patients to active tDCS (n = 10) vs. sham tDCS (n = 10) vs. fluoxetine 20 mg (n = 11, not blinded) and showed faster improvements in the tDCS group compared to the fluoxetine group, as well as the same Beck Depression Inventory (BDI) improvement 6 weeks later in the tDCS and fluoxetine groups, both of which were significantly superior to the sham tDCS group.

In the four-arm factorial SELECT-TDCS study, 120 patients were randomized to four groups combining active tDCS—F3 anode, F4 cathode, 10 sessions of 30 min per day over 2 weeks, then one session in each of weeks 3 and 4, all at 2 mA, 25 cm^2—or sham tDCS with sertraline 50 mg or placebo sertraline. Active tDCS + sertraline had better results than the other groups, and the half-active groups (placebo sertraline + active tDCS and active sertraline + sham tDCS) had similar results, but these two groups were also superior to placebo sertraline + sham tDCS.

Palm et al. [101] suggested that the combination of tDCS with antidepressants may have led to improved results as they may reach all cortico-limbic circuits involved in depressive disorders. Yet, a meta-analysis by Meron et al. [105], which showed that active tDCS was superior to sham, also showed that tDCS effects were attenuated by antidepressant co-medications and cognitive control training.

These same authors [101] also reported on open-label studies reporting relapses over time. Martin et al. [106] showed a relapse rate of 16% during weekly tDCS over a 3-month duration, which rose to 49% during biweekly tDCS over another 3 months. Valiengo et al. [107], in a follow-up of the SELECT-TDCS study, reported a 40% relapse rate during biweekly tDCS (cathode F4 25 cm^2) in the initial 3 months of follow-up, and a total relapse rate of 53% in the whole 6-month follow-up period, which included monthly tDCS in the last 3 months. The relapse rate was higher in cases with treatment resistance diagnoses on enrollment. Meanwhile, Dell'Osso et al. [108] showed positive after-effects in nearly half the sample for 3 months after stimulation, despite a progressive loss of study adherence.

Overall, tDCS has been found to be safe and well tolerated at standard stimulation parameters, cost-effective, and blinding appears to be feasible. However, recent studies [109, 110] showed that higher current intensities (e.g., 2 mA) lead to more sensory side effects and erythema than sham, which may be mitigated by using skin cream. Additionally, a recent meta-analysis [111] evaluated treatment-emergent mania/hypomania during tDCS antidepressant treatment, and found that active tDCS was not associated with a significantly higher number of treatment-emergent mania/hypomania episodes compared to sham.

However, long-term data on tDCS in depression is lacking overall, and there is a need for more data on its effects on neuropsychological testing and interventions in patients with depression compared to healthy controls, and on its modulation by psychotropic drugs [112]. Further high quality multicentric studies are needed to optimize stimulation parameters, particularly for treatment-resistant cases, as well as identify outcome predictors. Al-Kaysi et al. [113] suggested that EEG-based classification may help tailor patient selection for tDCS depression therapy, with frontal channels being especially informative for outcome prediction.

tDCS does not have FDA approval for treatment of depression at this time, although it can be used off-label in specialized centers.

Chronic Neuropathic Pain

The investigation of NIBS techniques for relieving neuropathic pain (NP), that is, pain resulting from injury to the nervous system, began after epidural motor cortex stimulation (EMCS) was proposed to have analgesic effects in patients with chronic NP [114, 115]. In EMCS, small electrodes are surgically placed on the dura overlying the primary motor cortex (M1), and a weak, subthreshold current is delivered [115]. A number of randomized clinical trials (RCT) and open-label studies proved the efficacy of EMCS in treating chronic NP during the 1990s [116–120]. rTMS later emerged as a non-invasive alternative, potentially producing similar analgesia. The first trial using rTMS was in 1998, and it showed that high-frequency (10 Hz) stimulation was able to relieve NP symptoms [121]. The following years witnessed a number of studies confirming the value of rTMS, while other studies investigated tDCS as another potential treatment for chronic NP.

In this section, we will summarize the main findings of current research on the therapeutic use of NIBS techniques on neuropathic pain.

Alterations Observed in Patients with Chronic Neuropathic Pain

Studies on patients with NP consistently show decreased metabolic activity in the thalamus contralateral to the side of ongoing pain [122–128]. This finding is consistent with other studies that show decreased gray matter volume, and biochemical changes signaling neuronal loss in the same location [129–131]. Moreover, studies using EEG revealed a shift of electrical brain activity towards lower frequencies (i.e., theta) in these patients [132, 133]. This phenomenon was proposed to be a manifestation of thalamocortical dysrhythmia, a process which involves increased bursting activity of thalamic nuclei, and which may represent a state of disinhibition [134]. Therefore, the current hypothesis among the scientific community is that these patients present an imbalance in the excitatory/inhibitory circuits that regulate thalamic processing of pain signals.

On the other hand, neuroimaging studies have shown that NP is associated with reduced gray matter volume in the prefrontal cortex (PFC) [135, 136]. This PFC atrophy is correlated with the duration of pain, and with altered connectivity between this region and the nucleus accumbens and insula, two areas of the brain related to the affective-emotional aspects of the pain experience [135, 137]. In this way, patients with NP present with alterations of varied areas within the pain matrix, which may be the reason they commonly have not only sensory-discriminative disturbances—such as hyperalgesia and allodynia—but also emotional disturbances, such as depression.

Mechanisms of Action of NIBS in Neuropathic Pain

Although M1 stimulation has been proven effective in reducing pain, the exact mechanism of action of this analgesic effect is still poorly understood. Here we will discuss consistent findings regarding the mechanism of action of these techniques across studies.

rTMS

High-frequency rTMS can elicit action potentials in superficially located horizontal interneurons when the figure-of-eight coil is placed over the M1 contralateral to the pain side, in an anteroposterior orientation [138]. This stimulation setting has been shown to reduce thalamic hyperactivity in NP patients, and the integrity of thalamocortical pathways is necessary for observing the analgesic effects of rTMS [138–142]. In this way, it is hypothesized that M1 stimulation produces antidromic modulation of thalamic activity, altering the processing of pain signals at a thalamic level [142]. On the other hand, this stimulation paradigm has also been shown to activate the prefrontal, orbitofrontal, and cingulate cortices, structures related to the affective-emotional aspects of pain processing [143–146]. Thus, the analgesic effects of rTMS appear to relate to the modulation of networks responsible for providing the sensory specificity (i.e., thalamus), and the emotional-affective valence of the pain experience.

Additionally, the effects of rTMS are also linked to changes in neurotransmitters. High-frequency rTMS has been shown to increase intracortical inhibition (ICI)—a physiological marker of GABAergic activity in the motor cortex—in correlation to the degree of analgesia [147–149]. This way, rTMS may function as an enhancer of inhibitory circuitries involved in the modulation of pain. On the other hand, rTMS has also been proposed to increase endogenous opioids, and, in fact, the analgesic effect of rTMS was blocked by naloxone administration in healthy volunteers [145]. Thus, it may also promote analgesia by increasing the release of endogenous opioids in important pain networks, including those in the descending modulation system.

tDCS

Anodal stimulation of M1 contralateral to the most painful side with 2 mA has also been shown to promote analgesia in patients with chronic NP. This low-intensity current delivered by tDCS is not sufficiently large to promote action potentials. Instead, it depolarizes neurons at the site of stimulation and in the connected areas, thus increasing the excitability of the neural networks connected to M1 [11, 150]. This change in excitability promotes transient activation of NMDA receptors, and changes in molecular cascades that ultimately result in modulation of synaptic plasticity [10, 32]. In addition, anodal tDCS over M1 has been shown to activate distant areas within the pain matrix that, like rTMS, involve sensory-discriminative and emotional-affective aspects of pain [20, 151].

tDCS has also been shown to promote changes in neurotransmitters. The stimulation paradigm with anodal tDCS over M1 has been associated with increased ICI, which pinpoints the modulation of GABAergic inhibitory systems within the motor cortex [152]. The observed increase in ICI after tDCS has also been correlated with the degree of analgesia [152]. Also, tDCS has been related to increases in endogenous opioids over the posterior thalamus, which points a possible mechanism for the analgesic effect of this technique [153].

Evidence of NIBS Efficacy on NP

rTMS

The efficacy of rTMS in treating neuropathic pain depends on a number of factors. Firstly, parameters of stimulation such as frequency, intensity, number of pulses delivered, cortical target, and coil orientation are highly determinant of analgesic effects. Moreover, other treatment protocol characteristics such as the number of sessions and intervals between them have also been shown to be crucial for treatment efficacy. Finally, anatomical variations across subjects and geometrical precision of stimulation are also important.

As to parameters of stimulation, studies comparing different frequencies of rTMS over M1 show that subthreshold stimulation with 10 Hz or 20 Hz is more effective than 5 Hz or 1 Hz [154–156]. Moreover, when comparing different types and orientation of coils, research has demonstrated that analgesic effects are only achieved when stimuli are delivered through a figure-of-eight coil, with the handle positioned in an anteroposterior orientation (i.e., parallel to mid-sagittal line) [138, 142]. Finally, studies have shown that at least 1000 pulses delivered per session suffice for promoting significant analgesic effects [157].

As to treatment protocol, single-session rTMS has been shown to provide only short-term analgesic effects, lasting 6–8 days [158, 159]. In comparison, protocols with 5–10 daily sessions are more effective, and promote pain relief that may last for at least 2 weeks beyond the stimulation [160–163]. One study testing optimal maintenance sessions indicated that the analgesia could last even longer when a sufficient number of sessions are in adequate intervals. A study by Mhalla et al. [149] tested a long-term protocol in 40 subjects with fibromyalgia and showed that pain relief lasted for 25 weeks. This protocol consisted of 14 sessions distributed in the following manner: 5 daily sessions for 1 week, followed by 1 weekly session for 1 month, 1 fortnightly session for 2 months, and 1 monthly session for 3 months, totaling more than 6 months of treatment. Two case series also demonstrated effects lasting for up to 6 months and 1 year, respectively [164, 165].

To summarize, rTMS is more effective in relieving NP when applied at high frequency (10 Hz or 20 Hz), with subthreshold intensity, using a figure-of-eight coil placed in an antero-posterior orientation over the M1 contralateral to the most painful side of the body. The duration of effects is dependent on the number and interval of sessions varying from 2 weeks for 5- to 10-session protocols, up to 1 year with a 14-session protocol. However, the optimal treatment protocol for NP is still under investigation and may vary with the disorder under investigation, patient comorbidities, and anatomical variations. In fact, regarding potential differences in anatomy, recent studies utilized imaging-guided rTMS in order to increase precision in the stimulation of the underlying cortex, with improved results [165]. Lastly, in terms of effect size, rTMS can reduce pain levels by 25–45% after stimulation, and achieve response rates of 35–60% (defined as percentage of subjects with at least 30% pain relief) when administered for at least 5 days of daily sessions with the optimized parameters discussed above [166].

tDCS

Similar to rTMS, the efficacy of tDCS in treating NP depends on various parameters, the most important ones being electrode montage, current intensity, electrode size, stimulation duration, and number of sessions. In the first clinical trial investigating the role of tDCS in relieving NP, Fregni et al. [167] randomized 17 patients with chronic NP secondary to spinal cord injury (SCI) to receive either anodal (2 mA, for 20 min) or sham stimulation over the M1 contralateral to the ongoing side of pain, for 5 consecutive days. Significant pain reduction was achieved after the active tDCS but not after sham stimulation, and the analgesic effects lasted for 16 days [167]. The same group compared this protocol (anodal M1, 2 mA, 20 min, for 5 days) with anodal stimulation of DLPFC in 32 patients with fibromyalgia and showed that anodal tDCS over M1 provided more pain relief, with effects lasting for 3 weeks [168]. Since then, this stimulation paradigm has been proven effective for treating NP in a number of other conditions [169–173], e.g., producing analgesic effects for up to 4 weeks in patients with NP due to multiple sclerosis [174].

On the other hand, a number of other tDCS trials have showed negative findings or only marginal effects [175–177]. These inconsistencies in clinical efficacy may be related to differences in study design, stimulation parameters, and disorder under study. For example, a recent trial showed tDCS to be ineffective in the treatment of patients with nonspecific chronic low-back pain [175]. Although the very same protocol used by Fregni et al. [167] in SCI was used in this condition, low-back pain is characterized by having a mix of nociceptive (i.e., pain elicited by detection of noxious or harmful stimuli by peripheral nociceptors) and neuropathic pain. In this way, the constant nociceptive component of this condition may have compromised the efficacy of tDCS. Nonetheless, better stimulation parameters and criteria for patient selection are still under investigation for this therapy.

In this context, some directions for improving the efficacy of tDCS in treating NP have been established in recent years. First, tDCS has been shown to provide greater analgesic effects when combined with concurrent treatments, such as visual illusion therapy. Soler et al. [178] showed that a protocol of ten sessions of anodal tDCS (2 mA, 20 min) over the right or left M1 combined with visual illusion therapy could provide better pain relief than each therapy alone in patients with SCI, and analgesic effects lasted up to 12 weeks [178]. Second, the low efficacy of tDCS has been associated with its diffuse brain current flow. In order to overcome this drawback, researchers developed High-Definition tDCS (HD-tDCS), with a 4 × 1 electrode montage (1 central anode and 4 encircling cathodes), which provides a non-invasive focal application of low-intensity direct current [179, 180]. The increased focality of HD-tDCS is believed to enhance the clinical effects of tDCS. In fact, a recent study assessed the necessary number of HD-tDCS sessions needed to achieve more than 50% pain relief in patients with fibromyalgia; a median of 15 sessions were necessary [181].

To conclude, tDCS has been shown to provide significant pain relief in patients with NP, whenever this population is carefully selected. Overall, repeated daily sessions of tDCS may promote more than 50% of pain relief in patients with NP, which is greater than the effect provided by rTMS. Additionally, the efficacy of tDCS can be enhanced when using this technique as an add-on to other behavioral or pharmacological therapies. Lastly, HD-tDCS emerges as a more efficacious treatment, and study protocols with extended numbers of sessions are under investigation.

TMS and tDCS in Pediatric Patients

Most clinical TMS and tDCS studies have focused on adults, and there is a great need for more research into their therapeutic uses in pediatric patients. Unlike adults, pediatric brains still have to go through various stages of neurodevelopment. They also have accelerated neuroplasticity compared to adults [182–184], which may be helpful for therapeutic purposes, but which may hypothetically harm brain development in unpredictable ways.

So far, both TMS and tDCS tend to be tolerated well by both children and adults. TMS can be used for both diagnostic and therapeutic purposes, and has been used for functional motor and language mapping prior to surgery in both children and adults [185–189]. EEG together with TMS further evaluates maturation and impaired cortical reactivity in children. Single- and paired-pulse TMS are cautiously considered safe in patients about the age of 2 years; under that age, specialized hearing protection is needed due to lack of evidence on risk of acoustic injury.

Quintana [190] reviewed 48 studies involving (single-pulse, paired, and repetitive) TMS in people less than 18 years of age ($n = 1036$, age range 2 months to 18 years). No major adverse effects (including seizures) were reported, even in children with epilepsy and cerebral palsy. However, rTMS had only been applied in seven studies ($n = 34$).

Overall, there is little safety data on rTMS use in pediatric populations [191], and while it is not believed to carry long-term adverse effects, it is unclear whether repeated rTMS over long periods of time may alter the maturing brain irreversibly. Therefore, rTMS should only be applied for clinical use when the benefit/risk ratio is potentially high, e.g., when there are no better treatments available.

There are unique issues surrounding the safety, applicability, and ethics of utilizing tDCS in pediatric populations. There are no longitudinal studies exploring tDCS' impact on the developing brain. The limited data available underscores some of the ethical questions arising from tDCS in children. Additionally, as RCTs offer therapy only to a subset of the population, new techniques are often tested only in compassionate use until found to be safe in pediatric populations. Just as recommendations on TMS in pediatric populations [21] were issued at a consensus conference, so consensus guidelines might help direct research on tDCS in pediatric populations as well.

Children's thinner skulls, the smaller distance between scalp and brain, and the gray-white matter differentiation differences led to studies addressing tDCS dosage in pediatrics [192, 193]. Several studies show higher peak current densities in children's brains compared to adults while using similar stimulation parameters [183, 194]. Computational models of current flow within the brain suggest that we should halve applied current strength in children compared to the amperage used on adults, though multiple studies have used higher intensities. Based on the results of a randomized crossover trial ($n = 19$) in 11–16-year-olds, Moliadze et al. [195] hypothesized that 1 mA could have a ceiling effect in children, and that 0.5 mA in children would probably be similar to 1 mA in adults.

In terms of safety, no severe adverse events have been reported in pediatric populations, and even in patients with epilepsy, seizures do not seem worse with tDCS. However, study designs for various disorders tend to be heterogeneous, and optimized stimulation protocols and dosages over different pediatric age groups are far from clear. Additionally, the delineation between childhood, adolescence, and adulthood is often undefined and can be variable between studies [196].

In a comprehensive review on tDCS in children and adolescents, Palm et al. [101] report that pediatric depression, unlike adult depression, is not covered by the literature, and that it is unclear whether tDCS could treat pediatric patients with affective disorders. There is some data on ADHD and autism treatment. Most pediatric placebo-controlled RCTs so far have been in movement disorders due to cerebral palsy.

tDCS is considered a potential therapy for some pediatric disorders, particularly when there are no other safe viable alternatives, but not for cognitive enhancement in healthy pediatric populations as that would raise ethical questions. In this pediatrics section, we focus on tDCS and TMS in epilepsy and cerebral palsy.

Epilepsy

tDCS in Pediatric Patients with Epilepsy

Animal models have supported the hypothesis that (cathodal) tDCS' neuromodulatory effects can raise the seizure threshold [197]. Its effects appear similar to those induced by rTMS [198, 199]. Palm et al. [187], in their review on tDCS in pediatrics, reported on two placebo-controlled RCTs [200, 201] and an open-label trial [201] on tDCS in children with epilepsy, all measuring seizure frequency (n = 59 overall, the highest number of subjects enrolled in studies on any of the disorders in this chapter).

In an open-label study, Shelyakin et al. [202] evaluated 4–8-year-olds (n = 18) with various syndromes (e.g., generalized epilepsy, cerebral palsy, and organic brain lesions). They placed the anode over the posterior temporal region, the cathode over the parietal cortex, and applied tDCS at 0.3–0.7 mA for 20–40 min, maximum 15 sessions. They found that seizure frequency improved in all the children, and there was a reduction in epileptiform discharges as well as slow wave activity. This is particularly interesting in view of its effects on patients with generalized epilepsy.

It is known that generalized seizures are not completely generalized; that is, while they may involve wide areas of both hemispheres, they do not affect the entire cortex. In invasive studies, secondarily generalized seizures do not involve all electrodes to an equal degree, or even all electrodes sampled [203]. Additionally, there have been a number of centers recording EEG with fMRI, revealing the involvement of multiple regions. For example, Gotman et al. [204] showed activation with generalized epileptic discharges that was bilateral and symmetric in the thalamus, mesial midfrontal cortex, insula, cerebellum, borders of the lateral ventricles, and deactivation that was also bilateral and symmetric in the anterior frontal and parietal cortices and in the posterior cingulate gyri as well as the left posterior temporal region; that is, there was a broad network involved, including areas of the default mode network, but not the whole cortex. Thus, focal stimulation with tDCS may be a potential therapy for generalized epilepsy syndromes, especially when we keep in mind that tDCS can also have broad network effects involving regions far from those directly stimulated.

The two sham-controlled RCTs reviewed by Palm et al. [101, 187] each applied stimulation at 1 mA for single active sessions of 20 min, with the cathode over the seizure focus. Auvichayapat et al. [200], which was the first RCT on children with focal epilepsy, aimed to investigate safety and tolerability of cathodal tDCS in this population and so used a single session (1 mA, 20 min, electrodes at 35 cm^2). They studied 6–15-year-olds (n = 36) with focal epilepsy of various etiologies, placed the cathode over the area of greatest spike amplitude and, unlike most studies, they placed the anode over the contralateral shoulder. Patients remained on their baseline antiepileptic drugs. The stimulation was well tolerated, with one case showing an erythematous rash lasting 2 h. Epileptiform discharges dropped to 43.5% of baseline immediately after stimulation ($p = 0.0002$), and remained at 57.6% of baseline 48 h later (p = 0.0014), but rose back to baseline levels at the 4-week follow-up. There was a small but statistically significant improvement in seizure frequency in the active group only (4.8%, $p = 0.0035$).

Varga et al. [201] was a crossover trial on 6–11-year-olds (n = 5) with refractory CSWSS (continuous spikes and waves during slow wave sleep) of focal etiology. The cathode was 25 cm^2, anode was 100 cm^2, intended to increase the focality of stimulation and to avoid the opposite effect under the reference. They placed the cathode over the seizure focus (peak negativity, area of epileptiform discharges as located on a 3D voltage map) and the anode over the area of peak positivity. The patients underwent sham stimulation in the first evening, and cathodal tDCS in the second evening. Patients and caretakers were blinded to active vs. sham sessions, with continuous monitoring by an unblinded physician. The ethics committee had approved five successive tDCS sessions as long as the first session reduced the spike-index (SI). However, while well tolerated, cathodal tDCS did not reduce the SI in any patient.

The authors recounted the work of Fregni et al. [50] on adults with malformations of cortical development and refractory epilepsy, where tDCS effect was strongest in patients with a single lesion; however, that study counted epileptiform discharges away from the focus; thus, Varga et al. [201] hypothesized that tDCS effects were mainly a result of reducing epileptiform discharge propagation rather than activity at the focus itself, and that by using a smaller cathode size on their CSWSS patients, they may have missed possible effects on propagation. They then found that the spikes in 3/5 patients appeared less propagated following cathodal stimulation. This finding, if supported by future RCTs, may suggest potential uses of tDCS in epilepsy, and may also suggest that it has limited applicability in seizures that remain localized, e.g., epilepsia partialis continua (EPC).

Faria et al. [205] took a different approach, testing a simultaneous tDCS and EEG system for tolerability on 15 healthy subjects, and for proof-of-principle on two patients with refractory epilepsy (CSWSS). They used a cap with electrodes in the 10-10 system; a single EEG electrode was used as cathode (placed at CP5 in the patients), and three EEG electrodes were shorted together as anodes (FP1, FPz, FP2), thereby making stimulation more focal and leading to higher current density under the cathode than the larger anode. The protocol began immediately after reaching stage II sleep, once weekly in three sessions of 30 min each. In patients 1 and 2, the number of epileptiform discharges decreased by about 40% and 50%, respectively, in the three sessions, and decreased by 10% in Patient 2 even after tDCS. The tDCS+EEG system was well tolerated, despite having a higher electric field in the scalp. Most of the healthy volunteers reported some sensation during active stimulation, so blinding was a concern.

In another study, Auvichayapat et al. [206] performed a pilot double-blind sham-controlled RCT on 4–9-year-old children (n = 22) with Lennox–Gastaut syndrome, a severe childhood epilepsy syndrome. Subjects received their routine antiepileptic drugs (AEDs) in addition to either cathodal tDCS (2 mA over M1, corresponding to C3; 35 cm^2) or sham tDCS in 20 min sessions for 5 consecutive days. Baseline seizure frequency in the active group was 80.67 ± 54.43 seizures/day, but seizure frequency (recorded in diaries) dropped daily during treatment, down to a 99.84% reduction on Day 5 of treatment. This slowly worsened to 55.96% reduction by the 4-week follow-up. All reductions relative to sham were significant (p ranging from <0.001 to $p = 0.004$).

While cathodal tDCS reduced seizure frequency by over 50% in all seizure types, this drop in mean seizure frequency was statistically significant only in tonic, atonic, and absence seizures, rather than myoclonic and partial seizures. Additionally, on visual EEG analysis, the baseline for epileptiform discharges in the active tDCS group was 640.13 ± 263.30 events/30 min awake EEG at baseline; this decreased by 76.48% immediately after stimulation. Reductions compared to sham were statistically significant immediately after each session up to the 3-week follow-up ($p < 0.001$ to $p = 0.005$). They considered that the longer duration of stimulation and higher current density in this study compared to the previous one [200] may explain the longer duration of antiepileptic effect.

Palm et al. [187] also reported on case reports: In Yook et al. [207], an 11-year-old with bilateral perisylvian focal cortical dysplasia with a baseline of 8 seizures/month who became seizure free during the 2 weeks of treatment had 6 seizures over the following 2 months, then 1 seizure over 2 months following a second tDCS course. This suggests that repeat courses may have a cumulative effect on seizure control.

San-Juan et al. [208] reported on two patients with atypical-onset Rasmussen's encephalitis (RE) with ongoing seizures in the affected hemisphere, one of whom was an adult and the other a 17-year-old; the latter received cathodal tDCS via a subdermal needle. Both patients improved in terms of seizures, language, motor function, and level of alertness. It is important to note that both patients tolerated a small needle electrode that lead to a charge density much greater than that in previously published studies.

Tekturk et al. [209] also reported on tDCS in five patients with RE, two of whom were children with left focal seizures and epilepsia partialis continua. One child received classic cathodal stimulation while the other received an amplitude-modulated form (a sinusoidal direct current with 0.85 mA peak-to-peak intensity was added to a 1.15 mA direct current); frequency was 12 Hz (intending to target normal surrounding cortical tissue and increase inhibitory connection effects to prevent seizure generation and spread). All patients except for one adult had a greater than 50% drop in seizure frequency, and the adult and child receiving modulated cathodal tDCS had better results, suggesting that this technique should be further investigated.

Drug Effects on tDCS

It is important to note the possible effects of drugs on cathodal tDCS. In Pineda et al. [210], the antidepressant citalopram led to the abolition of cathodal tDCS-induced inhibition, changing it to facilitation. Carbamazepine and flunarizine did not affect cathodal tDCS' excitability reduction in drug studies [31, 32]. NMDA receptor antagonism blocked long-term after-effects irrespective of directionality. Lorazepam (a GABA-A agonist) had no effect on cathodal tDCS-induced diminution of excitability. However, lorazepam selectively modulated anodal tDCS effects; it delayed then selectively increased and prolonged excitability enhancements induced by anodal tDCS, an effect that was temporarily disrupted by repeating anodal tDCS stimulation. The delay was likely due to lorazepam abolishing the intracortical neuroplastic excitability enhancements induced by anodal tDCS, and the prolonged enhancement of excitability may have resulted from more remote mechanisms modulating motor cortical excitability [211]. There is a theoretical concern that cathodal tDCS may decrease the effects of GABAergics [211] and other medications.

Overall, tDCS may be considered a potential therapy for pediatric patients with various forms of epilepsy, and may be particularly useful for refractory epilepsy. Additionally, in a letter, Scorza and Brunoni [212] suggested that tDCS may potentially help prevent sudden unexpected death in epilepsy (SUDEP), e.g., by reducing generalized tonic-clonic seizures, or aborting them with home tDCS-EEG. However, more sham-controlled double-blind RCTs assessing specific outcomes are needed before we can make any definitive determinations on the efficacy of tDCS in epilepsy.

TMS in Pediatric Patients with Epilepsy

TMS measures have been used to investigate patients with epilepsy (including epileptic myoclonus), for presurgical evaluations, cortical mapping, and in evaluating the acute effects of AEDs, and their effects on MT [213–216]. Electroconvulsive therapy (ECT) has been used to terminate status epilepticus in adults and children, so there is an interest in rTMS as an alternative that is less invasive [217, 218].

A meta-analysis [219] on antiepileptic effects of low-frequency rTMS concluded that it significantly reduced seizure frequency (effect size 0.34, 95% CI 0.10–0.57), especially in neocortical epilepsy and cortical dysplasia cases (effect size 0.71, 95% CI 0.3–1.12, vs. an effect size of 0.22 in other epileptic disorders), and that the effects could last at least 2–4 weeks using the paradigm of 1–2-week stimulation. Of note, an effect size of greater than 0.5 is considered clinically meaningful [220]. The pooled effect sizes were nonsignificant for other measures such as EEG spike number, duration of epileptiform abnormalities and rMT, none of which had been tested in most studies. Overall, 11 papers (n = 164) had been included in the analysis, with 10 of them focused on medically intractable epilepsy. The studies were mostly on adults, and they also noted limitations of the analysis such as the methodological heterogeneity among the different trials, their small sample sizes, the difficulty of estimating possible confounders (e.g., AEDs) and that the analysis was on data from only active rTMS but not sham.

There have been no studies on rTMS use as a therapeutic for pediatric epilepsy patients, presumably due to the higher likelihood of risks with rTMS, leading to its use only in compelling clinical pediatric cases. Some cases are described in the literature, with variable parameters showing mixed results. A 14-year-old with RE and EPC had transient improvements in clinical and EEG seizures during rTMS application over 9 days, but returned to baseline 30 min afterward each day [221].

Rotenberg et al. [222] reported disruption of ongoing seizures by rTMS in 5/7 cases, one of which was the case above; the others were adults. They also summarized published EPC cases of various etiologies treated by rTMS (at the site of seizure focus) by then, four of whom were children. Two children received single rTMS sessions: one had seizure cessation within 24 h lasting 2 weeks, while the other had subjective clinical seizure improvement with decreased spikes on EEG [223]. Both had reduced perfusion on single-photon emission computed tomography (SPECT) in areas of rTMS application and in distal regions; Graff-Guerrero et al. [223] believed the reduction reflected decreased metabolic demands in those areas due to transient reduction of focal epileptic activity, probably due to rTMS direct effects as well synaptic connections to more distal regions [224–227]. They noted that the mechanisms of low- and high-frequency rTMS are not known, and may lead to LTD or LTP, respectively. They also suggested that low-frequency rTMS may help maintain clinical improvement but not acutely interfere with epileptic activity, as it is unlikely to give the (low frequency) pulse at the exact time that could cause a switch from a synchronized to a desynchronized state. Considering this, as well as animal studies, direct cortical stimulation and ECT where high-frequency stimulation was used to switch from a synchronized to a desynchronized state, they had decided to go with high-frequency (20 Hz) stimulation for their patients.

The two other children summarized by Rotenberg et al. [222] had EPC, and one of them had a figure-of-eight coil navigation to the fMRI-visualized seizure focus; however, neither responded to rTMS. Morales et al. [228] suggested that AEDs likely interfered with the actions of rTMS.

Rotenberg et al. [222] noted that in all the above cases, when clinical benefits did last days or longer, they were associated with low-frequency rTMS trains (0.5–1 Hz). They did not find evidence of worsening clinical or EEG seizures or epileptiform discharges with ictal rTMS overall.

There are no studies reporting on rTMS safety specifically in pediatric epilepsy cases. Pereira et al.'s [229] systematic review concluded that rTMS had only a small likelihood of inducing seizures in patients with epilepsy, and that the risk of other adverse events was similar to that of rTMS in other populations, including healthy subjects. Seynaeve and Van Paesschen [230] responded to the review by reporting on an rTMS trial on patients with refractory focal epilepsy that was unpublished at the time of review; one of the 11 patients had a rebound in seizure frequency, and another patient's seizures increased by a magnitude of 4 after active stimulation [231]. This report suggests we should exercise extra caution in pediatric patients, who tend to have greater excitability overall [190]. On the other hand, rTMS effects on the developing fetus are unknown, so in females of child-bearing age, pretreatment pregnancy tests as well as confirming abstinence or effective birth control would be prudent.

It is important to note that there are some clues that different parts of the cerebral cortex might require different types of rTMS treatment. Large, multicenter sham-controlled RCTs on rTMS (preferably combined with EEG) are thus needed to better elicit the stimulation parameters that are safe and efficacious in various epilepsy populations, and to clarify the effects of high vs. low-frequency rTMS. Additionally, the penetration of TMS tends to be more superficial than that of tDCS; therefore the selection of NIBS modes of therapy will depend greatly on the extent of the involved cortex and how well it can be targeted [232].

Movement Disorders (in Cerebral Palsy)

tDCS in Pediatric Patients with Cerebral Palsy

Stroke is the most common cause of hemiparetic cerebral palsy (CP), which is the commonest term-born CP [233–235]; motor deficits are the most disabling and prominent finding [236–238]. Newborns in the first week since birth have the highest risk of ischemic stroke, much higher than that of adults with multiple stroke risk factors; another 50% of perinatal stroke occurs later during infancy, and perinatal stroke is the top cause of hemiplegic CP [239–244]. There are two types of perinatal stroke, both leading to hemiplegic CP: arterial ischemic strokes (following major artery occlusions) and periventricular venous infarctions (subcortical white matter lesions occurring in utero before 34 weeks gestation, following germinal matrix bleeds with subsequent medullary venous infarcts).

Most pediatric placebo-controlled tDCS RCTs in pediatric populations so far have been in movement disorders due to CP. They show largely positive data on the efficacy of tDCS combined with physiotherapy.

Palm et al. [187] noted that there were several early studies utilizing pulsed transcranial electrical stimulation (electric stimuli for milliseconds with intervals in between) for CP in pediatric populations, all reporting improvement in physiotherapeutic training in active vs. sham groups, and the stimulation was tolerated well. However, the pulsed TES was no longer assessed in Europe or the USA. Recent research utilized RCTs to evaluate tDCS combined with physiotherapeutic training.

Palm et al. [187] reported on six RCTs ($n = 161$ overall) and an open-label trial ($n = 21$) on tDCS in treatment of CP. As a rehabilitative intervention, 2/6 RCTs added treadmill training, 2/6 added virtual reality (mobility training game) and 2/6 as well as the open-label trial had no training. Sham-control was utilized in 5/6 RCTs. All of the RCTs in their review placed the anode at C3 and 5/6 placed the cathode over the right supraorbital region, while 1/6 placed it on the right shoulder. They reported overall improved mobility, gait distance, body sway velocity, balance, and spasticity following anodal tDCS (over the primary motor cortex of the more affected hemisphere) combined with either standard physiotherapeutic training or as monotherapy. This effect lasted a short period after a single tDCS session, but was more sustained after a series of sessions, lasting several weeks to a few months. Collange Grecco et al. [245] reported on a sham-controlled RCT in spastic diparetic CP and noted increased MEP amplitudes after active tDCS.

An early open-label study [246] studied 21 patients 6–18 years old with a hyperkinetic form of infantile CP. They applied the anode at F1, and cathode at either C3 or the mastoid; stimulation parameters were 0.2–0.8 mA over 20–50 min, for 7–15 sessions. They reported improved proprioception, decreased postural tonic reflexes and hyperkinesia, stable for 3–5 months. Additionally, there were reduced amplitudes on resting EMG.

Overall, they found some evidence that combined tDCS and physiotherapeutics improve motor functioning; however, the studies were heterogeneous in design with short follow-ups, and longer studies with more consistent protocols are needed.

Grecco et al. [247] evaluated data from three of their previous 7-week-long double-blind sham-controlled RCTs on children aged 5–10 years with spastic hemiparetic or diparetic CP who had independent gait for a year or more. These trials combined tDCS (anode over primary motor cortex between Cz and C3 or C4, cathode over contralateral supraorbital region, 1 mA active/sham stimulation over 20 min for ten sessions over 2 weeks) with either treadmill training or gait training with virtual reality. Treadmill training had significantly better results in both active and sham groups on the 6 min walk test, walking velocity and gait profile score ($p < 0.05$ on all analyses). This was an exploratory study using a secondary analysis of previous trial data to evaluate the influence of neurophysiologic and neuroanatomic biomarkers on the results of physiotherapeutic training combined with tDCS. They found that the presence of MEP was associated with functional variables (e.g., 6 min walk test and gait speed), while the presence of subcortical injury was associated with specific variables such as gait kinematics. They also noted that in the literature, a significant number of patients with hemiparetic CP have cortical motor representations that are ipsilateral to movement, while diparetic CP cases can have ipsilateral or contralateral representations [248–250], therefore, anode placement over the more affected primary motor cortex may not be ideal. However, the groups receiving active tDCS with gait training in their trials had significant improvements; they hypothesized that the current and effects were distributed between the anode and cathode (based on modeling studies) rather than anode only, so the lower limb area may have been affected by stimulation. They concluded that there is a need for controlled trials to allow further exploration into the effects of MEPs, injury location, and the cortical representations of movement with regard to tDCS responsiveness.

Finally, we would like to mention the case of a girl who responded well to ten sessions of anodal tDCS over the latter half of speech therapy, despite poor response to traditional speech therapy over prior years [251].

To conclude, combined tDCS and physiotherapeutics have been shown to improve motor functioning in pediatric CP in heterogeneous studies, including multiple RCTs, and early literature may support well-designed trials investigating the effects of combined tDCS with speech therapy aiming to improve speech.

TMS in Pediatric Patients with Cerebral Palsy

Similar to epilepsy, therapeutic TMS/rTMS has not been well investigated in pediatric patients with CP. D'Agati et al. [252] reviewed English-language studies on rTMS in patients under 18 years of age; 6 published reports met their criteria, involving a total of 19 cases receiving rTMS at >1 Hz (including 5 with spastic CP, average age 9.8 years). Valle et al. [253] studied 17 patients (average age 9.1 years) with spastic quadriplegic CP in a double-blind sham-controlled RCT. They were randomized to either 1 or 5 Hz rTMS and received 1500 pulses/session at intensity 90% of MT, using a figure-of-eight coil; however, the pulses were applied in a continuous train in the 1 Hz group, while the 5 Hz group had the pulses divided in 5 of 1 min trains with 2 min intervals in between. A sham coil was used for the sham group ($n = 5$), half of which received 5 Hz parameters, while the other half received 1 Hz parameters.

They had hypothesized that increasing motor cortical activity would increase inhibitory input to the corticospinal tract and decrease gamma and alpha neuron hyperactivity. Quartarone et al. [254] had suggested that 5 Hz at 90% MT can increase inhibitory input to alpha motoneurons, and 1 Hz was used as a comparison to see if rTMS effects on spasticity were specific for stimulation frequency. The therapeutic effects of 5 Hz rTMS on spasticity in CP patients were modest (evaluated 2 h after the last treatment session), and were not significant in all joints and tests; however, the effects were specific to stimulation frequency (5 Hz had the largest effect), suggesting that this frequency may be beneficial. No adverse effects were encountered, and importantly, no seizures were induced by either high- or low-frequency rTMS in the patients with epilepsy.

Gupta et al. [255] reported assigning 20 pediatric patients with CP (mean age about 8 years) to either an rTMS or a control group (ten subjects in each group). The therapeutic group received rTMS at 5 Hz and 10 Hz for 15 min daily followed by 1 h of standard therapy over 20 days; the control group received the same standard therapy but no rTMS. On statistical analysis of pre- and post-therapy Modified Ashworth Scale scores, they found that the rTMS group showed a significant decrease in muscle tightness for all muscles selected for therapy ($p < 0.05$), while few muscles showed tightness reduction in the control group, suggesting that rTMS combined with therapy was potentially beneficial.

Guo et al. [256] reported on a 6-year-old with mild ataxia CP (hypoxic ischemic encephalopathy on MRI) who received rTMS to the right DLPFC 5 consecutive days/week for a total of 8 months, and had a resting-state fMRI before and after each month of rTMS. Overall, there were improvements in motor and cognitive functions on both clinical assessment and fMRI after rTMS treatment.

There is very limited data on the efficacy of rTMS in pediatric patients with CP; however, based on what we have, it may worthwhile to design RCTs evaluating high-frequency rTMS in therapy of motor function, and long-term low-frequency rTMS in therapy of motor and/or cognitive functions.

Conclusion

Various modes of non-invasive brain stimulation show promise in the treatment of neurological disorders in adults and children. The strongest evidence of therapeutic efficacy lies in rTMS treatment of major depressive disorder in adults, which has FDA approval. The heterogeneity of studies on tDCS and other forms of TMS (such as deep TMS) in therapy of various neurologic disorders (e.g., chronic pain, epilepsy, cerebral palsy) in adult and pediatric patients represents a major challenge that necessitates more well-designed sham-controlled RCTs with larger sample sizes and greater protocol standardization in order to confirm efficacy of each protocol.

While TMS and tDCS tend to be well tolerated in adult and pediatric populations overall, long-term data is rather limited, and caution is particularly important in applying rTMS to pediatric populations. Overall, the potential for NIBS to safely improve neuroplasticity and treat many neurologic disorders, particularly when added to rehabilitative therapy, is very encouraging. We look forward to enhancing our understanding of neural networks and how to treat their pathological states in future studies utilizing cutting-edge NIBS techniques.

Acknowledgement The authors would like to acknowledge Anthony T. O'Brien, MD for assistance with references.

References

1. Largus S. De compositionibus medicamentorum. In: Ruello J, editor. De compositionibus medicamentorum. Liber unus. Paris: Wechel; 1529.
2. Pascual-Leone A, Wagner T. A brief summary of the history of noninvasive brain stimulation. Supplementary appendix. Annu Rev Biomed Eng. 2007;9:1–7. https://doi.org/10.1146/annurev.bioeng.9.06.
3. Galvani A. De Viribus Electricitatis in Motu Musculari. Bologna; 1791.
4. Galvani A Memorie sull'elettricita' animale (lettera a L. Spallanzani). Bologna; 1797.
5. Lippold OC, Redfearn JW. Mental changes resulting from the passage of small direct currents through the human brain. Br J Psychiatry. 1964;110:768–72. https://doi.org/10.1192/bjp.110.469.768.
6. Sheffield LJ, Mowbray RM. The effects of polarization on normal subjects. Br J Psychiatry. 1968;114(507):225–32. https://doi.org/10.1192/bjp.114.507.225.
7. Dymond AM, Coger RW, Serafetinides EA. Intracerebral current levels in man during electrosleep therapy. Biol Psychiatry. 1975;10(1):101–4.
8. Hall KM, Hicks RA, Hopkins HK. The effects of low level DC scalp positive and negative current on the performance of various tasks. Br J Psychiatry. 1970;117(541):689–91. https://doi.org/10.1192/bjp.117.541.689.
9. Jaeger D, Elbert T, Lutzenberger W, Birbaumer N.The effects of externally applied transcephalic weak direct currents on lateralization in choice reaction tasks. J Psychophysiol. 1987;1(2):127–33.
10. Nitsche MA, Paulus W. Sustained excitability elevations induced by transcranial DC motor cortex stimulation in humans. Neurology. 2001;57(10):1899–901. http://www.ncbi.nlm.nih.gov/pubmed/11723286.
11. Nitsche MA, Paulus W. Excitability changes induced in the human motor cortex by weak transcranial direct current stimulation. J Physiol. 2000;527 Pt 3:633–9. http://doi.org/PHY_1055 [pii].
12. Priori A, Berardelli A, Rona S, Accornero N, Manfredi M. Polarization of the human motor cortex through the scalp. Neuroreport. 1998;9(10):2257–60. https://doi.org/10.1097/00001756-199807130-00020.
13. Nitsche MA, Cohen LG, Wassermann EM, Priori A, Lang N, Antal A, et al. Transcranial direct current stimulation: state of the art 2008. Brain Stimul. 2008;1(3):206–23. https://doi.org/10.1016/j.brs.2008.06.004.
14. Bickford RG, Freeming BD . Non-invasive magnetic stimulation of the human motor cortex. In: Digest of the 6th international conference of medical electronics in biology and engineering; 1965, p. 112.
15. Epstein CM, Schwartzberg DG, Davey KR, Sudderth DB. Localizing the site of magnetic brain stimulation in humans. Neurology. 1990;40(4):666–70. https://doi.org/10.1212/WNL.40.4.666.
16. Merton PA, Morton HB. Stimulation of the cerebral cortex in the intact human subject. Nature. 1980;285:22.

17. Pascual-Leone A, Gates JR, Dhuna A. Induction of speech arrest and counting errors with rapid-rate transcranial magnetic stimulation. Neurology. 1991;41(5):697–702. https://doi.org/10.1212/WNL.41.5.697.
18. Pascual-Leone A, Valls-Solé J, Wassermann EM, Hallett M. Responses to rapid-rate transcranial stimulation of the human motor cortex. Brain. 1994;117:847–58.
19. Rothwell JC, Thompson PD, Day BL, Boyd S, Marsden CD. Stimulation of the human motor cortex through the scalp. Exp Physiol. 1991;76:159–200.
20. Werhahn KJ, Fong JKY, Meyer BU, Priori A, Rothwell JC, Day BL, Thompson PD. The effect of magnetic coil orientation on the latency of surface EMG and single motor unit responses in the first dorsal interosseous muscle. Electroencephalogr Clin Neurophysiol. 1994;93(2):138–46. https://doi.org/10.1016/0168-5597(94)90077-9.
21. Rossi S, Hallett M, Rossini PM, Pascual-Leone A, Safety of TMS Consensus Group. Safety, ethical considerations, and application guidelines for the use of transcranial magnetic stimulation in clinical practice and research. Clin Neurophysiol. 2009;120(12):2008–39. https://doi.org/10.1016/j.clinph.2009.08.016.
22. Roth Y, Zangen A. Protocol for depression treatment utilizing H-coil deep brain stimulation. In: Rotenberg A, Horvath J, Pascual-Leone A, editors. Transcranial magnetic stimulation. Neuromethods, vol. 89. New York: Springer; 2014. p. 313–36. http://link.springer.com/10.1007/978-1-4939- 0879-0_15. [cited 2017 Dec 29].
23. Faraday M. Experimental researches in electricity. Thirtieth series. Philos Trans R Soc Lond. 1856;3:8–546. https://doi.org/10.1098/rstl.1856.0011.
24. Deng Z-D, Lisanby SH, Peterchev AV. Electric field depth-focality tradeoff in transcranial magnetic stimulation: simulation comparison of 50 coil designs. Brain Stimul. 2013;6(1):1–13. https://doi.org/10.1016/j.brs.2012.02.005.
25. Amassian VE, Eberle L, Maccabee PJ, Cracco RQ. Modelling magnetic coil excitation of human cerebral cortex with a peripheral nerve immersed in a brain-shaped volume conductor: the significance of fiber bending in excitation. Electroencephalogr Clin Neurophysiol. 1992;85(5):291–301. http://www.ncbi.nlm.nih.gov/pubmed/1385089.
26. Roth Y, Amir A, Levkovitz Y, Zangen A. Three-dimensional distribution of the electric field induced in the brain by transcranial magnetic stimulation using figure-8 and deep H-coils. J Clin Neurophys. 2007;24(1):31–8. https://doi.org/10.1097/WNP.0b013e31802fa393.
27. Wagner TA, Zahn M, Grodzinsky AJ, Pascual-Leone A. Three-dimensional head model simulation of transcranial magnetic stimulation. IEEE Trans Biomed Eng. 2004;51(9):1586–98. https://doi.org/10.1109/TBME.2004.827925.
28. Hamada M, Galea JM, Di Lazzaro V, Mazzone P, Ziemann U, Rothwell JC. Two distinct interneuron circuits in human motor cortex are linked to different subsets of physiological and behavioral plasticity. J Neurosci. 2014;34(38):12837–49. https://doi.org/10.1523/JNEUROSCI.1960-14.2014.
29. Mu M, Murphy SC, Palmer LM, Nyffeler T. Transcranial magnetic stimulation (TMS) inhibits cortical dendrites. Elife. 2016;5. pii: e13598. https://doi.org/10.7554/eLife.13598.
30. Zaghi S, Acar M, Hultgren B, Boggio PS, Fregni F. Noninvasive brain stimulation with low-intensity electrical currents: putative mechanisms of action for direct and alternating current stimulation. Neuroscientist. 2010;16(3):285–307. https://doi.org/10.1177/1073858409336227.
31. Liebetanz D, Nitsche MA, Tergau F, Paulus W. Pharmacological approach to the mechanisms of transcranial DC-stimulation-induced after-effects of human motor cortex excitability. Brain. 2002;125(Pt 10):2238–47. http://www.ncbi.nlm.nih.gov/pubmed/12244081.
32. Nitsche MA, Fricke K, Henschke U, Schlitterlau A, Liebetanz D, Lang N, et al. Pharmacological modulation of cortical excitability shifts induced by transcranial direct current stimulation in humans. J Physiol. 2003;553(Pt 1):293–301. https://doi.org/10.1113/jphysiol.2003.049916.
33. Boros K, Poreisz C, Münchau A, Paulus W, Nitsche MA. Premotor transcranial direct current stimulation (tDCS) affects primary motor excitability in humans. Eur J Neurosci. 2008;27(5):1292–300. https://doi.org/10.1111/j.1460-9568.2008.06090.x.
34. Vines BW, Cerruti C, Schlaug G. Dual-hemisphere tDCS facilitates greater improvements for healthy subjects' non-dominant hand compared to uni-hemisphere stimulation. BMC Neurosci. 2008;9(1):103. https://doi.org/10.1186/1471-2202-9-103.
35. Ardolino G, Bossi B, Barbieri S, Priori A. Non-synaptic mechanisms underlie the after-effects of cathodal transcutaneous direct current stimulation of the human brain. J Physiol. 2005;568(Pt 2):653–63. https://doi.org/10.1113/jphysiol.2005.088310.
36. Kwon YH, Ko M-H, Ahn SH, Kim Y-H, Song JC, Lee C-H, et al. Primary motor cortex activation by transcranial direct current stimulation in the human brain. Neurosci Lett. 2008;435(1):56–9. https://doi.org/10.1016/j.neulet.2008.02.012.
37. Lang N, Siebner HR, Ward NS, Lee L, Nitsche MA, Paulus W, et al. How does transcranial DC stimulation of the primary motor cortex alter regional neuronal activity in the human brain? Eur J Neurosci. 2005;22(2):495–504. https://doi.org/10.1111/j.1460-9568.2005.04233.x.
38. Marshall L, Mölle M, Hallschmid M, Born J. Transcranial direct current stimulation during sleep improves declarative memory. J Neurosci. 2004;24(44):9985–92. https://doi.org/10.1523/JNEUROSCI.2725-04.2004.

39. Monte-Silva K, Kuo M-F, Hessenthaler S, Fresnoza S, Liebetanz D, Paulus W, Nitsche MA. Induction of late LTP-like plasticity in the human motor cortex by repeated non-invasive brain stimulation. Brain Stimul. 2013;6(3):424–32. https://doi.org/10.1016/j.brs.2012.04.011.
40. Nitsche MA, Nitsche MS, Klein CC, Tergau F, Rothwell JC, Paulus W. Level of action of cathodal DC polarisation induced inhibition of the human motor cortex. Clin Neurophysiol. 2003;114(4):600–4. https://doi.org/10.1016/S1388-2457(02)00412-1.
41. Monte-Silva K, Kuo M-F, Liebetanz D, Paulus W, Nitsche MA. Shaping the optimal repetition interval for cathodal transcranial direct current stimulation (tDCS). J Neurophysiol. 2010;103(4):1735–40. https://doi.org/10.1152/jn.00924.2009.
42. Wankerl K, Weise D, Gentner R, Rumpf JJ, Classen J. L-type voltage-gated Ca^{2+} channels: a single molecular switch for long-term potentiation/long-term depression-like plasticity and activity-dependent metaplasticity in humans. J Neurosci. 2010;30(18):6197–204. https://doi.org/10.1523/JNEUROSCI.4673-09.2010.
43. Furubayashi T, Terao Y, Arai N, Okabe S, Mochizuki H, Hanajima R, et al. Short and long duration transcranial direct current stimulation (tDCS) over the human hand motor area. Exp Brain Res. 2008;185(2):279–86. https://doi.org/10.1007/s00221-007-1149-z.
44. Datta A, Bansal V, Diaz J, Patel J, Reato D, Bikson M. Gyri-precise head model of transcranial direct current stimulation: improved spatial focality using a ring electrode versus conventional rectangular pad. Brain Stimul. 2009;2(4):201–7, 207.e1. https://doi.org/10.1016/j.brs.2009.03.005.
45. Paulus W. Transcranial electrical stimulation (tES – tDCS; tRNS , tACS) methods. Neuropsychol Rehabil. 2011;21(5):602–17. https://doi.org/10.1080/09602011.2011.557292.
46. Wagner T, Fregni F, Fecteau S, Grodzinsky A, Zahn M, Pascual-Leone A. Transcranial direct current stimulation: a computer-based human model study. NeuroImage. 2007;35(3):1113–24. https://doi.org/10.1016/j.neuroimage.2007.01.027.
47. Poreisz C, Boros K, Antal A, Paulus W. Safety aspects of transcranial direct current stimulation concerning healthy subjects. Brain Res Bull. 2007;72(4–6):208–14.
48. Brunoni AR, Amadera J, Berbel B, Volz MS, Rizzerio BG, Fregni F. A systematic review on reporting and assessment of adverse effects associated with transcranial direct current stimulation. Int J Neuropsychopharmacol. 2011;14(8):1133–45. https://doi.org/10.1017/S1461145710001690.
49. Fregni F, Nitsche MA, Loo CK, Brunoni AR, Marangolo P, Leite J, et al. Regulatory considerations for the clinical and research use of transcranial direct current stimulation (tDCS): review and recommendations from an expert panel. Clin Res Regul Aff. 2015;32(1):22–35. https://doi.org/10.3109/10601333.2015.980944.
50. Fregni F, Thome-Souza S, Nitsche MA, Freedman SD, Valente KD, Pascual-Leone A. A controlled clinical trial of cathodal DC polarization in patients with refractory epilepsy. Epilepsia. 2006;47(2):335–42. https://doi.org/10.1111/j.1528-1167.2006.00426.x.
51. Muszkat D, Polanczyk GV, Dias TGC, Brunoni AR. Transcranial direct current stimulation in child and adolescent psychiatry. J Child Adolesc Psychopharmacol. 2016;26(7):590–7. https://doi.org/10.1089/cap.2015.0172.
52. Reardon JPO, Solvason HB, Janicak PG, Sampson S, Isenberg KE, Nahas Z, et al. Efficacy and safety of transcranial magnetic stimulation in the acute treatment of major depression: a multisite randomized controlled trial. Biol Psychiatry. 2007;62(11):1208–16. https://doi.org/10.1016/j.biopsych.2007.01.018.
53. Wassermann EM. Risk and safety of repetitive transcranial magnetic stimulation: report and suggested guidelines from the International Workshop on the Safety of Repetitive Transcranial Magnetic Stimulation, June 5-7, 1996. Electroencephalogr Clin Neurophysiol. 1998;108(1):1–16. https://doi.org/10.1016/S0168-5597(97)00096-8.
54. Machii K, Cohen D, Ramos-Estebanez C, Pascual-Leone A. Safety of rTMS to non-motor cortical areas in healthy participants and patients. Clin Neurophysiol. 2006;117(2):455–71. https://doi.org/10.1016/j.clinph.2005.10.014.
55. Counter SA, Borg E, Lofqvist L, Brismar T. Hearing loss from the acoustic artifact of the coil used in extracranial magnetic stimulation. Neurology. 1990;40(8):1159–62. https://doi.org/10.1212/WNL.40.8.1159.
56. Pascual-Leone A, Cohen LG, Shotland LI, Dang N, Pikus A, Wassermannn EM, et al. No evidence of hearing loss in humans due to transcranial magnetic stimulation. Neurlology. 1992;42:647–51.
57. Loo C, Sachdev P, Elsayed H, McDarmont B, Mitchell P, Wilkinson M, et al. Effects of a 2- to 4-week course of repetitive transcranial magnetic stimulation (rTMS) on neuropsychologic functioning, electroencephalogram, and auditory threshold in depressed patients. Biol Psychiatry. 2001;49(7):615–23. https://doi.org/10.1016/S0006-3223(00)00996-3.
58. Folmer RL, Carroll JR, Rahim A, Shi Y, Hal Martin W. Effects of repetitive transcranial magnetic stimulation (rTMS) on chronic tinnitus. Acta Otolaryngol Suppl. 2006;(556):96–101. https://doi.org/10.1080/03655230600895465.
59. Collado-Corona MA, Mora-Magana I, Cordero GL, Toral-Martinon R, Shkurovich-Zaslavsky M, Ruiz-Garcia M, Gonzalez-Astiazaran A. Transcranial magnetic stimulation and acoustic trauma or hearing loss in children. Neurol Res. 2001;23(4):343–6. https://doi.org/10.1179/016164101101198532.
60. Bae EH, Schrader LM, Machii K, Alonso-Alonso M, Riviello JJ Jr, Pascual-Leone A, Rotenberg A. Safety and tolerability of repetitive transcranial magnetic

stimulation in patients with epilepsy: a review of the literature. Epilepsy Behav. 2007;10(4):521–8.

61. Rossi S, Pasqualetti P, Rossini PM, Feige B, Ulivelli M, Glocker FX, et al. Effects of repetitive transcranial magnetic stimulation on movement-related cortical activity in humans. Cereb Cortex. 2000;10(8):802–8. https://doi.org/10.1093/cercor/10.8.802.
62. Hansenne M, Laloyaux O, Mardaga S, Ansseau M. Impact of low frequency transcranial magnetic stimulation on event-related brain potentials. Biol Psychol. 2004;67(3):331–41. https://doi.org/10.1016/j.biopsycho.2004.01.004.
63. Holler I, Siebner HR, Cunnington R, Gerschlager W. 5 Hz repetitive TMS increases anticipatory motor activity in the human cortex. Neurosci Lett. 2006;392(3):221–5. https://doi.org/10.1016/j.neulet.2005.09.018.
64. Loo CK, McFarquhar TF, Mitchell PB. A review of the safety of repetitive transcranial magnetic stimulation as a clinical treatment for depression. Int J Neuropsychopharmacol. 2008;11(1):131–47. https://doi.org/10.1017/S1461145707007717.
65. Zwanzger P, Ella R, Keck ME, Rupprecht R, Padberg F. Occurrence of delusions during repetitive transcranial magnetic stimulation (rTMS) in major depression. Biol Psychiatry. 2002;51(7):602–3. http://doi.org/S0006322301013695 [pii].
66. Janicak PG, O'Reardon JP, Sampson SM, Husain MM, Lisanby SH, Rado JT, et al. Transcranial magnetic stimulation in the treatment of major depressive disorder: a comprehensive summary of safety experience from acute exposure, extended exposure, and during reintroduction treatment. J Clin Psychiatry. 2008;69(2):222–32. http://doi.org/ej07m03619 [pii].
67. Xia G, Gajwani P, Muzina DJ, Kemp DE, Gao K, Ganocy SJ, Calabrese JR. Treatment-emergent mania in unipolar and bipolar depression: focus on repetitive transcranial magnetic stimulation. Int J Neuropsychopharmacol. 2008;11(1):119–30. https://doi.org/10.1017/S1461145707007699.
68. McClintock SM, Freitas C, Oberman L, Lisanby SH, Pascual-Leone A. Transcranial magnetic stimulation: a neuroscientific probe of cortical function in schizophrenia. Biol Psychiatry. 2011;70(1):19–27. https://doi.org/10.1016/j.biopsych.2011.02.031.
69. Bruckmann S, Hauk D, Roessner V, Resch F, Freitag CM, Kammer T, et al. Cortical inhibition in attention deficit hyperactivity disorder: new insights from the electroencephalographic response to transcranial magnetic stimulation. Brain. 2012;135(Pt 7):2215–30. https://doi.org/10.1093/brain/aws071.
70. Jackson SR, Parkinson A, Manfredi V, Millon G, Hollis C, Jackson GM. Motor excitability is reduced prior to voluntary movements in children and adolescents with Tourette syndrome. J Neuropsychol. 2013;7(1):29–44. https://doi.org/10.1111/j.1748-6653.2012.02033.x.
71. Vry J, Linder-Lucht M, Berweck S, Bonati U, Hodapp M, Uhl M, et al. Altered cortical inhibitory function in children with spastic diplegia: a TMS study. Exp Brain Res. 2008;186(4):611–8. https://doi.org/10.1007/s00221-007-1267-7.
72. Garvey MA, Mall V. Transcranial magnetic stimulation in children. Clin Neurophysiol. 2008;119(5):973–84. https://doi.org/10.1016/j.clinph.2007.11.048.
73. Benali A, Trippe J, Weiler E, Mix A, Petrasch-Parwez E, Girzalsky W, et al. Theta-burst transcranial magnetic stimulation alters cortical inhibition. J Neurosci. 2011;31(4):1193–203. https://doi.org/10.1523/JNEUROSCI.1379-10.2011.
74. Stagg CJ, Wylezinska M, Matthews PM, Johansen-Berg H, Jezzard P, Rothwell JC, Bestmann S. Neurochemical effects of theta burst stimulation as assessed by magnetic resonance spectroscopy. J Neurophysiol. 2009;101(6):2872–7. https://doi.org/10.1152/jn.91060.2008.
75. Horvath JC, Najib U, Press D. Transcranial magnetic stimulation (TMS) clinical applications: therapeutics. 2014. https://doi.org/10.1007/978-1-4939-0879-0_12.
76. Burt T, Lisanby SH, Sackeim HA. Neuropsychiatric applications of transcranial magnetic stimulation: a meta analysis. Int J Neuropsychopharmacol. 2002;5(1):73–103.https://doi.org/10.1017/S1461145702002791.
77. Herrmann LL, Ebmeier KP. Factors modifying the efficacy of transcranial magnetic stimulation in the treatment of depression: a review. J Clin Psychiatry. 2006;67(12):1870–6. http://www.ncbi.nlm.nih.gov/pubmed/17194264.
78. Holtzheimer PE, Russo J, Avery DH. A meta-analysis of repetitive transcranial magnetic stimulation in the treatment of depression. Psychopharmacol Bull. 2001;35(4):149–69. http://www.ncbi.nlm.nih.gov/pubmed/12397863.
79. Martin JLR, Barbanoj MJ, Schlaepfer TE, Thompson E, Pérez V, Kulisevsky J. Repetitive transcranial magnetic stimulation for the treatment of depression. Systematic review and meta-analysis. Br J Psychiatry. 2003;182:480–91. http://www.ncbi.nlm.nih.gov/pubmed/12777338.
80. McNamara B, Ray JL, Arthurs OJ, Boniface S. Transcranial magnetic stimulation for depression and other psychiatric disorders. Psychol Med. 2001;31(7):1141–6. http://www.ncbi.nlm.nih.gov/pubmed/11681540.
81. Schutter DJLG. Antidepressant efficacy of high-frequency transcranial magnetic stimulation over the left dorsolateral prefrontal cortex in double-blind sham-controlled designs: a meta-analysis. Psychol Med. 2009;39(1):65–75. https://doi.org/10.1017/S0033291708003462.
82. Slotema CW, Blom JD, Hoek HW, Sommer IEC. Should we expand the toolbox of psychiatric treatment methods to include Repetitive Transcranial Magnetic Stimulation (rTMS)? A meta-analysis of the efficacy of rTMS in psychiatric disorders. J Clin Psychiatry. 2010;71(7):873–84. https://doi.org/10.4088/JCP.08m04872gre.

83. Greden JF. The burden of disease for treatment-resistant depression. J Clin Psychiatry. 2001;62(Suppl 16):26–31. http://www.ncbi.nlm.nih.gov/pubmed/11480881.
84. Horvath JC, Najib U, Press D. Transcranial magnetic stimulation (TMS) clinical applications: therapeutics. In: Rotenberg A, Horvath J, Pascual-Leone A, editors. Transcranial magnetic stimulation. Neuromethods, vol. 89. New York: Springer. https://doi.org/10.1007/978-1-4939-0879-0_14.
85. George MS, Lisanby SH, Avery D, McDonald WM, Durkalski V, Pavlicova M, et al. Daily left prefrontal transcranial magnetic stimulation therapy for major depressive disorder: a sham-controlled randomized trial. Arch Gen Psychiatry. 2010;67(5):507–16. https://doi.org/10.1001/archgenpsychiatry.2010.46.
86. Rosenberg PB, Mehndiratta RB, Mehndiratta YP, Wamer A, Rosse RB, Balish M. Repetitive transcranial magnetic stimulation treatment of comorbid posttraumatic stress disorder and major depression. J Neuropsychiatry Clin Neurosci. 2002;14(3):270–6. https://doi.org/10.1176/jnp.14.3.270.
87. Levkovitz Y, Isserles M, Padberg F, Lisanby SH, Bystritsky A, Xia G, et al. Efficacy and safety of deep transcranial magnetic stimulation for major depression: a prospective multicenter randomized controlled trial. World Psychiatry. 2015;14(1):64–73. https://doi.org/10.1002/wps.20199.
88. Fox MD, Buckner RL, White MP, Greicius MD, Pascual-Leone A. Efficacy of transcranial magnetic stimulation targets for depression is related to intrinsic functional connectivity with the subgenual cingulate. Biol Psychiatry. 2012;72(7):595–603. https://doi.org/10.1016/j.biopsych.2012.04.028.
89. Fox MD, Halko MA, Eldaief MC, Pascual-Leone A. Measuring and manipulating brain connectivity with resting state functional connectivity magnetic resonance imaging (fcMRI) and transcranial magnetic stimulation (TMS). NeuroImage. 2012;62(4):2232–43. https://doi.org/10.1016/j.neuroimage.2012.03.035.
90. Mayberg HS, Lozano AM, Voon V, McNeely HE, Seminowicz D, Hamani C, et al. Deep brain stimulation for treatment-resistant depression. Neuron. 2005;45(5):651–60. https://doi.org/10.1016/j.neuron.2005.02.014.
91. Roth Y, Pell GS, Chistyakov AV, Sinai A, Zangen A, Zaaroor M. Motor cortex activation by H-coil and figure-8 coil at different depths. Combined motor threshold and electric field distribution study. Clin Neurophysiol. 2014;125(2):336–43. https://doi.org/10.1016/j.clinph.2013.07.013.
92. Roth Y, Zangen A, Hallett M. A coil design for transcranial magnetic stimulation of deep brain regions. J Clin Neurophysiol. 2002;19(4):361–70. http://www.ncbi.nlm.nih.gov/pubmed/12436090.
93. Zangen A, Roth Y, Voller B, Hallett M. Transcranial magnetic stimulation of deep brain regions: evidence for efficacy of the H-coil. Clin Neurophysiol. 2005;116(4):775–9. https://doi.org/10.1016/j.clinph.2004.11.008.
94. Kedzior KK, Gellersen HM, Brachetti AK, Berlim MT. Deep transcranial magnetic stimulation (DTMS) in the treatment of major depression: An exploratory systematic review and meta-analysis. J Affect Disord. 2015;187:73–83. https://doi.org/10.1016/j.jad.2015.08.033.
95. Berlim MT, Van den Eynde F, Tovar-Perdomo S, Chachamovich E, Zangen A, Turecki G. Augmenting antidepressants with deep transcranial magnetic stimulation (DTMS) in treatment-resistant major depression. World J Biol Psychiatry. 2014;15(7):570–8. https://doi.org/10.3109/15622975.2014.925141.
96. Bersani FS, Minichino A, Enticott PG, Mazzarini L, Khan N, Antonacci G, et al. Deep transcranial magnetic stimulation as a treatment for psychiatric disorders: a comprehensive review. Eur Psychiatry. 2013;28(1):30–9. https://doi.org/10.1016/j.eurpsy.2012.02.006.
97. Fournier JC, DeRubeis RJ, Hollon SD, Dimidjian S, Amsterdam JD, Shelton RC, Fawcett J. Antidepressant drug effects and depression severity: a patient-level meta-analysis. JAMA. 2010;303(1):47–53. https://doi.org/10.1001/jama.2009.1943.
98. Levkovitz Y, Harel EV, Roth Y, Braw Y, Most D, Katz LN, et al. Deep transcranial magnetic stimulation over the prefrontal cortex: evaluation of antidepressant and cognitive effects in depressive patients. Brain Stimul. 2009;2(4):188–200. https://doi.org/10.1016/j.brs.2009.08.002.
99. Minichino A, Bersani FS, Capra E, Pannese R, Bonanno C, Salviati M, et al. ECT, rTMS, and deepTMS in pharmacoresistant drug-free patients with unipolar depression: a comparative review. Neuropsychiatr Dis Treat. 2012;8:55–64. https://doi.org/10.2147/NDT.S27025.
100. Rosenberg O, Isserles M, Levkovitz Y, Kotler M, Zangen A, Dannon PN. Effectiveness of a second deep TMS in depression: a brief report. Prog Neuropsychopharmacol Biol Psychiatry. 2011;35(4):1041–4. https://doi.org/10.1016/j.pnpbp.2011.02.015.
101. Palm U, Hasan A, Strube W, Padberg F. tDCS for the treatment of depression: a comprehensive review. Eur Arch Psychiatry Clin Neurosci. 2016;266(8):681–94. https://doi.org/10.1007/s00406-016-0674-9.
102. Boggio PS, Rigonatti SP, Ribeiro RB, Myczkowski ML, Nitsche MA, Pascual-Leone A, Fregni F. A randomized, double-blind clinical trial on the efficacy of cortical direct current stimulation for the treatment of major depression. Int J Neuropsychopharmacol. 2008;11(2):249–54. https://doi.org/10.1017/S1461145707007833.
103. Rigonatti SP, Boggio PS, Myczkowski ML, Otta E, Fiquer JT, Ribeiro RB, et al. Transcranial direct stimulation and fluoxetine for the treatment of depression. Eur Psychiatry. 2008;23(1):74–6. https://doi.org/10.1016/j.eurpsy.2007.09.006.
104. Brunoni AR, Valiengo L, Baccaro A, Zanão TA, de Oliveira JF, Goulart A, et al. The sertraline vs. electrical current therapy for treating depression clinical

study: results from a factorial, randomized, controlled trial. JAMA Psychiatry. 2013;70(4):383–91. https://doi.org/10.1001/2013.jamapsychiatry.32.

105. Meron D, Hedger N, Garner M, Baldwin DS. Transcranial direct current stimulation (tDCS) in the treatment of depression: systematic review and meta-analysis of efficacy and tolerability. Neurosci Biobehav Rev. 2015;57:46–62. https://doi.org/10.1016/j.neubiorev.2015.07.012.
106. Martin DM, Alonzo A, Ho K-A, Player M, Mitchell PB, Sachdev P, Loo CK. Continuation transcranial direct current stimulation for the prevention of relapse in major depression. J Affect Disord. 2013;144(3):274–8. https://doi.org/10.1016/j.jad.2012.10.012.
107. Valiengo L, Benseñor IM, Goulart AC, de Oliveira JF, Zanao TA, Boggio PS, et al. The sertraline versus electrical current therapy for treating depression clinical study (select-TDCS): results of the crossover and follow-up phases. Depress Anxiety. 2013;30(7):646–53. https://doi.org/10.1002/da.22079.
108. Dell'Osso B, Oldani L, Camuri G, Dobrea C, Cremaschi L, Benatti B, et al. Augmentative repetitive Transcranial Magnetic Stimulation (rTMS) in the acute treatment of poor responder depressed patients: a comparison study between high and low frequency stimulation. Eur Psychiatry. 2015;30(2):271–6. https://doi.org/10.1016/j.eurpsy.2014.12.001.
109. O'Connell NE, Cossar J, Marston L, Wand BM, Bunce D, Moseley GL, De Souza LH. Rethinking clinical trials of transcranial direct current stimulation: participant and assessor blinding is inadequate at intensities of 2mA. PLoS One. 2012;7(10):e47514. https://doi.org/10.1371/journal.pone.0047514.
110. Palm U, Reisinger E, Keeser D, Kuo M-F, Pogarell O, Leicht G, et al. Evaluation of sham transcranial direct current stimulation for randomized, placebo-controlled clinical trials. Brain Stimul. 2013;6(4):690–5. https://doi.org/10.1016/j.brs.2013.01.005.
111. Brunoni AR, Moffa AH, Sampaio-Júnior B, Gálvez V, Loo CK. Treatment-emergent mania/hypomania during antidepressant treatment with transcranial direct current stimulation (tDCS): a systematic review and meta-analysis. Brain Stimul. 2017;10(2):260–2. https://doi.org/10.1016/j.brs.2016.11.005.
112. Nitsche MA, Müller-Dahlhaus F, Paulus W, Ziemann U. The pharmacology of neuroplasticity induced by non-invasive brain stimulation: building models for the clinical use of CNS active drugs. J Physiol. 2012;590(19):4641–62. https://doi.org/10.1113/jphysiol.2012.232975.
113. Al-Kaysi AM, Al-Ani A, Loo CK, Breakspear M, Boonstra TW, Al-Kaysi AM, et al. Predicting brain stimulation treatment outcomes of depressed patients through the classification of EEG oscillations. In: Conference proceedings: ... annual international conference of the IEEE Engineering in Medicine and Biology Society. IEEE Engineering in Medicine and Biology Society. Annual conference; 2016, p. 5266–9. https://doi.org/10.1109/EMBC.2016.7591915.
114. Tsubokawa T, Katayama Y, Yamamoto T, Hirayama T, Koyama S. Treatment of thalamic pain by chronic motor cortex stimulation. Pacing Clin Electrophysiol. 1991;14(1):131–4. https://doi.org/10.1111/j.1540-8159.1991.tb04058.x.
115. Tsubokawa T, Katayama Y, Yamamoto T, Hirayama T, Koyama S. Chronic motor cortex stimulation for the treatment of central pain. Acta Neurochir Suppl. 1991;52:137–9.
116. Lefaucheur J-P, Drouot X, Cunin P, Bruckert R, Lepetit H, Creange A, et al. Motor cortex stimulation for the treatment of refractory peripheral neuropathic pain. Brain. 2009;132(Pt 6):1463–71.
117. Nguyen J-P, Velasco F, Brugieres P, Velasco M, Keravel Y, Boleaga B, et al. Treatment of chronic neuropathic pain by motor cortex stimulation: results of a bicentric controlled crossover trial. Brain Stimul. 2008;1(2):89–96. https://doi.org/10.1016/j.brs.2008.03.007.
118. Velasco F, Argüelles C, Carrillo-Ruiz JD, Castro G, Velasco AL, Jiménez F, Velasco M. Efficacy of motor cortex stimulation in the treatment of neuropathic pain: a randomized double-blind trial. J Neurosurg. 2008;108(4):698–706.
119. Nizard J, Raoul S, Nguyen J-P, Lefaucheur J-P. Invasive stimulation therapies for the treatment of refractory pain. Discov Med. 2012;14(77):237–46.
120. Nguyen JP, Lefaucheur JP, Raoul S, Roualdes V, Péréon Y, Keravel Y. Motor cortex stimulation for the treatment of neuropathic pain. Neuromodulation. 2009;1:515–26. https://doi.org/10.1016/B978-0-12-374248-3.00041-0.
121. Lefaucheur JP, Nguyen JP, Drouot X, Pollin B, Keravel Y, H. A. Chronic pain treated by rTMS of motor cortex. Electroencephalogr Clin Neurophysiol. 1998;107:92.
122. Cahana A, Carota A, Annoni JM. The long-term effect of repeated intravenous lidocaine on central pain and possible correlation in positron emission tomography measurements. Anesth Analg. 2004;98(6):1581–4. https://doi.org/10.1213/01.ANE.0000113258.31039.C8.
123. De Salles AAF, Bittar GT. Thalamic pain syndrome: anatomic and metabolic correlation. Surg Neurol. 1994;41(2):147–51. https://doi.org/10.1016/0090-3019(94)90113-9.
124. Di Piero V, Jones AKP, Iannotti F, Powell M, Perani D, Lenzi GL, Frackowiak RSJ. Chronic pain: a PET study of the central effects of percutaneous high cervical cordotomy. Pain. 1991;46(1):9–12. https://doi.org/10.1016/0304-3959(91)90026-T.
125. Garcia-Larrea L, Maarrawi J, Peyron R, Costes N, Mertens P, Magnin M, Laurent B. On the relation between sensory deafferentation, pain and thalamic activity in Wallenberg's syndrome: a PET-scan study before and after motor cortex stimulation. Eur J Pain. 2006;10(8):677–88. https://doi.org/10.1016/j.ejpain.2005.10.008.

126. Henderson LA, Peck CC, Petersen ET, Rae CD, Youssef AM, Reeves JM, et al. Chronic pain: lost inhibition? J Neurosci. 2013;33(17):7574–82. https://doi.org/10.1523/JNEUROSCI.0174-13.2013.
127. Hirato M, Horikoshi S, Kawashima Y, Satake K, Shibasaki T, Ohye C. The possible role of the cerebral cortex adjacent to the central sulcus for the genesis of central (thalamic) pain—a metabolic study. Acta Neurochir Suppl. 1993;58:141–4.
128. Hirato M, Kawashima Y, Shibazaki T, Shibasaki T, Ohye C. Pathophysiology of central (thalamic) pain: a possible role of the intralaminar nuclei in superficial pain. Acta Neurochir Suppl. 1991;52:133–6.
129. Baliki MN, Apkarian AV. Nociception, pain, negative moods, and behavior selection. Neuron. 2015;87(3):474–91. https://doi.org/10.1016/j.neuron.2015.06.005.
130. Gustin SM, Wrigley PJ, Siddall PJ, Henderson LA. Brain anatomy changes associated with persistent neuropathic pain following spinal cord injury. Cereb Cortex. 2010;20(6):1409–19. https://doi.org/10.1093/cercor/bhp205.
131. Pattany PM, Yezierski RP, Widerstrom-Noga EG, Bowen BC, Martinez-Arizala A, Garcia BR, Quencer RM. Proton magnetic resonance spectroscopy of the thalamus in patients with chronic neuropathic pain after spinal cord injury. AJNR Am J Neuroradiol. 2002;23(6):901–5.
132. Ngernyam N, Jensen MP, Arayawichanon P, Auvichayapat N, Tiamkao S, Janjarasjitt S, et al. The effects of transcranial direct current stimulation in patients with neuropathic pain from spinal cord injury. Clin Neurophysiol. 2015;126(2):382–90. https://doi.org/10.1016/j.clinph.2014.05.034.
133. Sarnthein J, Jeanmonod. High thalamocortical theta coherence in patients with neurogenic pain. NeuroImage. 2008;39(4):1910–7.
134. Llinás RR, Ribary U, Jeanmonod D, Kronberg E, Mitra PP. Thalamocortical dysrhythmia: a neurological and neuropsychiatric syndrome characterized by magnetoencephalography. Proc Natl Acad Sci U S A.1999;96(26):15222–7. https://doi.org/10.1073/pnas.96.26.15222.
135. Geha PY, Baliki MN, Harden RN, Bauer WR, Parrish TB, Apkarian AV. The brain in chronic CRPS pain: abnormal gray-white matter interactions in emotional and autonomic regions. Neuron. 2008;60(4):570–81. https://doi.org/10.1016/j.neuron.2008.08.022.
136. Kucyi A, Moayedi M, Weissman-Fogel I, Goldberg MB, Freeman BV, Tenenbaum HC, Davis KD. Enhanced medial prefrontal-default mode network functional connectivity in chronic pain and its association with pain rumination. J Neurosci. 2014;34(11):3969–75. https://doi.org/10.1523/JNEUROSCI.5055-13.2014.
137. Hashmi JA, Baliki MN, Huang L, Baria AT, Torbey S, Hermann KM, et al. Shape shifting pain: chronification of back pain shifts brain representation from nociceptive to emotional circuits. Brain. 2013;136(Pt 9):2751–68. https://doi.org/10.1093/brain/awt211.
138. André-Obadia N, Mertens P, Gueguen A, Peyron R, Garcia-Larrea L. Pain relief by rTMS: differential effect of current flow but no specific action on pain subtypes. Neurology. 2008;71(11):833–40. https://doi.org/10.1212/01.wnl.0000325481.61471.f0.
139. Goto T, Saitoh Y, Hashimoto N, Hirata M, Kishima H, Oshino S, et al. Diffusion tensor fiber tracking in patients with central post-stroke pain; correlation with efficacy of repetitive transcranial magnetic stimulation. Pain. 2008;140(3):509–18. https://doi.org/10.1016/j.pain.2008.10.009.
140. Lefaucheur J-P, Drouot X, Menard-Lefaucheur I, Zerah F, Bendib B, Cesaro P, et al. Neurogenic pain relief by repetitive transcranial magnetic cortical stimulation depends on the origin and the site of pain. J Neurol Neurosurg Psychiatry. 2004;75(4):612–6. https://doi.org/10.1136/jnnp.2003.022236.
141. Lefaucheur J-P, Drouot X, Ménard-Lefaucheur I, Keravel Y, Nguyen J-P. Motor cortex rTMS in chronic neuropathic pain: pain relief is associated with thermal sensory perception improvement. J Neurol Neurosurg Psychiatry. 2008;79(9):1044–9. https://doi.org/10.1136/jnnp.2007.135327.
142. Lefaucheur JP, Holsheimer J, Goujon C, Keravel Y, Nguyen JP. Descending volleys generated by efficacious epidural motor cortex stimulation in patients with chronic neuropathic pain. Exp Neurol. 2010;223(2):609–14.
143. Ahmed MA, Mohamed SA, Sayed D. Long-term antalgic effects of repetitive transcranial magnetic stimulation of motor cortex and serum beta-endorphin in patients with phantom pain. Neurol Res. 2011;33(9):953–8. https://doi.org/10.1179/1743132811Y.0000000045.
144. Tamura Y, Okabe S, Ohnishi T, Saito DN, Arai N. Effects of 1-Hz repetitive transcranial magnetic stimulation on acute pain induced by capsaicin. Prog Brain Res. 2004;107:107–15. https://doi.org/10.1016/j.pain.2003.10.011.
145. Taylor JJ, Borckardt JJ, Canterberry M, Li X, Hanlon CA, Brown TR, George MS. Naloxone-reversible modulation of pain circuitry by left prefrontal rTMS. Neuropsychopharmacology. 2013;38(7):1189–97. https://doi.org/10.1038/npp.2013.13.
146. Taylor JJ, Borckardt JJ, George MS. Endogenous opioids mediate left dorsolateral prefrontal cortex rTMS-induced analgesia. Pain. 2012;153(6):1219–25. https://doi.org/10.1016/j.pain.2012.02.030.
147. Fierro B, De TM, Giglia F, Giglia G, Palermo A, Brighina F. Repetitive transcranial magnetic stimulation (rTMS) of the dorsolateral prefrontal cortex (DLPFC) during capsaicin-induced pain: modulatory effects on motor cortex excitability. Exp Brain Res. 2010;203(1):31–8.
148. Lefaucheur JP, Ayache SS, Sorel M, Farhat WH, Zouari HG, Ciampi De Andrade D, et al. Analgesic effects of repetitive transcranial magnetic stimulation of the motor cortex in neuropathic pain: influence of theta burst stimulation priming.

Eur J Pain. 2012;16(10):1403–13. https://doi.org/10.1002/j.1532-2149.2012.00150.x.

149. Mhalla A, Baudic S, Ciampi D, Andrade D, Gautron M, Perrot S, et al. Long-term maintenance of the analgesic effects of transcranial magnetic stimulation in fibromyalgia. Pain. 2011;152(7):1478–85. https://doi.org/10.1016/j.pain.2011.01.034.

150. Wagner T, Valero-Cabre A, Pascual-Leone A. Noninvasive human brain stimulation. Annu Rev Biomed Eng. 2007;9:527–65. https://doi.org/10.1146/annurev.bioeng.9.061206.133100.

151. Yoon E, Kim Y, Kim H. Transcranial direct current stimulation to lessen neuropathic pain after spinal cord injury a mechanistic PET study. Neurorehabil Neural Repair. 2014;28:250–9.

152. Antal A, Terney D, Kühnl S, Paulus W. Anodal transcranial direct current stimulation of the motor cortex ameliorates chronic pain and reduces short intracortical inhibition. J Pain Symptom Manage. 2010;39(5):890–903. https://doi.org/10.1016/j.jpainsymman.2009.09.023.

153. DosSantos MF, Love TM, Martikainen IK, Nascimento TD, Fregni F, Cummiford C, et al. Immediate effects of tDCS on the μ-opioid system of a chronic pain patient. Front Psychiatry. 2012;3:93. https://doi.org/10.3389/fpsyt.2012.00093.

154. Andre-Obadia N, Peyron R, Mertens P, Mauguiere F, Laurent B, Garcia-Larrea L. Transcranial magnetic stimulation for pain control. Double-blind study of different frequencies against placebo, and correlation with motor cortex stimulation efficacy. Clin Neurophysiol. 2006;117:1536–44.

155. Lefaucheur JP, Drouot X, Keravel Y, Nguyen JP. Pain relief induced by repetitive transcranial magnetic stimulation of precentral cortex. Neuroreport. 2001;12(13):2963–5. https://doi.org/10.1097/00001756-200109170-00041.

156. Saitoh Y, Hirayama A, Kishima H, Shimokawa T, Oshino S, Hirata M, et al. Reduction of intractable deafferentation pain due to spinal cord or peripheral lesion by high-frequency repetitive transcranial magnetic stimulation of the primary motor cortex. J Neurosurg. 2007;107(3):555–9. https://doi.org/10.3171/JNS-07/09/0555.

157. Lefaucheur J, André-Obadia N. Evidence-based guidelines on the therapeutic use of repetitive transcranial magnetic stimulation (rTMS). Clin Neurophysiol. 2014;125:1250–06.

158. Lefaucheur JP, Drouot X, Nguyen JP. Interventional neurophysiology for pain control: duration of pain relief following repetitive transcranial magnetic stimulation of the motor cortex. Neurophysiol Clin. 2001;31(4):247–52. https://doi.org/10.1016/S0987-7053(01)00260-X.

159. Rollnik JD, Wustefeld S, Dauper J, Karst M, Fink M, Kossev A, Dengler R. Repetitive transcranial magnetic stimulation for the treatment of chronic pain—a pilot study. Eur Neurol. 2002;48:6–10.

160. Fricova J, Klirova M, Masopust V, Novak T, Verebova K, Rokyta R. Repetitive transcranial magnetic stimulation in the treatment of chronic orofacial pain. Physiol Res. 2013;62(Suppl 1):S125–34.

161. Hosomi K, Shimokawa T, Ikoma K, Nakamura Y, Sugiyama K, Ugawa Y, et al. Daily repetitive transcranial magnetic stimulation of primary motor cortex for neuropathic pain: a randomized, multicenter, double-blind, crossover, sham-controlled trial. Pain. 2013;154(7):1065–72. https://doi.org/10.1016/j.pain.2013.03.016.

162. Khedr EM, Kotb HI, Mostafa MG, Mohamad MF, Amr SA, Ahmed MA, Karim AA. Repetitive transcranial magnetic stimulation in neuropathic pain secondary to malignancy: a randomized clinical trial. Eur J Pain. 2015;19:519–27. https://doi.org/10.1002/ejp.576.

163. Khedr EM, Kotb H, Kamel NF, Ahmed MA, Sadek R, Rothwell JC. Longlasting antalgic effects of daily sessions of repetitive transcranial magnetic stimulation in central and peripheral neuropathic pain. J Neurol Neurosurg Psychiatry. 2005;76(6):833–8. https://doi.org/10.1136/jnnp.2004.055806.

164. Hodaj H, Alibeu J-P, Payen J-F, Lefaucheur J-P. Treatment of chronic facial pain including cluster headache by repetitive transcranial magnetic stimulation of the motor cortex with maintenance sessions: a naturalistic study. Brain Stimul. 2015;8(4):801–7. https://doi.org/10.1016/j.brs.2015.01.416.

165. Pommier B, Créac'h C, Beauvieux V, Nuti C, Vassal F, Peyron R. Robot-guided neuronavigated rTMS as an alternative therapy for central (neuropathic) pain: clinical experience and long-term follow-up. Eur J Pain. 2016;20(6):907–16. https://doi.org/10.1002/ejp.815.

166. Lefaucheur J-P. Cortical neurostimulation for neuropathic pain. Pain. 2016;157:S81–9. https://doi.org/10.1097/j.pain.0000000000000401.

167. Fregni F, Boggio PS, Lima MC, Ferreira MJL, Wagner T, Rigonatti SP, et al. A sham-controlled, phase II trial of transcranial direct current stimulation for the treatment of central pain in traumatic spinal cord injury. Pain. 2006;122(1–2):197–209. https://doi.org/10.1016/j.pain.2006.02.023.

168. Fregni F, Gimenes R, Valle AC. A randomized, sham-controlled, proof of principle study of transcranial direct current stimulation for the treatment of pain in fibromyalgia. Arthritis Rheum. 2006;54(12):3988–98.

169. Bolognini N, Olgiati E, Maravita A, Ferraro F, Fregni F. Motor and parietal cortex stimulation for phantom limb pain and sensations. Pain. 2013;154:1274–80.

170. Hagenacker T, Bude V, Naegel S, Holle D, Katsarava Z, Diener H-C, Obermann M. Patient-conducted anodal transcranial direct current stimulation of the motor cortex alleviates pain in trigeminal neuralgia. J Headache Pain. 2014;15(1):78. https://doi.org/10.1186/1129-2377-15-78.

171. Knotkova H, Portenoy RK, Cruciani RA. Transcranial direct current stimulation (tDCS) relieved itching in a patient with chronic neuropathic pain. Clin J Pain. 2013;29(7). https://doi.org/10.1097/AJP.0b013e31826b1329.

172. Morishita T, Hyakutake K, Saita K, Takahara M, Shiota E, Inoue T. Pain reduction associated with improved functional interhemispheric balance following transcranial direct current stimulation for post-stroke central pain: a case study. J Neurol Sci. 2015;358(1–2):484–5. https://doi.org/10.1016/j.jns.2015.08.1551.
173. Zaghi S, DaSilva A, Acar M, Lopes M, Fregni F. One-year rTMS treatment for refractory trigeminal neuralgia. J Pain Symptom Manage. 2009;38:e1–5.
174. Mori F, Codecà C, Kusayanagi H, Monteleone F, Buttari F, Fiore S, et al. Effects of anodal transcranial direct current stimulation on chronic neuropathic pain in patients with multiple sclerosis. J Pain. 2010;11(5):436–42. https://doi.org/10.1016/j.jpain.2009.08.011.
175. Luedtke K, Rushton A, Wright C, Jürgens T, Polzer A, Mueller G, May A. Effectiveness of transcranial direct current stimulation preceding cognitive behavioural management for chronic low back pain: sham controlled double blinded randomised controlled trial. BMJ. 2015;350(18):h1640. https://doi.org/10.1136/bmj.h1640.
176. O'Connell NE, Cossar J, Marston L, Wand BM, Bunce D, De Souza LH, et al. Transcranial direct current stimulation of the motor cortex in the treatment of chronic nonspecific low back pain. Clin J Pain. 2013;29(1):26–34. https://doi.org/10.1097/AJP.0b013e318247ec09.
177. Wrigley PJ, Gustin SM, McIndoe L, Chakiath RJ, Henderson LA, Siddall PJ. Longstanding neuropathic pain after spinal cord injury is refractory to transcranial direct current stimulation: a randomized controlled trial. Pain. 2013;154(10):2178–84.
178. Soler MD, Kumru H, Pelayo R, Vidal J, Tormos JM, Fregni F, et al. Effectiveness of transcranial direct current stimulation and visual illusion on neuropathic pain in spinal cord injury. Brain. 2010;133(9):2565–77. https://doi.org/10.1093/brain/awq184.
179. Donnell A, Nascimento TD, Lawrence M, Gupta V, Zieba T, Truong DQ, et al. High-definition and non-invasive brain modulation of pain and motor dysfunction in chronic TMD. Brain Stimul. 2015;8(6):1085–92. https://doi.org/10.1016/j.brs.2015.06.008.
180. Villamar M, Wivatvongvana P, Patumanond J. Focal modulation of the primary motor cortex in fibromyalgia using 4× 1-ring high-definition transcranial direct current stimulation (HD-tDCS): immediate and delayed. J Pain. 2013;14(4):371–83.
181. Castillo-Saavedra L, Gebodh N, Bikson M, Diaz-Cruz C, Brandao R, Coutinho L, et al. Clinically effective treatment of fibromyalgia pain with high-definition transcranial direct current stimulation: phase II open-label dose optimization. J Pain. 2016;17(1):14–26. https://doi.org/10.1016/j.jpain.2015.09.009.
182. Brunoni AR, Ferrucci R, Fregni F, Boggio PS, Priori A. Transcranial direct current stimulation for the treatment of major depressive disorder: a summary of preclinical, clinical and translational findings. Prog Neuropsychopharmacol Biol Psychiatry. 2012;39(1):9–16. https://doi.org/10.1016/j.pnpbp.2012.05.016.
183. Kolb B, Teskey GC. Age, experience, injury, and the changing brain. Dev Psychobiol. 2012;54(3):311–25. https://doi.org/10.1002/dev.20515.
184. Stortelder F, Ploegmakers-Burg M. Adolescence and the reorganization of infant development: a neuro-psychoanalytic model. J Am Acad Psychoanal Dyn Psychiatry. 2010;38(3):503–31. https://doi.org/10.1521/jaap.2010.38.3.503.
185. Eldaief MC, Press DZ, Pascual-Leone A. Transcranial magnetic stimulation in neurology: a review of established and prospective applications. Neurol Clin Pract. 2013;3(6):519–26. https://doi.org/10.1212/01.CPJ.0000436213.11132.8e.
186. Klein MM, Treister R, Raij T, Pascual-Leone A, Park L, Nurmikko T, et al. Transcranial magnetic stimulation of the brain: guidelines for pain treatment research. Pain. 2015;156(9):1601–14. https://doi.org/10.1097/j.pain.0000000000000210.
187. Palm U, Segmiller FM, Epple AN, Freisleder F-J, Koutsouleris N, Schulte-Körne G, Padberg F. Transcranial direct current stimulation in children and adolescents: a comprehensive review. J Neural Transm (Vienna). 2016;123(10):1219–34. https://doi.org/10.1007/s00702-016-1572-z.
188. Rajapakse T, Kirton A. Non-invasive brain stimulation in children: applications and future directions. Transl Neurosci. 2013;4(2). https://doi.org/10.2478/s13380-013-0116-3.
189. Schwedt TJ, Vargas B. Neurostimulation for treatment of migraine and cluster headache. Pain Med. 2015;16(9):1827–34. https://doi.org/10.1111/pme.12792.
190. Quintana H. Transcranial magnetic stimulation in persons younger than the age of 18. J Ect. 2005;21(2):88–95. https://doi.org/10.1097/01.yct.0000162556.02720.58.
191. Gilbert DL, Garvey MA, Bansal AS, Lipps T, Zhang J, Wassermann EM. Should transcranial magnetic stimulation research in children be considered minimal risk? Clin Neurophysiol. 2004;115(8):1730–9. https://doi.org/10.1016/j.clinph.2003.10.037.
192. Beauchamp MS, Beurlot MR, Fava E, Nath AR, Parikh NA, Saad ZS, et al. The developmental trajectory of brain-scalp distance from birth through childhood: Implications for functional neuroimaging. PLoS One. 2011;6(9):e24981. https://doi.org/10.1371/journal.pone.0024981.
193. Brain Development Cooperative Group. Total and regional brain volumes in a population-based normative sample from 4 to 18 years: the NIH MRI Study of Normal Brain Development. Cereb Cortex. 2012;22(1):1–12. https://doi.org/10.1093/cercor/bhr018.
194. Reiner PB. Comment on "Can transcranial electrical stimulation improve learning difficulties in atypical brain development? A future possibility for cognitive training" by Krause and Cohen Kadosh. Dev Cogn

Neurosci. 2013;6:195–6. https://doi.org/10.1016/j.dcn.2013.05.002.

195. Moliadze V, Andreas S, Lyzhko E, Schmanke T, Gurashvili T, Freitag CM, Siniatchkin M. Ten minutes of 1 mA transcranial direct current stimulation was well tolerated by children and adolescents: self-reports and resting state EEG analysis. Brain Res Bull. 2015;119(Pt A):25–33. https://doi.org/10.1016/j.brainresbull.2015.09.011.
196. Krishnan C, Santos L, Peterson MD, Ehinger M. Safety of noninvasive brain stimulation in children and adolescents. Brain Stimul. 2015;8(1):76–87. https://doi.org/10.1016/j.brs.2014.10.012.
197. Liebetanz D, Klinker F, Hering D, Koch R, Nitsche MA, Potschka H, et al. Anticonvulsant effects of transcranial direct-current stimulation (tDCS) in the rat cortical ramp model of focal epilepsy. Epilepsia. 2006;47(7):1216–24. https://doi.org/10.1111/j.1528-1167.2006.00539.x.
198. Gangitano M, Valero-Cabré A, Tormos JM, Mottaghy FM, Romero JR, Pascual-Leone A. Modulation of input-output curves by low and high frequency repetitive transcranial magnetic stimulation of the motor cortex. Clin Neurophysiol. 2002;113(8):1249–57. http://www.ncbi.nlm.nih.gov/pubmed/12140004.
199. Maeda F, Keenan JP, Tormos JM, Topka H, Pascual-Leone A. Modulation of corticospinal excitability by repetitive transcranial magnetic stimulation. Clin Neurophysiol. 2000;111(5):800–5. http://www.ncbi.nlm.nih.gov/pubmed/10802449.
200. Auvichayapat N, Rotenberg A, Gersner R, Ngodklang S, Tiamkao S, Tassaneeyakul W, Auvichayapat P. Transcranial direct current stimulation for treatment of refractory childhood focal epilepsy. Brain Stimul. 2013;6(4):696–700. https://doi.org/10.1016/j.brs.2013.01.009.
201. Varga ET, Terney D, Atkins MD, Nikanorova M, Jeppesen DS, Uldall P, et al. Transcranial direct current stimulation in refractory continuous spikes and waves during slow sleep: a controlled study. Epilepsy Res. 2011;97(1–2):142–5. https://doi.org/10.1016/j.eplepsyres.2011.07.016.
202. Shelyakin AM, Preobrazhenskaya IG, Kassil' MV, Bogdanov OV. The effects of transcranial micropolarization on the severity of convulsive fits in children. Neurosci Behav Physiol. 2001;31(5):555–60. http://www.ncbi.nlm.nih.gov/pubmed/11693481.
203. Schindler K, Leung H, Lehnertz K, Elger CE. How generalised are secondarily "generalised" tonic–clonic seizures? J Neurol Neurosurg Psychiatry. 2007;78(9):993–6. https://doi.org/10.1136/jnnp.2006.108753.
204. Gotman J, Grova C, Bagshaw A, Kobayashi E, Aghakhani Y, Dubeau F. Generalized epileptic discharges show thalamocortical activation and suspension of the default state of the brain, (Track II). Proc Natl Acad Sci U S A. 2005;102(42):15236–40.
205. Faria P, Fregni F, Sebastião F, Dias AI, Leal A. Feasibility of focal transcranial DC polarization with simultaneous EEG recording: preliminary assessment in healthy subjects and human epilepsy. Epilepsy Behav. 2012;25(3):417–25. https://doi.org/10.1016/j.yebeh.2012.06.027.
206. Auvichayapat N, Sinsupan K, Tunkamnerdthai O, Auvichayapat P. Transcranial direct current stimulation for treatment of childhood pharmacoresistant Lennox-Gastaut syndrome: a pilot study. Front Neurol. 2016;7:66. https://doi.org/10.3389/fneur.2016.00066.
207. Yook S-W, Park S-H, Seo J-H, Kim S-J, Ko M-H. Suppression of seizure by cathodal transcranial direct current stimulation in an epileptic patient—a case report. Ann Rehabil Med. 2011;35(4):579. https://doi.org/10.5535/arm.2011.35.4.579.
208. San-Juan D, Del Castillo Calcáneo JD, González-Aragón MF, Bermúdez Maldonado L, Moreno Avellán Á, Gómez Argumosa EV, Fregni F. Transcranial direct current stimulation in adolescent and adult Rasmussen's encephalitis. Epilepsy Behav. 2011;20(1):126–31. https://doi.org/10.1016/j.yebeh.2010.10.031.
209. Tekturk P, Erdogan ET, Kurt A, Kocagoncu E, Kucuk Z, Kinay D, et al. Transcranial direct current stimulation improves seizure control in patients with Rasmussen encephalitis. Epileptic Disord. 2016;18(1):58–66. https://doi.org/10.1684/epd.2016.0796.
210. Pineda E, Shin D, Sankar R, Mazarati AM. Comorbidity between epilepsy and depression: experimental evidence for the involvement of serotonergic, glucocorticoid, and neuroinflammatory mechanisms. Epilepsia. 2010;51(Suppl 3):110–4. https://doi.org/10.1111/j.1528-1167.2010.02623.x.
211. Nitsche MA, Liebetanz D, Schlitterlau A, Henschke U, Fricke K, Frommann K, et al. GABAergic modulation of DC stimulation-induced motor cortex excitability shifts in humans. Eur J Neurosci. 2004;19(10):2720–6. https://doi.org/10.1111/j.0953-816X.2004.03398.x.
212. Scorza FA, Brunoni AR. Transcranial direct current stimulation against sudden unexpected death in epilepsy: press that button again, please. Brain Stimul. 2015;8(4):839–40. https://doi.org/10.1016/j.brs.2015.04.006.
213. Hufnagel A, Elger CE, Marx W, Ising A. Magnetic motor-evoked potentials in epilepsy: effects of the disease and of anticonvulsant medication. Ann Neurol. 1990;28(5):680–6. https://doi.org/10.1002/ana.410280513.
214. Michelucci R, Passarelli D, Riguzzi P, Buzzi AM, Gardella E, Tassinari CA. Transcranial magnetic stimulation in partial epilepsy: drug-induced changes of motor excitability. Acta Neurol Scand. 1996;94(1):24–30. http://www.ncbi.nlm.nih.gov/pubmed/8874589.
215. Michelucci R, Valzania F, Tassinari CA. Chapter 62 Transcranial magnetic stimulation in epilepsy and Parkinson's disease: drug induced changes in motor excitability. Suppl Clin Neurophysiol.

2002;54:416–21. https://doi.org/10.1016/S1567-424X(09)70482-9.
216. Cantello R, Civardi C, Cavalli A, Varrasi C, Tarletti R, Monaco F, Migliaretti G. Cortical excitability in cryptogenic localization-related epilepsy: interictal transcranial magnetic stimulation studies. Epilepsia. 2000;41(6):694–704. http://www.ncbi.nlm.nih.gov/pubmed/10840401.
217. Griesemer DA, Kellner CH, Beale MD, Smith GM. Electroconvulsive therapy for treatment of intractable seizures. Initial findings in two children. Neurology. 1997;49(5):1389–92. http://www.ncbi.nlm.nih.gov/pubmed/9371927.
218. Lisanby SH, Bazil CW, Resor SR, Nobler MS, Finck DA, Sackeim HA. ECT in the treatment of status epilepticus. J ECT. 2001;17(3):210–5. http://www.ncbi.nlm.nih.gov/pubmed/11528315.
219. Hsu W-Y, Cheng C-H, Lin M-W, Shih Y-H, Liao K-K, Lin Y-Y. Antiepileptic effects of low frequency repetitive transcranial magnetic stimulation: a meta-analysis. Epilepsy Res. 2011;96(3):231–40. https://doi.org/10.1016/j.eplepsyres.2011.06.002.
220. Sloan JA, Cella D, Hays RD. Clinical significance of patient-reported questionnaire data: another step toward consensus. J Clin Epidemiol. 2005;58(12):1217–9. https://doi.org/10.1016/j.jclinepi.2005.07.009.
221. Rotenberg A, Depositario-cabacar D, Hyunji E. Transient suppression of seizures by repetitive transcranial magnetic stimulation in a case of Rasmussen's encephalitis. Epilepsy Behav. 2008;13:260–2. https://doi.org/10.1016/j.yebeh.2007.12.022.
222. Rotenberg A, Bae E, Takeoka M, Tormos J, Schachter S, Pascual-Leone A. Repetitive transcranial magnetic stimulation in treatment of epilepsia partialis continua. Epilepsy Behav. 2009;14(1):253–7. https://doi.org/10.1016/j.yebeh.2008.09.007.
223. Graff-Guerrero A, Olvera J, Ruiz-García M, Avila-Ordoñez U, Vaugier V, García-Reyna JC. rTMS reduces focal brain hyperperfusion in two patients with EPC. Acta Neurol Scand. 2004;109(4):290–6. https://doi.org/10.1046/j.1600-0404.2003.00222.x.
224. Kimbrell TA, Dunn RT, George MS, Danielson AL, Willis MW, Repella JD, et al. Left prefrontal-repetitive transcranial magnetic stimulation (rTMS) and regional cerebral glucose metabolism in normal volunteers. Psychiatry Res. 2002;115(3):101–13. http://www.ncbi.nlm.nih.gov/pubmed/12208488.
225. Paus T, Jech R, Thompson CJ, Comeau R, Peters T, Evans AC. Transcranial magnetic stimulation during positron emission tomography: a new method for studying connectivity of the human cerebral cortex. J Neurosci. 1997;17(9):3178–84. http://www.ncbi.nlm.nih.gov/pubmed/9096152.
226. Siebner HR, Peller M, Willoch F, Minoshima S, Boecker H, Auer C, et al. Lasting cortical activation after repetitive TMS of the motor cortex: a glucose metabolic study. Neurology. 2000;54(4):956–63. http://www.ncbi.nlm.nih.gov/pubmed/10690992.
227. Stallings L, Speer A, Spicer K, Cheng K, George M. Combining SPECT and repetitive transcranial magnetic stimulation (rTMS)–left prefrontal stimulation decreases relative perfusion locally in a dose dependent manner (abstract). Neuroimage. 1997;5:S521. https://www.scienceopen.com/document?vid=6bbc2130-d492-4ec3-961d-1700d30df2c9.
228. Morales OG, Henry ME, Nobler MS, Wassermann EM, Lisanby SH. Electroconvulsive therapy and repetitive transcranial magnetic stimulation in children and adolescents: a review and report of two cases of epilepsia partialis continua. Child Adolesc Psychiatr Clin North Am. 2005;14(1 SPEC.ISS.):193–210. https://doi.org/10.1016/j.chc.2004.07.010.
229. Pereira LS, Müller VT, da Mota Gomes M, Rotenberg A, Fregni F. Safety of repetitive transcranial magnetic stimulation in patients with epilepsy: a systematic review. Epilepsy Behav. 2016;57:167–76. https://doi.org/10.1016/j.yebeh.2016.01.015.
230. Seynaeve L, Van Paesschen W. Response to "Safety of repetitive transcranial magnetic stimulation in patients with epilepsy: a systematic review" by Luisa Santos Pereira and colleagues. Epilepsy Behav. 2016;62:308. https://doi.org/10.1016/j.yebeh.2016.07.002.
231. Seynaeve L, Devroye A, Dupont P, Van Paesschen W. Randomized crossover sham-controlled clinical trial of targeted low-frequency transcranial magnetic stimulation comparing a figure-8 and a round coil to treat refractory neocortical epilepsy. Epilepsia. 2016;57(1):141–50. https://doi.org/10.1111/epi.13247.
232. Post RM, Kimbrell T, Frye M, George M, McCann U, Little J, et al. Implications of kindling and quenching for the possible frequency dependence Of rTMS. CNS Spectrums. 1997;2(1):54–60. https://doi.org/10.1017/S1092852900004508.
233. Hagberg B, Hagberg G, Beckung E, Uvebrant P. Changing panorama of cerebral palsy in Sweden. VIII. Prevalence and origin in the birth year period 1991-94. Acta Paediatr. 2001;90(3):271–7. http://www.ncbi.nlm.nih.gov/pubmed/11332166.
234. Mercuri E, Rutherford M, Cowan F, Pennock J, Counsell S, Papadimitriou M, et al. Early prognostic indicators of outcome in infants with neonatal cerebral infarction: a clinical, electroencephalogram, and magnetic resonance imaging study. Pediatrics. 1999;103(1):39–46. http://www.ncbi.nlm.nih.gov/pubmed/9917437.
235. Mercuri E, Barnett A, Rutherford M, Guzzetta A, Haataja L, Cioni G, et al. Neonatal cerebral infarction and neuromotor outcome at school age. Pediatrics. 2004;113(1 Pt 1):95–100. http://www.ncbi.nlm.nih.gov/pubmed/14702455.
236. de Veber G, Andrew M, Adams C, Bjornson B, Booth F, Buckley DJ, et al. Cerebral sinovenous thrombosis in children. N Engl J Med. 2001;345(6):417–23. https://doi.org/10.1056/NEJM200108093450604.

237. Nelson KB. Can we prevent cerebral palsy? N Engl J Med. 2003;349(18):1765–9. https://doi.org/10.1056/NEJMsb035364.
238. Nelson KB, Lynch JK. Stroke in newborn infants. Lancet Neurol. 2004;3(3):150–8. https://doi.org/10.1016/S1474-4422(04)00679-9.
239. deVeber GA, MacGregor D, Curtis R, Mayank S. Neurologic outcome in survivors of childhood arterial ischemic stroke and sinovenous thrombosis. J Child Neurol. 2000;15(5):316–24. https://doi.org/10.1177/088307380001500508.
240. Mercuri E, Cowan F, Gupte G, Manning R, Laffan M, Rutherford M, et al. Prothrombotic disorders and abnormal neurodevelopmental outcome in infants with neonatal cerebral infarction. Pediatrics. 2001;107(6):1400–4. http://www.ncbi.nlm.nih.gov/pubmed/11389264.
241. Mineyko A, Kirton A. The black box of perinatal ischemic stroke pathogenesis. J Child Neurol. 2011;26(9):1154–62. https://doi.org/10.1177/0883073811408312.
242. Petty GW, Brown RD, Whisnant JP, Sicks JD, O'Fallon WM, Wiebers DO. Ischemic stroke subtypes: a population-based study of incidence and risk factors. Stroke. 1999;30(12):2513–6. http://www.ncbi.nlm.nih.gov/pubmed/10582970.
243. Raju TNK, Nelson KB, Ferriero D, Lynch JK, NICHD-NINDS Perinatal Stroke Workshop Participants. Ischemic perinatal stroke: summary of a workshop sponsored by the National Institute of Child Health and Human Development and the National Institute of Neurological Disorders and Stroke. Pediatrics. 2007;120(3):609–16. https://doi.org/10.1542/peds.2007-0336.
244. Sreenan C, Bhargava R, Robertson CM. Cerebral infarction in the term newborn: clinical presentation and long-term outcome. J Pediatr. 2000;137(3):351–5. https://doi.org/10.1067/mpd.2000.107845.
245. Collange Grecco LA, de Almeida Carvalho Duarte N, Mendonça ME, Galli M, Fregni F, Oliveira CS. Effects of anodal transcranial direct current stimulation combined with virtual reality for improving gait in children with spastic diparetic cerebral palsy: a pilot, randomized, controlled, double-blind, clinical trial. Clin Rehabil. 2015;29(12):1212–23. https://doi.org/10.1177/0269215514566997.
246. Bogdanov OV, Pinchuk DY, Pisar'kova EV, Shelyakin AM, Sirbiladze KT. The use of the method of transcranial micropolarization to decrease the severity hyperkineses in patients with infantile cerebral palsy. Neurosci Behav Physiol. 1994;24(5):442–5. http://www.ncbi.nlm.nih.gov/pubmed/7838369.
247. Grecco LAC, Oliveira CS, Galli M, Cosmo C, Duarte NAC, Zanon N, et al. Spared primary motor cortex and the presence of MEP in cerebral palsy dictate the responsiveness to tDCS during gait training. Front Human Neurosci. 2016;10:1–11. https://doi.org/10.3389/fnhum.2016.00361.
248. Kesar TM, Sawaki L, Burdette JH, Cabrera MN, Kolaski K, Smith BP, et al. Motor cortical functional geometry in cerebral palsy and its relationship to disability. Clin Neurophysiol. 2012;123(7):1383–90. https://doi.org/10.1016/j.clinph.2011.11.005.
249. Mackey A, Stinear C, Stott S, Byblow WD. Upper limb function and cortical organization in youth with unilateral cerebral palsy. Front Neurol. 2014;5:117. https://doi.org/10.3389/fneur.2014.00117.
250. Pihko E, Nevalainen P, Vaalto S, Laaksonen K, Mäenpää H, Valanne L, Lauronen L. Reactivity of sensorimotor oscillations is altered in children with hemiplegic cerebral palsy: a magnetoencephalographic study. Human Brain Mapping. 2014;35(8):4105–17. https://doi.org/10.1002/hbm.22462.
251. Carvalho Lima VLC, Collange Grecco LA, Marques VC, Fregni F, Brandão de Ávila CR. Transcranial direct current stimulation combined with integrative speech therapy in a child with cerebral palsy: a case report. J Bodyw Mov Ther. 2016;20(2):252–7. https://doi.org/10.1016/j.jbmt.2015.03.007.
252. D'Agati D, Bloch Y, Levkovitz Y, Reti I. rTMS for adolescents: safety and efficacy considerations. Psychiatry Res. 2010;177(3):280–5. https://doi.org/10.1016/j.psychres.2010.03.004.
253. Valle AC, Dionisio K, Pitskel NB, Pascual-Leone A, Orsati F, Ferreira MJL, et al. Low and high frequency repetitive transcranial magnetic stimulation for the treatment of spasticity. Dev Med Child Neurol. 2007;49(7):534–8. https://doi.org/10.1111/j.1469-8749.2007.00534.x.
254. Quartarone A, Bagnato S, Rizzo V, Morgante F, Sant'angelo A, Battaglia F, et al. Distinct changes in cortical and spinal excitability following high-frequency repetitive TMS to the human motor cortex. Exp Brain Res. 2005;161(1):114–24. https://doi.org/10.1007/s00221-004-2052-5.
255. Gupta M, Lal Rajak B, Bhatia D, Mukherjee A. Effect of r-TMS over standard therapy in decreasing muscle tone of spastic cerebral palsy patients. J Med Eng Technol. 2016;40(4):210–6. https://doi.org/10.3109/03091902.2016.1161854.
256. Guo Z, Xing G, He B, Chen H, Ou J, McClure MA, et al. Dynamic modulation of rTMS on functional connectivity and functional network connectivity to children with cerebral palsy: a case report. Neuroreport. 2016;27(4):284–8. https://doi.org/10.1097/WNR.0000000000000534.

The Future of Neuromodulation 13

Kenneth M. Peters, Laura N. Nguyen, and Larry T. Sirls

Neuromodulation has long been used to restore physiologic function to patients with overactive bladder, urinary retention, pain, and fecal symptoms. Despite the commercial availability of neuromodulation for almost 20 years, only minimal technical advances have been made in the field. Approved targets for neuromodulation in urology are limited to the sacral and tibial nerves. Pudendal neuromodulation has been described, but is not FDA-approved (Fig. 13.1). Approved urologic indications for sacral neuromodulation are urgency incontinence, overactive bladder, and nonobstructive urinary retention. Tibial neuromodulation is approved only for overactive bladder. In recent years, numerous innovative devices designed to address the limitations of currently available products have been investigated. The emergence of new technologies, and the development of novel nerve targets, may significantly expand the clinical application of neuromodulation in the near future.

K. M. Peters (✉) · L. N. Nguyen · L. T. Sirls
Department of Urology, Beaumont Health, Royal Oak, MI, USA
e-mail: kenneth.peters@beaumont.edu; lauranguyen@icloud.com; laura.nguyen@beaumont.org; larry.sirls@beaumont.edu

Sacral Nerve

When introduced in 1997, sacral neuromodulation was an invasive procedure requiring an open sacral incision, incising the dorsolumbar fascia, identifying the foramen, placing a lead adjacent to the S3 sacral nerve, and securing the lead to the sacral periosteum (Fig. 13.2). The lead required an implantable pulse generator (IPG) placed subcutaneously in the upper buttock. Prior to undergoing this relatively invasive procedure that required inpatient hospitalization, a peripheral nerve evaluation (PNE) was done in the office by placing a percutaneous monopolar sacral lead for several days while stimulating the nerve with an external generator. The PNE test had several limitations including poor placement of the lead, early migration, and overall poor clinical response [1, 2]. It wasn't until 2002 that a tined lead was introduced making lead placement truly a percutaneous procedure. This minimally invasive approach allowed for the development of a staged test where the permanent lead was placed and externalized for up to 2 weeks. This increased the amount of time the patient had to determine the efficacy of the device, allowed for reprogramming and improved clinical outcomes [3, 4]. The only other technical update to sacral neuromodulation since its approval was in 2007 when the implantable pulse generator was reduced in size from 42 to 22 g [5, 6]. This improved patient

J. P. Gilleran, S. A. Alpert (eds.), *Adult and Pediatric Neuromodulation*,
https://doi.org/10.1007/978-3-319-73266-4_13

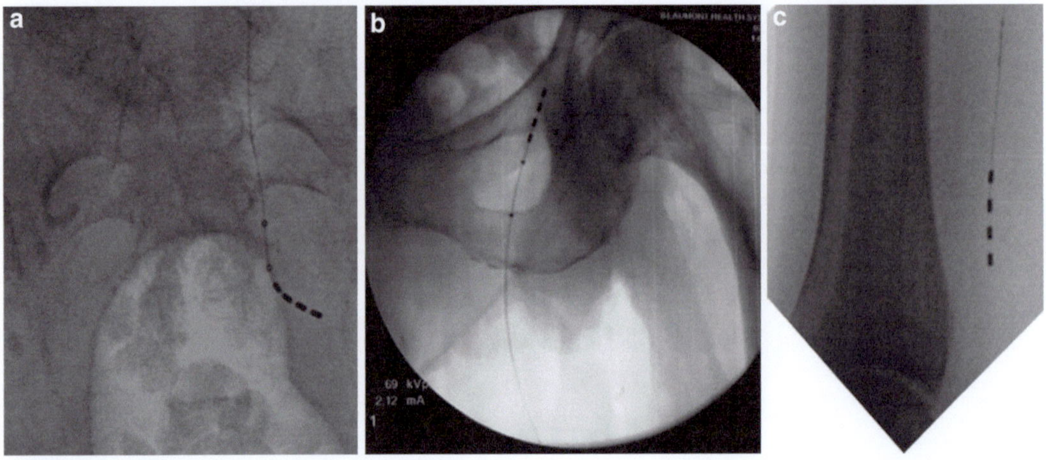

Fig. 13.1 Fluoroscopic images of leads placed percutaneously at the (**a**) S3 sacral nerve, (**b**) pudendal nerve, and (**c**) posterior tibial nerve

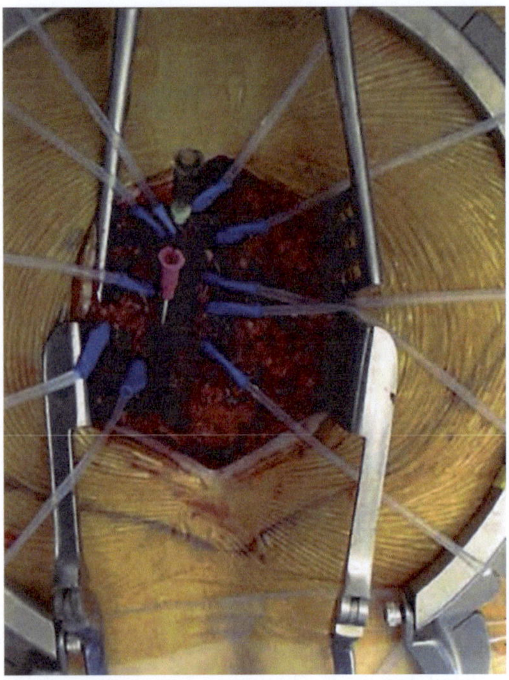

Fig. 13.2 The first implantable neuromodulation system was more invasive than the percutaneous methods used today. An insulated needle in the S3 foramen during placement of the first generation InterStim® (Medtronic, Inc.) via paramedian sacral incision. Reproduced with permission from AK Das et al. [76]. Sacral nerve modulation for the management of voiding dysfunction. Rev. Urol. 2000; 2: 43–52, 60. Reviews in Urology is a copyrighted publication of MedReviews®, LLC.

satisfaction and reduced complaints of pain at the IPG site, but increased the cost of the device as the battery life was reduced from 8 to 4 years requiring additional surgery and replacement costs. Finally, in 2011 sacral neuromodulation was approved for fecal incontinence [7], though this had been described since 1995 [8], ending further development of the technology.

While sacral neuromodulation (InterStim®, Medtronic, Inc.) is safe and effective, it has several limitations. First, implantation of a neurostimulator requires at least one (if successful PNE), but usually two procedures (staged approach) under sedation in the operating room. The implantable pulse generator is still bulky in size and may cause site symptoms requiring reoperation and, importantly, is non-rechargeable requiring surgery every 4–5 years to replace. Another major limitation is that the leads and generators are not compatible with magnetic resonance imaging (MRI). The potential need for MRI can limit the number of patients who may otherwise benefit from this therapy and may require the removal of a very expensive device if MRI is required. Finally, the cost of sacral neuromodulation to the healthcare system is high as there are no competitors on the market to drive competitive pricing.

The currently available system relies on decades-old technology. New technologies with modern capabilities are under investigation with a focus on decreasing cost, patient burden, and invasiveness of the treatment, while maintaining or improving efficacy. In the past few years, several new technologies have been in development including longer lasting and rechargeable batteries, wireless charging and power sources, advances in programming, reducing the invasiveness with a single-stage rather than a two-stage procedure, or by simply developing new devices to provide a more competitive pricing environment.

Improved Battery Technology and External Power Sources

Cutaneously rechargeable battery technology has the ability to reduce the size of the IPG, improving patient comfort and extending battery life. The Axonics® Sacral Neuromodulation System is 60% smaller than the Medtronic InterStim® II device and has a CE mark in Europe, but is not yet available in the USA. The battery life is 15 years, compared to 4–5 years for the InterStim® product (see Fig. 13.3) [9]. The system is wirelessly and transcutaneously rechargeable and is expected to require charging for less than 2 h every 1–3 weeks. The patient remote is the size of a key fob and controls the intensity of stimulation and notifies the patient when charging is required. The clinician programmer has a graphic interface and allows for EMG input to enhance programming parameters. A clinical trial is currently underway in Europe [10].

Several other technologies that use external power sources are currently also in development, including the StimWave® and StimGuard® devices. StimWave is currently approved for peripheral nerve pain including the pudendal nerve, dorsal root ganglion (T7-S1), and for spinal cord stimulation (T7-L5). StimGuard is studying a percutaneously implanted lead for chronic stimulation of posterior tibial nerve and sacral nerve for voiding dysfunction. We discuss these technologies in more detail later in this chapter.

Programming

There is minimal data on programming parameters with sacral neuromodulation. Continuous stimulation is typically used, but cycling, intermittent, or on-demand use of the InterStim® neurostimulator device may improve battery life and reduce “nerve fatigue” leading to reduced efficacy. Small studies have demonstrated comparable symptom score outcomes with use of on-demand [11] and intermittent [12] sacral neuromodulation. More studies are needed to evaluate different programming strategies to understand the ideal settings that may improve efficacy and prolong battery life.

Boost Technology

Another new approach to improve clinical efficacy would be to modify the energy delivery by transmitting surges of higher amplitude energy when there are symptoms of an impending incontinent episode [13, 14]. Theoretically, either the patient controller or a dedicated smaller key-fob type device could be used to deliver a burst of stimulation to suppress oncoming urge symptoms of detrusor overactivity. Several small studies suggest that conditional stimulation may be effective in reducing detrusor overactivity.

Staging of the Procedure

The issue of patient burden and system cost may be addressed by moving from a two-stage to a single-stage procedure. The single-stage procedure would consist only of implantation of the lead and generator in the operating room without a testing phase, followed by an extended (several weeks or months) trial with optimization of programming. The device would be removed in a second procedure if ineffective after this trial. Nikolavsky et al. found that 90.3% of patients in their study would benefit from a single-stage procedure, reducing operative and anesthesia risks, time lost from work, and burden on patients and

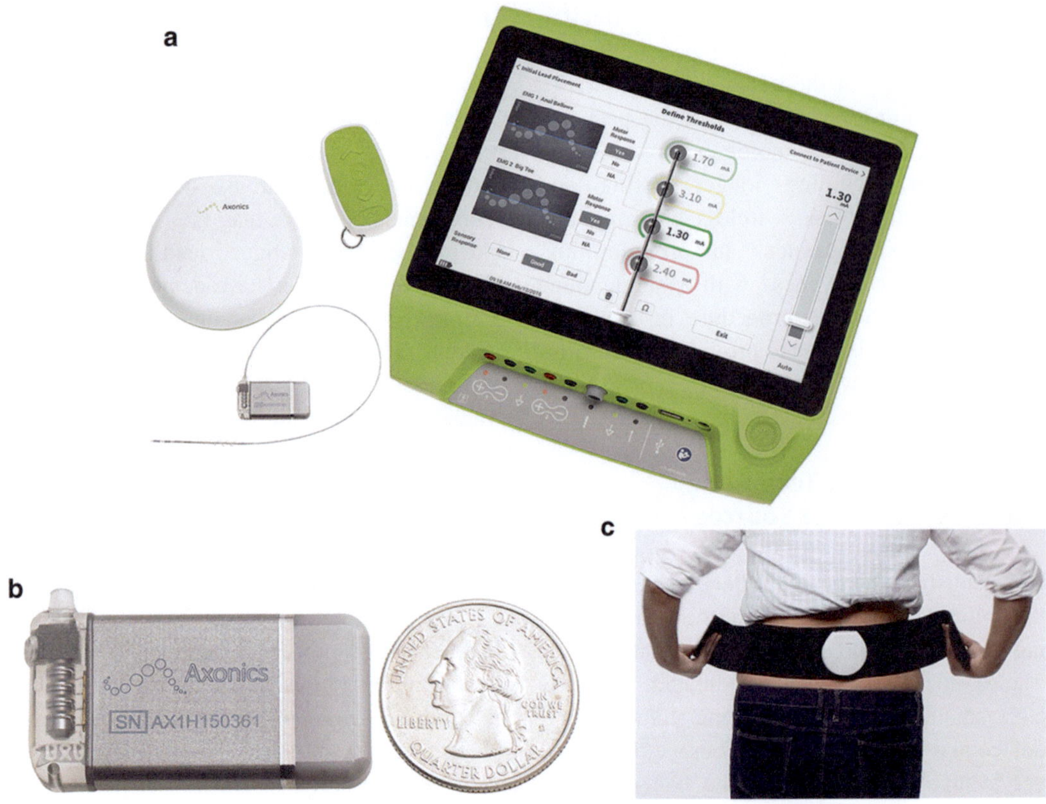

Fig. 13.3 The Axonics sacral neuromodulation (**a**) full system, (**b**) implantable pulse generator with rechargeable battery, and (**c**) wearable flexible belt with recharging device in dock. Reproduced with permission from Axonics Modulation Technologies, Inc.

providers [15]. A single-stage approach was also found to decrease cost with Blue Cross/Blue Shield reimbursement (overall average savings of $3655/patient), but not with Medicare (overall average loss of $806/patient) due to differences in payment structure. The cost-effectiveness of a staged procedure in the operating room has also been shown to save $1050 compared to PNE in the office followed by placement of a permanent lead and generator in the operating room [16].

Improving Lead Placement at Implantation

Further improvements may also be directed at enhanced precision of nerve identification during neurostimulator implantation. In 2014, Jacobs et al. demonstrated improved lead placement with a curved over a straight stylet, achieving a motor response at lower amplitude at the deepest leads and a lower combined altitude over all leads [17]. In addition to the use of anatomic and fluoroscopic landmarks and motor and sensory response, use of intraoperative electromyography (EMG) may improve the ability of clinicians to accurately pinpoint the location of the targeted nerve. Studies are underway to evaluate whether EMG guided programming is superior to the standard sensory programming

Additional Nerve Targets

Currently, the S3 sacral nerve is the only FDA-approved site for the treatment of bladder and bowel dysfunction using an implantable device. Neuromodulation is thought to improve symptoms by afferent stimulation to the central nervous system. Other nerve targets such as the pudendal nerve (S2, S3, and S4) and the tibial nerve (L4, L5, S1, S2, and S3) are proving to be alternative sites for implantable technologies.

Pudendal Nerve

Pudendal neuromodulation for bladder and bowel dysfunction is not FDA approved and there have been no industry-sponsored studies to assess the efficacy of this nerve target. However, there have been numerous single-site publications using the current InterStim® device at the pudendal nerve. The first studies showing efficacy of this technique were published in 2005 [18, 19]. Spinelli et al. studied 15 patients with neurogenic overactive bladder with urge incontinence refractory to medical therapy, who underwent pudendal InterStim® lead placement via perineal or posterior approach [18]. Of these patients, three had had prior sacral neuromodulation with inadequate results. After first-stage lead placement, 12/15 patients proceeded to second-stage IPG placement. Of these, eight patients were completely continent during the screening phase; two had greater than 80% improvement in number of incontinent episodes per day; and two had greater than 50% improvement in number of incontinent episodes per day. Objective urodynamic parameters also improved in all seven patients who had 6-month follow-up with increase in maximal cystometric capacity and decrease in maximal detrusor pressure.

The same year, Peters et al. reported on the results of a single-blinded randomized clinical trial of sacral vs. pudendal neuromodulation in a non-neurogenic population (n = 30) with idiopathic overactive bladder [19]. These patients were all implanted with both sacral and pudendal leads and blinded to lead location during the screening phase. The majority of patients had a chief complaint of urgency/frequency (n = 22), with the remaining patients urge incontinence and urinary retention (n = 5 and n = 3, respectively). Time to place leads was similar between sacral and pudendal sites. After lead placement, the patients were randomized to begin pudendal or sacral stimulation for the initial 7 days, and then switched to the other lead for the next 7 days. Twenty-four patients had a significant benefit and went on to undergo the second-stage procedure. Sixty-nine percent found the pudendal lead more efficacious and underwent permanent implantation. The remaining responders were implanted with sacral neuromodulation. This study suggested that pudendal neuromodulation might be more efficacious than sacral neuromodulation.

Dedicated Product Development

Despite the first report of pudendal neuromodulation in 2005, there have been no attempts by industry to complete appropriate clinical trials for FDA approval. The currently available InterStim® product has been used at the pudendal nerve. Migration of the lead is more common (6%) than sacral neuromodulation due to the placement of the lead in the ischiorectal space [19, 20]. However, no dedicated product development has been done to reduce lead migration, enhance lead positioning or to evaluate patient selection. One of the more common uses of pudendal neuromodulation has been for pelvic pain or pudendal neuropathy associated with voiding dysfunction [20, 21]. Recently, Stimwave Technologies, Inc. received approval for peripheral nerve stimulation for pain using their novel, wireless electrode. This electrode is placed through a tiny skin nick and has an integrated, programmable receiver with adjustable length. The energy is delivered via a small rechargeable battery and antenna that is placed near the receiver either over or under the clothing. This system is now being used for pudendal neuromodulation for pudendal neuropathy, but is not approved for voiding or bowel dysfunction, although likely will result in secondary improvement of these symptoms. With the approval of this wireless system, the use of pudendal neuromodulation may expand for those suffering from pudendal nerve directed pain.

Tibial Nerve

The tibial nerve has been investigated as a neuromodulation target since the 1980s for treatment of overactive bladder. Peripheral tibial nerve stimulation (PTNS) had been shown to improve urgency, frequency, and number of urge incontinent episodes as early as 2001, but these were uncontrolled clinical trials [22, 23]. Randomized controlled trials established efficacy compared to both pharmacologic therapy and sham treatment in 2009 and 2010, respectively. Level 1 evidence of the efficacy of PTNS was established and published compared to both pharmacologic therapy and sham in 2009 and 2010, in the Overactive Bladder Innovative Therapy (OrBIT) [24] and Study of Urgent® PC versus sham effectiveness in overactive bladder Treatment (SUmiT) [25] trials, respectively. In the OrBIT trial, 100 adults with urinary frequency were randomized 1:1 to 12 weekly of treatments of PTNS or to 4 mg daily extended-release tolterodine. Both arms had statistically significant improvements in symptoms, although PTNS had a 79.5% cure/improvement versus 54.8% with tolterodine. In the SUmiT trial, 220 patients were randomized to PTNS or validated sham over 12 weeks of therapy. At 13 weeks, there was a reported 54.5% improved response compared to 20.9% in the sham. Follow-up of the patients in both of these pivotal trials confirmed a maintained response with continued monthly treatments out to 36 months [26, 27]. Following these trials, PTNS has become a standard third-line treatment for overactive bladder and the associated symptoms of frequency, urgency, and urge incontinence, and a category I CPT code was approved by the Centers for Medicare and Medicaid Services (effective Jan. 1, 2011).

PTNS, while less invasive than implantable neurostimulators, requires frequent weekly visits for the initial period then monthly stimulation visits indefinitely. Space limitations in the lower limb do not allow for implantation of a power source. All treatments must take place in the office, creating patient burden that can affect treatment compliance [26]. While PTNS has been shown to be more cost-effective than other options including pharmacotherapy [28], the cost of frequent visits and indefinite office follow-up is a barrier.

Noninvasive Leads and Home Stimulation Devices

The Biowave PTNS System is under investigation for use in patients with overactive bladder symptoms as an alternative to traditional PTNS. Rather than inserting a 35-gauge needle to the tibial nerve, stimulation is delivered by a less invasive, microneedle skin patch (that is a percutaneous electrode array) to allow stimulation of the tibial nerve (see Fig. 13.4). Biowave has a patented technology allowing easy passage of the energy through the impedance of the skin and has been shown to activate the tibial nerve. A recent pilot study treating eight women with overactive bladder with twelve 30-min weekly sessions [29] showed significant decreases in Overactive Bladder Questionnaire Symptom Score and Health-Related Quality of Life, and Urogenital Distress Inventory 6 (UDI-6) [29]. This technology is currently used for treatment of pelvic and groin pain (applied over the sacrum), as well as many other types of pain. As a patch electrode with a home stimulation unit, the Biowave potentially could be used for in-home patient-controlled chronic stimulation.

External Power Sources

The availability of wireless technology with an implantable electrode and receiver and an external rechargeable energy source and antenna could render implantable generators and intermittent percutaneous needle placement obsolete. With external wireless power sources, leads can be smaller and be used to precisely modulate new nerve targets. An implantable tibial nerve stimulator made up of a 4 cm electromagnetic receiver composed of two platinum electrodes, called Urgent-SQ, had been studied in eight patients [30, 31]. The external generator transmits radiofrequency electromagnetic pulses to the electrodes, creating pulses, stimulating the tibial nerve [30, 31]. Patients first underwent PTNS

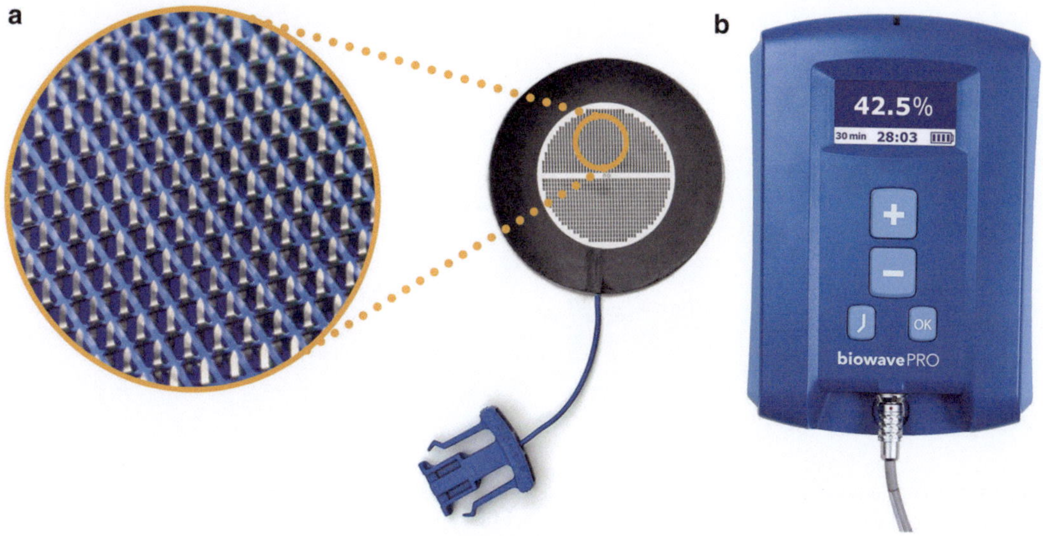

Fig. 13.4 The Biowave Percutaneous Electrical Nerve Stimulation device has a (**a**) percutaneous electrode array and (**b**) patient-controlled home stimulation unit. Reproduced with permission from Biowave Corporation

and were evaluated by questionnaires and voiding diaries, then PTNS was stopped and all patients returned to baseline symptomatology prior to implantation. Implantation required a two-day hospital admission with bed rest [30]. Patients were stimulated at home three times weekly for 30-min duration, and four of the eight patients met the primary outcome of significantly improved symptoms as measured by voiding diaries and quality of life at 12-month follow-up [30]. Adverse events included difficulties walking, urinary tract infection, and spontaneous sensory response; one of the eight patients had the device explanted within the first year [30]. Nine-year follow-up was recently published and showed persistent efficacy in three of the remaining patients [31]. Although older technology, this early studied suggested that implantable devices at the tibial nerve may be effective.

With the advent of smaller devices, BlueWind, a compact tibial neurostimulator placed via an open surgical technique, has demonstrated safety and efficacy in a small group presented at the International Continence Society Annual Meeting 2015 (see Fig. 13.5) [32]. This lead is placed in the lower limb adjacent to the tibial nerve via a cut-down technique. Early results in the first 12 patients treated with BlueWind demonstrated that 58% had at least a 50% improvement in overactive bladder symptoms. This device is undergoing trials in patients with overactive bladder and pelvic pain [33, 34].

StimGuard is studying a small, implantable neuromodulation electrode with integrated circuitry and receiver that can be placed percutaneously at the tibial nerve in the office. This new wireless technology provides patient-controlled chronic stimulation for overactive bladder and was presented at the International Continence Society Annual Meeting 2016 (see Fig. 13.6) [35]. Efficacy was also demonstrated with data presented at the same conference describing two patients with refractory urge incontinence who were completely dry within 48 h after implantation [36]. This device has a rechargeable external power source and integrated antennas that is worn an ankle wrap around the leg at the site of the subcutaneous receiver. Patients can stimulate on demand and can titrate their stimulation frequency based on clinical response. The minimally invasive nature of this device and the ability to implant this in an office setting has the potential to ease the burden of currently available PTNS, improve clinical outcomes, and reduce the cost associated with implantable sacral neuromodulation. A randomized trial comparing StimGuard to traditional PTNS is currently underway [37].

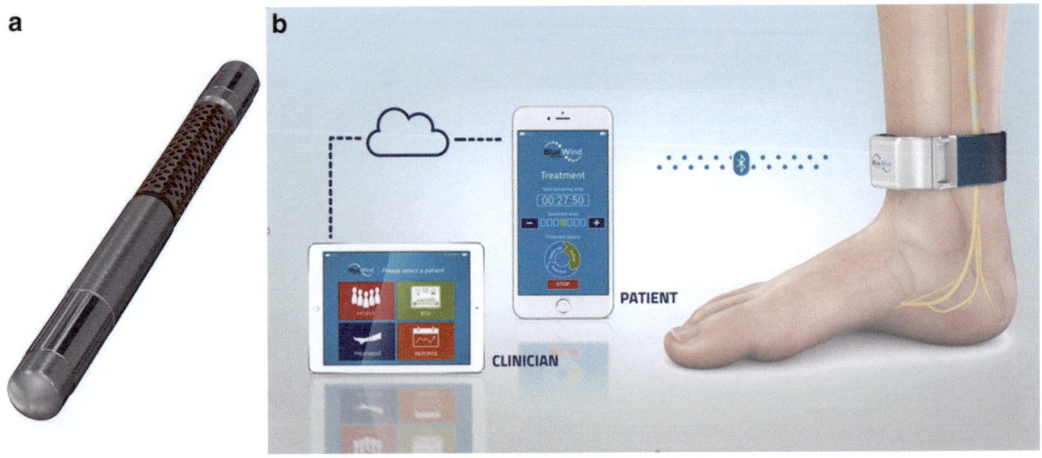

Fig. 13.5 The BlueWind wireless tibial nerve stimulator (**a**) implantable device, (**b**) wearable patient-controlled system. Reproduced with permission from BlueWind Medical, Ltd

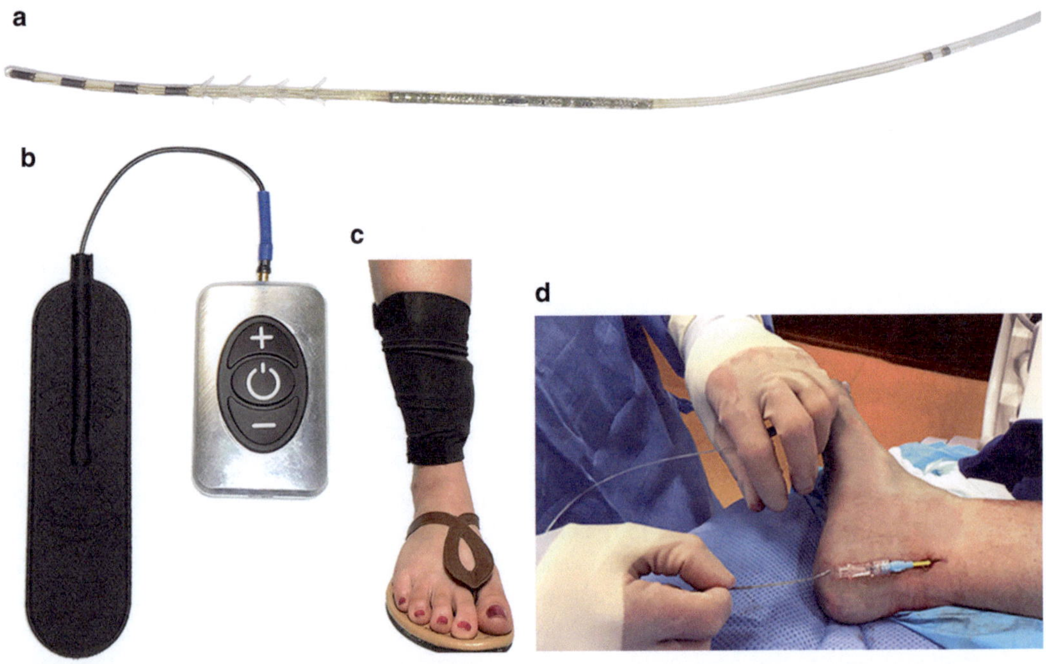

Fig. 13.6 The StimGuard percutaneously implantable wireless tibial nerve stimulator (**a**) tined lead, (**b**) patient controller, (**c**) wearable energy source. The device can be (**d**) placed percutaneously in a retrograde fashion under local anesthetic. Reproduced with permission from StimGuard, LLC

Potential Undertreatment

The currently available paradigm for PTNS is once weekly for 30 min. There is no data to suggest that this is the ideal treatment interval, rather it is based on convenience to the patient and the physician. Some have shown that daily stimulation leads to more rapid and robust symptom improvement [38]. Minimally invasive chronic leads with external power sources like the BlueWind and StimGuard devices could advance tibial nerve neuromodulation by easing patient burden and potentially improving outcomes through daily stimulation.

Cavernous Nerve Stimulation for Erectile Dysfunction

Erectile dysfunction is common in men and increases with age [39, 40]. The Massachusetts Male Aging Study reported rates of mild, moderate, and complete erectile dysfunction in 17%, 25%, and 10% of men, respectively [39]. The National Health and Social Life Survey study of men aged 18–59 reported that 10.2% of the 1244 men had difficulty achieving or maintaining an erection [40]. Treatment of these patients with oral phosphodiesterase type 5 inhibitors has 65–70% efficacy and tolerability [41], yet fewer than half of those patients renewed their prescriptions 6–12 months after the initial visit [42]. Following oral therapy, patients progress to intracavernous injections or penile implants. Intracavernous injections have response rates of 70–92%, with potential adverse events including fibrosis, pain, and priapism [41]. Though penile implantation provides high satisfaction rates, there is surgical morbidity including infection and potential irreversible erectile dysfunction [43, 44].

Penile tumescence and erectile response with electrical stimulation of the cavernous nerves have been demonstrated in canine, primate, and rat models in the 1980s and 1990s [45–47]. These findings were extrapolated to a clinical setting by stimulating the cavernous nerve intraoperatively during radical retropubic prostatectomy or penile surgery for venous leakage, with erection induced in 8/16 and 5/6 patients, respectively [48].

Shafik studied stimulation at the cavernous nerve in animal and human models since the 1990s for treatment of erectile dysfunction [49–51]. Stimulating the cavernous nerves via an extrapelvic subpubic approach using a bipolar platinum electrode and radiofrequency receiver at a frequency of 60 Hz caused full erections in dogs [49]. He repeated this in 15 human patients with erectile dysfunction with a similar device, using a parapenile incision to expose the cavernous nerve [50]. With similar stimulation frequency, he again was able to induce full erection in all patients. Another study evaluated noninvasive magnetic stimulation of the cavernous nerve by placing a magnetic coil over the dorsal penis [51]. In 30 men with erectile dysfunction, the coil was activated, while in 15 control patients it was placed but not activated. All patients in the treatment group reproducibly achieved full erections, while none in the control group had any change in intracavernous pressure or tumescence. While these findings have not been reproduced, further investigation of external stimulation of the cavernous nerve is warranted. Currently, a trial is ongoing evaluating early cavernous nerve stimulation via an implantable neurostimulator to enhance nerve erectile recovery after radical prostatectomy [52].

Expanding Indications and Novel Nerve Targets

Dozens of articles have shown that sacral, pudendal, and tibial nerve stimulation may provide secondary gain in the treatment of pelvic pain, vulvodynia, persistent genital arousal disorder, neurogenic bladder, irritable bowel syndrome, chronic constipation, female sexual dysfunction, and dysfunctional elimination syndrome in children [21, 53–69]. However, these are mostly single-center, noncontrolled case reports. The dorsal genital nerve (branch of the pudendal) has been shown to be a potential site of stimulation for overactive bladder and neurogenic detrusor overactivity [70–74]. Robust, well-controlled trials are needed to study other indications to potentially expand our current indications for neuromodulation.

Not only is research on new nerve targets and clinical indications needed, there is data suggesting that stimulation of different regions of the same nerve may impact the clinical effect. Grinberg et al. examined the effect of perineural thickness, fascicular diameter, and fascicle position on axonal excitation thresholds and adjacent fascicular recruitment [75]. His findings demonstrated that increased perineural thickness and fascicular diameter increase axonal excitation thresholds, and that size of neighboring fascicles affected recruitment (e.g., small fascicles were recruited at lower thresholds than larger fascicles, large fascicles caused large changes in activation threshold of adjacent small fascicles). They concluded that studying individual nerve targets would thus allow for accurate models to improve design of neurostimulators and ultimately clinical outcomes.

Conclusion

Neuromodulation is changing the future of medicine. Treatment of voiding dysfunction and likely other disorders such as pelvic pain, sexual dysfunction, and bowel disorders will no longer rely only on medications with moderate efficacy and multiple side effects, or destructive and reconstructive surgeries that are plagued by significant complications. Rather, by modulating the nerves, the clinician will be able to treat these disorders in a minimally invasive and effective fashion. Advances in neuromodulation technology will allow easier integration of this treatment into patients' lives. Rechargeable and wireless technologies and new, minimally invasive nerve targets should reduce the cost to the healthcare system and expand availability worldwide.

References

1. Peters KM, Carey JM, Konstandt DB. Sacral neuromodulation for the treatment of refractory interstitial cystitis: outcomes based on technique. Int Urogynecol J Pelvic Floor Dysfunct. 2003;14(4):223–8; discussion 8. https://doi.org/10.1007/s00192-003-1070-3.
2. Spinelli M, Weil E, Ostardo E, Del Popolo G, Ruiz-Cerda JL, Kiss G, et al. New tined lead electrode in sacral neuromodulation: experience from a multicentre European study. World J Urol. 2005;23(3):225–9. https://doi.org/10.1007/s00345-005-0502-8.
3. Borawski KM, Foster RT, Webster GD, Amundsen CL. Predicting implantation with a neuromodulator using two different test stimulation techniques: a prospective randomized study in urge incontinent women. Neurourol Urodyn. 2007;26(1):14–8. https://doi.org/10.1002/nau.20332.
4. Leong RK, De Wachter SG, Nieman FH, de Bie RA, van Kerrebroeck PE. PNE versus 1st stage tined lead procedure: a direct comparison to select the most sensitive test method to identify patients suitable for sacral neuromodulation therapy. Neurourol Urodyn. 2011;30(7):1249–52. https://doi.org/10.1002/nau.20979.
5. Amend B, Khalil M, Kessler TM, Sievert KD. How does sacral modulation work best? Placement and programming techniques to maximize efficacy. Curr Urol Rep. 2011;12(5):327–35. https://doi.org/10.1007/s11934-011-0204-2.
6. Le NB, Kim JH. Expanding the role of neuromodulation for overactive bladder: new indications and alternatives to delivery. Curr Bladder Dysfunct Rep. 2011;6(1):25–30. https://doi.org/10.1007/s11884-010-0074-3.
7. Alavi K, Chan S, Wise P, Kaiser AM, Sudan R, Bordeianou L. Fecal incontinence: etiology, diagnosis, and management. J Gastrointest Surg. 2015;19(10):1910–21. https://doi.org/10.1007/s11605-015-2905-1.
8. Matzel KE, Stadelmaier U, Hohenfellner M, Gall FP. Electrical stimulation of sacral spinal nerves for treatment of faecal incontinence. Lancet. 1995;346(8983):1124–7.
9. Cohn JA, Kowalik CG, Kaufman MR, Reynolds WS, Milam DF, Dmochowski RR. Evaluation of the axonics modulation technologies sacral neuromodulation system for the treatment of urinary and fecal dysfunction. Expert Rev Med Devices. 2017;14(1):3–14. https://doi.org/10.1080/17434440.2017.1268913.
10. Axonics Modulation Technologies I. Treatment of REfractory Overactive BLadder With the AXonics Sacral Neuromodulation System. 2016. https://ClinicalTrials.gov/show/NCT02620410.
11. Oerlemans DJ, van Voskuilen AC, Marcelissen T, Weil EH, de Bie RA, Van Kerrebroeck PE. Is on-demand sacral neuromodulation in patients with OAB syndrome a feasible therapy regime? Neurourol Urodyn. 2011;30(8):1493–6. https://doi.org/10.1002/nau.21070.
12. 't Hoen LA, Groen J, Scheepe JR, Blok BF. Intermittent sacral neuromodulation for idiopathic urgency urinary incontinence in women. Neurourol Urodyn. 2015. https://doi.org/10.1002/nau.22938.
13. Fjorback MV, Rijkhoff N, Petersen T, Nohr M, Sinkjaer T. Event driven electrical stimulation of the dorsal penile/clitoral nerve for management of neurogenic detrusor overactivity in multiple sclerosis. Neurourol Urodyn. 2006;25(4):349–55. https://doi.org/10.1002/nau.20170.
14. Opisso E, Borau A, Rodriguez A, Hansen J, Rijkhoff NJ. Patient controlled versus automatic stimulation of pudendal nerve afferents to treat neurogenic detrusor overactivity. J Urol. 2008;180(4):1403–8. https://doi.org/10.1016/j.juro.2008.06.023.
15. Nikolavsky D, Killinger K, Boura J, Peters K. Comparison of patients undergoing a two-stage

sacral nerve stimulation procedure: is there a cost benefit for a single-stage procedure? Int Urol Nephrol. 2011;43(4):997–1002. https://doi.org/10.1007/s11255-011-9919-8.
16. Baxter C, Kim JH. Contrasting the percutaneous nerve evaluation versus staged implantation in sacral neuromodulation. Curr Urol Rep. 2010;11(5):310–4. https://doi.org/10.1007/s11934-010-0128-2.
17. Jacobs SA, Lane FL, Osann KE, Noblett KL. Randomized prospective crossover study of interstim lead wire placement with curved versus straight stylet. Neurourol Urodyn. 2014;33(5):488–92. https://doi.org/10.1002/nau.22437.
18. Spinelli M, Malaguti S, Giardiello G, Lazzeri M, Tarantola J, Van Den Hombergh U. A new minimally invasive procedure for pudendal nerve stimulation to treat neurogenic bladder: description of the method and preliminary data. Neurourol Urodyn. 2005;24(4):305–9. https://doi.org/10.1002/nau.20118.
19. Peters KM, Feber KM, Bennett RC. Sacral versus pudendal nerve stimulation for voiding dysfunction: a prospective, single-blinded, randomized, crossover trial. Neurourol Urodyn. 2005;24(7):643–7. https://doi.org/10.1002/nau.20174.
20. Peters KM, Killinger KA, Boguslawski BM, Boura JA. Chronic pudendal neuromodulation: expanding available treatment options for refractory urologic symptoms. Neurourol Urodyn. 2010;29(7):1267–71. https://doi.org/10.1002/nau.20823.
21. Peters KM, Killinger KA, Jaeger C, Chen C. Pilot study exploring chronic pudendal neuromodulation as a treatment option for pain associated with pudendal neuralgia. Low Urin Tract Symptoms. 2015;7(3):138–42. https://doi.org/10.1111/luts.12066.
22. Govier F, Litwiller S, Nitti V, Kreder KJ, Rosenblatt P. Percutaneous afferent neuromodulation for the refractory overactive bladder: results of a multicenter study. J Urol. 2001;165:1193–8.
23. van Balken MR, Vandoninck V, Gisolf KW, Vergunst H, Kiemeney LA, Debruyne FM, et al. Posterior tibial nerve stimulation as neuromodulative treatment of lower urinary tract dysfunction. J Urol. 2001;166(3):914–8.
24. Peters KM, Macdiarmid SA, Wooldridge LS, Leong FC, Shobeiri SA, Rovner ES, et al. Randomized trial of percutaneous tibial nerve stimulation versus extended-release tolterodine: results from the overactive bladder innovative therapy trial. J Urol. 2009;182(3):1055–61. https://doi.org/10.1016/j.juro.2009.05.045.
25. Peters KM, Carrico DJ, Perez-Marrero RA, Khan AU, Wooldridge LS, Davis GL, et al. Randomized trial of percutaneous tibial nerve stimulation versus Sham efficacy in the treatment of overactive bladder syndrome: results from the SUmiT trial. J Urol. 2010;183(4):1438–43. https://doi.org/10.1016/j.juro.2009.12.036.
26. MacDiarmid SA, Peters KM, Shobeiri SA, Wooldridge LS, Rovner ES, Leong FC, et al. Long-term durability of percutaneous tibial nerve stimulation for the treatment of overactive bladder. J Urol. 2010;183(1):234–40. https://doi.org/10.1016/j.juro.2009.08.160.
27. Peters KM, Carrico DJ, Wooldridge LS, Miller CJ, MacDiarmid SA. Percutaneous tibial nerve stimulation for the long-term treatment of overactive bladder: 3-year results of the STEP study. J Urol. 2013;189(6):2194–201. https://doi.org/10.1016/j.juro.2012.11.175.
28. Chen HW, Bercik RS, Werner EF, Thung SF. Cost-effectiveness of percutaneous tibial nerve stimulation versus extended release tolterodine for overactive bladder. J Urol. 2012;187(1):178–84. https://doi.org/10.1016/j.juro.2011.09.052.
29. Peters KM. Pilot clinical trial on BiowavePTNS (Percutnaeous Tibial Nerve Stimulation) for the treatment of OAB. (Unpublished).
30. van der Pal F, van Balken MR, Heesakkers JP, Debruyne FM, Bemelmans BL. Implant-driven tibial nerve stimulation in the treatment of refractory overactive bladder syndrome: 12-month follow-up. Neuromodulation. 2006;9(2):163–71. https://doi.org/10.1111/j.1525-1403.2006.00056.x.
31. Janssen DA, Farag F, Heesakkers JP. Urgent-SQ implant in treatment of overactive bladder syndrome: 9-year follow-up study. Neurourol Urodyn. 2013;32(5):472–5. https://doi.org/10.1002/nau.22322.
32. Elneil S, Digesu A, van Breda H, Heesakkers J, Van Kerrebroeck P. Safety and performance of a wireless implantable tibial nerve stimulator device for the treatment of patients with overactive bladder (OAB). Neurourol Urodyn. 2016;35(Suppl 4):S45–S6. https://doi.org/10.1002/nau.23074.
33. BlueWind Medical, Rainbow Medical. BlueWind reprieve system for the treatment of PNP. 2014. https://ClinicalTrials.gov/show/NCT02209896.
34. Rainbow Medical, BlueWind Medical. Overactive bladder posterior tibial implantable MIcro STimulator-1. 2017. https://ClinicalTrials.gov/show/NCT03019094.
35. Sirls L, Peters K. A cadaver model describing a novel retrograde approach for percutaneous placement of an implantable tibial nerve stimulation lead. In: International Continence Society Annual Meeting 2016, Tokyo, Japan; 13–16 Sept 2016.
36. Kessler TM, Knuepfer S, De Wachter S, Kozomara M, Sievert K. Tibial neuromodulation: novel chronic implantable device achieves urinary continence in initial cases. In: International Continence Society Annual Meeting 2016, Tokyo, Japan; 13–16 Sept 2016.
37. StimGuard, LLC. CAN-stim compared to PTNS in treatment of urinary urgency incontinence with wireless neuromodulation technology. 2016. https://ClinicalTrials.gov/show/NCT02577302.

38. Thomas GP, Dudding TC, Bradshaw E, Nicholls RJ, Vaizey CJ. A pilot study to compare daily with twice weekly transcutaneous posterior tibial nerve stimulation for faecal incontinence. Color Dis. 2013;15(12):1504–9. https://doi.org/10.1111/codi.12428.
39. Feldman HA, Goldstein I, Hatzichristou DG, Krane RJ, McKinlay JB. Impotence and its medical and psychosocial correlates: results of the Massachusetts Male Aging Study. J Urol. 1994;151(1):54–61.
40. Laumann EO, Paik A, Rosen RC. Sexual dysfunction in the United States: prevalence and predictors. JAMA. 1999;281(6):537–44.
41. McMahon CN, Smith CJ, Shabsigh R. Treating erectile dysfunction when PDE5 inhibitors fail. BMJ. 2006;332(7541):589–92. https://doi.org/10.1136/bmj.332.7541.589.
42. Fagelman E, Fagelman A, Shabsigh R. Efficacy, safety, and use of sildenafil in urologic practice. Urology. 2001;57(6):1141–4. https://doi.org/10.1016/s0090-4295(01)00984-0.
43. Kucuk EV, Tahra A, Bindayi A, Onol FF. Erectile dysfunction patients are more satisfied with penile prosthesis implantation compared with tadalafil and intracavernosal injection treatments. Andrology. 2016;4(5):952–6. https://doi.org/10.1111/andr.12237.
44. Hatzimouratidis K, Amar E, Eardley I, Giuliano F, Hatzichristou D, Montorsi F, et al. Guidelines on male sexual dysfunction: erectile dysfunction and premature ejaculation. Eur Urol. 2010;57(5):804–14. https://doi.org/10.1016/j.eururo.2010.02.020.
45. Lue TF, Schmidt RA, Tanagho EA. Electrostimulation and penile erection. Urol Int. 1985;40(1):60–4.
46. Mueller SC, Aboseif S, Fahey MR, Lue TF, Tanagho EA. Spinal anesthesia and electroerection in dogs and monkeys. J Urol. 1989;142(1):171–5.
47. Martinez-Pineiro L, Brock G, Trigo-Rocha F, Hsu GL, Lue TF, Tanagho EA. Rat model for the study of penile erection: pharmacologic and electrical-stimulation parameters. Eur Urol. 1994;25(1):62–70.
48. Lue TF, Gleason CA, Brock GB, Carroll PR, Tanagho EA. Intraoperative electrostimulation of the cavernous nerve: technique, results and limitations. J Urol. 1995;154(4):1426–8.
49. Shafik A. Cavernous nerve stimulation through an extrapelvic subpubic approach: role in penile erection. Eur Urol. 1994;26(1):98–102.
50. Shafik A. Extrapelvic cavernous nerve stimulation in erectile dysfunction. Human study. Andrologia. 1996;28(3):151–6.
51. Shafik A, el-Sibai O, Shafik AA. Magnetic stimulation of the cavernous nerve for the treatment of erectile dysfunction in humans. Int J Impot Res. 2000;12(3):137–41; discussion 41–2.
52. Peters KM. A pilot study of the feasibility of chronic cavernous nerve stimulation to promote regeneration and erectile function. https://ClinicalTrials.gov/show/NCT02006927.
53. Marcelissen T, Van Kerrebroeck P, de Wachter S. Sacral neuromodulation as a treatment for neuropathic clitoral pain after abdominal hysterectomy. Int Urogynecol J. 2010;21(10):1305–7. https://doi.org/10.1007/s00192-010-1145-x.
54. Jones CL, Fischer JR, Hernandez SL. Sacral neuromodulation for the treatment of persistent genital arousal disorder. Obstet Gynecol. 2016;128(2):321–3. https://doi.org/10.1097/AOG.0000000000001452.
55. Hill AJ, Paraiso MF. Resolution of chronic vulvar pruritus with replacement of a neuromodulation device. J Minim Invasive Gynecol. 2015;22(5):889–91. https://doi.org/10.1016/j.jmig.2015.02.020.
56. Ramsay LB, Wright J Jr, Fischer JR. Sacral neuromodulation in the treatment of vulvar vestibulitis syndrome. Obstet Gynecol. 2009;114(2 Pt 2):487–9. https://doi.org/10.1097/AOG.0b013e3181af5f80.
57. Krames E, Mousad DG. Spinal cord stimulation reverses pain and diarrheal episodes of irritable bowel syndrome: a case report. Neuromodulation. 2004;7(2):82–8. https://doi.org/10.1111/j.1094-7159.2004.04011.x.
58. Canbaz Kabay S, Kabay S, Mestan E, Cetiner M, Ayas S, Sevim M, et al. Long term sustained therapeutic effects of percutaneous posterior tibial nerve stimulation treatment of neurogenic overactive bladder in multiple sclerosis patients: 12-months results. Neurourol Urodyn. 2017;36(1):104–10. https://doi.org/10.1002/nau.22868.
59. Lombardi G, Musco S, Celso M, Del Corso F, Del Popolo G. Sacral neuromodulation for neurogenic non-obstructive urinary retention in incomplete spinal cord patients: a ten-year follow-up single-centre experience. Spinal Cord. 2014;52(3):241–5. https://doi.org/10.1038/sc.2013.155.
60. Wosnitzer MS, Walsh R, Rutman MP. The use of sacral neuromodulation for the treatment of non-obstructive urinary retention secondary to Guillain-Barre syndrome. Int Urogynecol J Pelvic Floor Dysfunct. 2009;20(9):1145–7. https://doi.org/10.1007/s00192-009-0826-9.
61. Guys JM, Haddad M, Planche D, Torre M, Louis-Borrione C, Breaud J. Sacral neuromodulation for neurogenic bladder dysfunction in children. J Urol. 2004;172(4 Pt 2):1673–6.
62. Marinkovic SP, Miller B, Hughes S, Marinkovic C, Gillen L. Successful bilateral pudendal neuromodulation to treat male detrusor areflexia following severe pubic symphysis fracture, a case report. BMC Urol. 2015;15:115. https://doi.org/10.1186/s12894-015-0108-4.
63. Baron M, Grynberg L, Delcourt C, Cornu JN, Grise P. [Does urinary sacral neuromodulation improve bowel symptoms other than fecal incontinence: a systematic review]. Prog Urol. 2016;26(7):395–400. https://doi.org/10.1016/j.purol.2016.01.007.
64. Killinger KA, Kangas JR, Wolfert C, Boura JA, Peters KM. Secondary changes in bowel function after successful treatment of voiding symptoms with neuro-

modulation. Neurourol Urodyn. 2011;30(1):133–7. https://doi.org/10.1002/nau.20975.
65. van der Wilt AA, van Wunnik BP, Sturkenboom R, Han-Geurts IJ, Melenhorst J, Benninga MA, et al. Sacral neuromodulation in children and adolescents with chronic constipation refractory to conservative treatment. Int J Color Dis. 2016;31(8):1459–66. https://doi.org/10.1007/s00384-016-2604-8.
66. Musco S, Serati M, Lombardi G, Lumi E, Parisi AI, Del Popolo G, et al. Percutaneous tibial nerve stimulation improves female sexual function in women with overactive bladder syndrome. J Sex Med. 2016;13(2):238–42. https://doi.org/10.1016/j.jsxm.2015.12.025.
67. Parnell BA, Howard JF Jr, Geller EJ. The effect of sacral neuromodulation on pudendal nerve function and female sexual function. Neurourol Urodyn. 2015;34(5):456–60. https://doi.org/10.1002/nau.22579.
68. Yih JM, Killinger KA, Boura JA, Peters KM. Changes in sexual functioning in women after neuromodulation for voiding dysfunction. J Sex Med. 2013;10(10):2477–83. https://doi.org/10.1111/jsm.12085.
69. Dwyer ME, Vandersteen DR, Hollatz P, Reinberg YE. Sacral neuromodulation for the dysfunctional elimination syndrome: a 10-year single-center experience with 105 consecutive children. Urology. 2014;84(4):911–7. https://doi.org/10.1016/j.urology.2014.03.059.
70. Goldman HB, Amundsen CL, Mangel J, Grill J, Bennett M, Gustafson KJ, et al. Dorsal genital nerve stimulation for the treatment of overactive bladder symptoms. Neurourol Urodyn. 2008;27(6):499–503. https://doi.org/10.1002/nau.20544.
71. Horvath EE, Yoo PB, Amundsen CL, Webster GD, Grill WM. Conditional and continuous electrical stimulation increase cystometric capacity in persons with spinal cord injury. Neurourol Urodyn. 2010;29(3):401–7. https://doi.org/10.1002/nau.20766.
72. Martens FM, Heesakkers JP, Rijkhoff NJ. Minimal invasive electrode implantation for conditional stimulation of the dorsal genital nerve in neurogenic detrusor overactivity. Spinal Cord. 2011;49(4):566–72. https://doi.org/10.1038/sc.2010.134.
73. Opisso E, Borau A, Rijkhoff NJ. Subject-controlled stimulation of dorsal genital nerve to treat neurogenic detrusor overactivity at home. Neurourol Urodyn. 2013;32(7):1004–9. https://doi.org/10.1002/nau.22359.
74. van Breda HM, Farag FF, Martens FM, Heesakkers JP, Rijkhoff NJ. Subject-controlled, on-demand, dorsal genital nerve stimulation to treat urgency urinary incontinence; a pilot. Front Neurosci. 2016;10:24. https://doi.org/10.3389/fnins.2016.00024.
75. Grinberg Y, Schiefer MA, Tyler DJ, Gustafson KJ. Fascicular perineurium thickness, size, and position affect model predictions of neural excitation. IEEE Trans Neural Syst Rehabil Eng. 2008;16(6):572–81. https://doi.org/10.1109/TNSRE.2008.2010348.
76. Das AK, White MD, Longhurst PA. Sacral nerve stimulation for the management of voiding dysfunction. Rev Urol. 2000;2(1):43–60.

Part II

Pediatrics

Pediatric Posterior Tibial Nerve Stimulation

14

Kassem Faraj, Chirag Dave, and Kevin M. Feber

Introduction

Non-neurogenic lower urinary tract dysfunction (LUTD) is common throughout the pediatric population, with nearly 40% of pediatric urology visits being related to voiding dysfunction [1]. This is thought to be related to delayed maturation or lack of inhibitory input from higher micturition centers [2]. LUTD can involve a combination of symptoms including increased/decreased urinary frequency, incontinence, urgency, nocturia, dysuria, straining, or intermittency [3]. LUTD has been shown to be associated with other non-urologic entities such as obstipation and behavioral problems, and therefore a multimodal approach must be taken [4].

On many occasions, these symptoms can resolve with age. For example, nocturnal enuresis has a 15% resolution rate per year and overall decrease in prevalence from 20 to 1% from ages 5–16 [5]. However, pediatric urologists still frequently encounter patients who require treatment. First-line treatment for non-neurogenic LUTD includes behavioral therapy (i.e., bladder training, pelvic floor exercises, biofeedback). Patients not responding to behavioral therapy may require medical therapy (i.e., anticholinergics, alpha-blockers). Although a combination of these treatment modalities have been shown to be very effective in managing these symptoms in the pediatric population, up to 20% of these patients will be refractory [6]. This introduces a conundrum for both patients and their physicians. In an attempt to manage patients who are resistant to conventional treatment methods, some unconventional approaches have been investigated. Neuromodulation, including posterior tibial nerve stimulation, has emerged as a safe and efficacious tool in the management of refractory voiding dysfunction and is well studied in the adult population. It has been increasingly studied for the management of pediatric LUTD. This chapter will discuss relevant literature and describe procedural techniques supporting the use of PTNS in a pediatric patient population.

History

Although neuromodulation has established a role in the management of adult voiding disorders, there were some initial reservations to performing these techniques in the pediatric population. It was thought that neuromodulation was too invasive for this population, thus potentially resulting in pain and noncompliance [7]. Tanagho

K. Faraj · C. Dave · K. M. Feber (✉)
Department of Urology, Beaumont Hospital/Oakland University William Beaumont School of Medicine, Royal Oak, MI, USA
e-mail: kfeber@urologist.org

J. P. Gilleran, S. A. Alpert (eds.), *Adult and Pediatric Neuromodulation*,
https://doi.org/10.1007/978-3-319-73266-4_14

was the first to assess the safety and efficacy of sacral neuromodulation in the pediatric population and he found that in addition to tolerating the procedures very well, most patients had improvement of their urinary symptoms after testing and many received implant of permanent electrodes as a result [8].

PTNS was first described in 1983 by McGuire and colleagues, where they showed that percutaneous stimulation of the tibial nerve was effective in treating patients with detrusor instability [9]. The idea behind stimulating nerves to control voiding dysfunction is one that goes back to traditional Chinese medicine and acupuncture, where various points are stimulated in an attempt to normalize voiding function [10]. One of the acupuncture points of interest is the Sanyinjiao (SP6), a point that is located 5 cm cephalad from the medial malleolus, which is the area of the tibial nerve [9]. Stimulation of the tibial nerve is thought to affect voiding function because it contains fibers that are of the same spinal segments as the parasympathetic nerves that innervate the bladder and thus, stimulation can modulate bladder activation [11].

Posterior Tibial Nerve Stimulation (PTNS) in Pediatrics

PTNS has gained increased popularity in recent years in the adult population, gaining approval from the Food and Drug Administration in 2000 for the management of overactive bladder. It was around this time that this procedure was introduced in the pediatric population. There are two PTNS approaches that have been described in the literature for the pediatric population: percutaneous and transcutaneous. Both will be discussed in this section.

Percutaneous PTNS

The percutaneous method was the first approach described for PTNS and requires a percutaneous electrical nerve stimulation device, which consists of the following: interface cable, surface electrode, percutaneous needle, portable stimulator (Fig. 14.2). The procedure is performed as follows [12]:

1. Insertion of the needle about 2 cm cephalad to the medial malleolus (Figs. 14.1 and 14.2)
2. Placement of the surface electrode on the medial side of the same foot
3. Adjust the portable stimulator to provide pulsations between the needle and electrode at 20 Hz
4. Ensure proper stimulation of the tibial nerve by observing flexion of the big toe and/or tingling sensation at the bottom of the foot
5. Adjust amplitude to just below the sensory threshold
6. Continue therapy for 30 min

A pilot study by Hoebeke and colleagues in 2002 prospectively looked at the utility of percutaneous PTNS in 32 children with mixed lower urinary tract symptoms (LUTS) who were resistant to conventional therapy [12]. Treatment sessions took place weekly, where needle stimulation was performed for 30 min. Children were evaluated at 6 weeks and therapy was continued for 12 additional sessions, if favorable results were observed. They found that there was resolution and improvement of urgency in 25% and 36% of the patients, respectively. Incontinence also resolved in 17% and improved in 63% of the patients. Of the patients who had disturbed voiding frequency (i.e., less than 4 or more than 8 voids daily), 84% achieved normal (4–6) frequency of voiding. There was also a statistically significant increase in mean bladder capacity from 185 to 279 cm^3 and 43% of patients had a normalized uroflowmetry curve after treatment sessions.

One of the perceived drawbacks of performing this procedure in the pediatric population is the pain associated with the needle. In the study by Hoebeke and colleagues, one patient discontinued stimulation therapy due to fear of the needle [12]. Another study by De Gennaro and colleagues looked at pain tolerability in addition to the efficacy of percutaneous PTNS in pediatric patients with refractory bladder dysfunction [13].

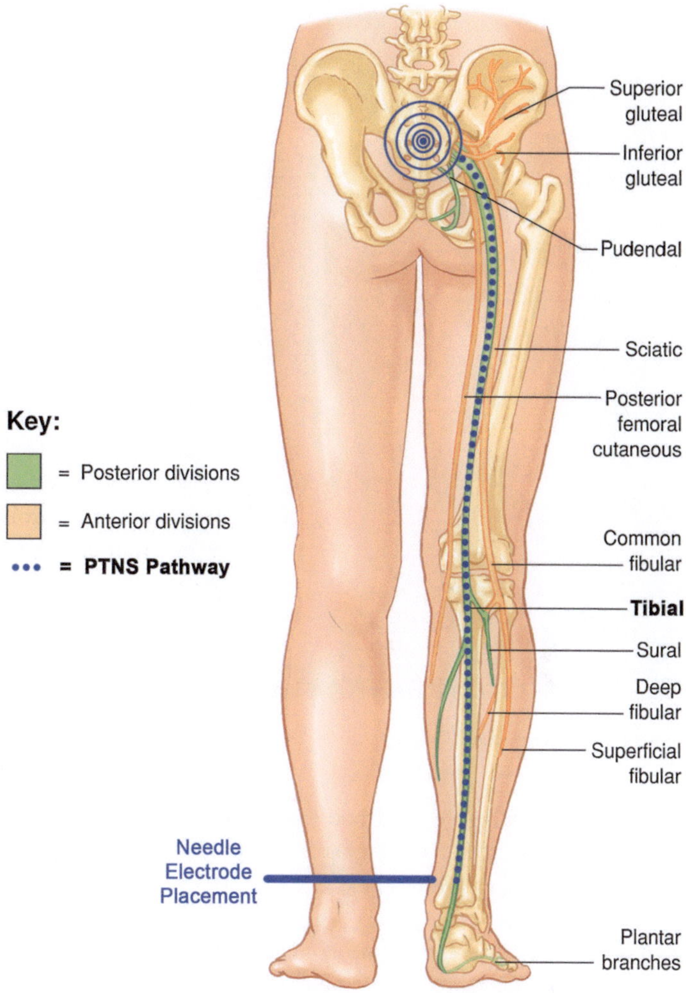

Fig. 14.1 PTNS needle placement. © Cogent Medical. All rights reserved

There were 23 patients with LUTS refractory to conventional treatment in this study and again PTNS was found to be effective in improving symptoms in 80% of those with overactive bladder and 71% of those with urinary retention. Incontinence was also cured in 56% of those affected. In addition, urodynamic studies showed improved detrusor pressure at maximum flow and improved flow rate, after stimulation. Pain was monitored in ten children at the first, sixth, and last sessions during needle insertion and electrical stimulation using various scoring systems (i.e., the faces pain rating scale, Children's Hospital of Eastern Ontario pain scale, visual analogue scale, Questionario Italiano del Dolore). These metrics demonstrated generally low levels of pain associated with needle insertion, which decreased significantly during the subsequent sessions. This suggests that this procedure is well-tolerated in the pediatric population, in spite of the use of a needle.

Transcutaneous PTNS

Boudaoud and colleagues first described the use of transcutaneous PTNS in the pediatric population in 2015. This group cited the following potential advantages to using the transcutaneous technique in the pediatric population: simplicity of use, noninvasiveness, decreased pain, and lack of reported adverse events. The equipment they

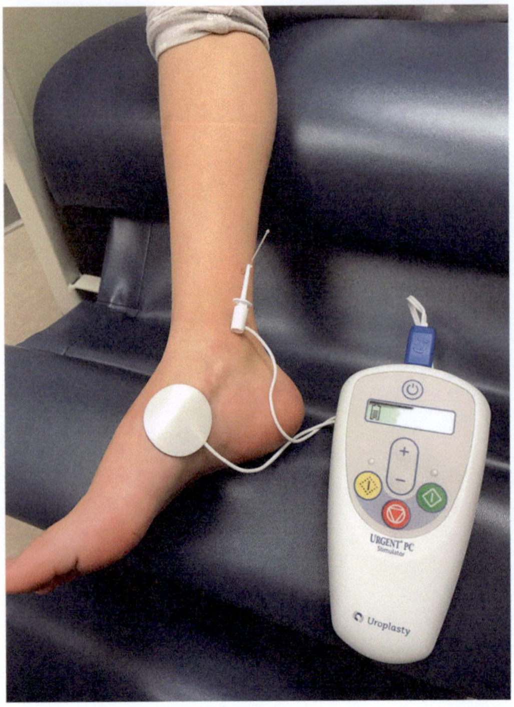

Fig. 14.2 Percutaneous PTNS

used included: adhesive electrode (3), electrical stimulator connected to a computer. The procedure is performed as follows [14]:

1. Two adhesive electrodes are connected to a stimulator (connected to a computer)
2. One electrode is placed above (positive) the medial malleolus and the other is placed below (negative) the medial malleolus on the same foot
3. A grounding electrode is placed along the path of the other electrodes, superior to the previous two
4. Current intensity is set below the pain threshold at 10 mA, frequency at 10 Hz, and continuous stimulation of 200 μs for 30 min

In the study by Boudaoud and colleagues, 20 children with overactive bladder were randomized in a double-blind, controlled manner. The treatment group received transcutaneous PTNS, while the control group received sham treatments. Treatments consisted of two weekly 30-min sessions for 12 weeks. The investigators found no difference in subjective clinical results (i.e., reported frequency of episodes, urgency, daytime continence, presence of nocturia) at the end of the study, as recorded by events in a bladder diary. They did, however, find significant improvement in the urodynamic tests measured in the treatment group, including a significant increase in the following: volume voided during urgency (184–265 mL), maximal cystometric volume (215–274 mL), volume at onset of first detrusor contraction (48–174 mL). The treatment group also experienced a significant decrease in the maximal bladder pressure during an overactive detrusor contraction (61–46). In addition, Patidar and colleagues performed a randomized sham controlled trial evaluating the efficacy of transcutaneous PTNS in the treatment of overactive bladder [15]. In contrast to the results of the study by Boudaoud and colleagues, this study found that with weekly 30-min treatments, the treatment group reported a significant subjective improvement of overactive bladder symptoms, as well as the number of daily voids, by the end of 12 weeks. In light of the results of these studies, the authors in both papers concluded that transcutaneous PTNS should be presented as an option for managing pediatric patients with overactive bladder refractory to conventional treatments.

The utility of transcutaneous PTNS for anatomical causes of bladder dysfunction has also been investigated. In a study by Lecompte and colleagues, eight children with fecal and urinary incontinence due to congenital intestinal diseases or medullary pathologies were managed with transcutaneous PTNS [16]. The equipment used included: autoadhesive electrode (2), electrical stimulation device (Urostim2®). Treatment was initiated with a visiting nurse at the patient's home, who instructed the patient on how to properly perform treatments. Sessions involved the following steps:

1. Two adhesive electrodes are connected to the stimulator
2. One electrode (positive) is placed 3–4 cm above the medial malleolus, the other (negative) is placed just underneath the medial malleolus of the same leg

3. The frequency was set to 10 Hz, with intensity adjusted until flexion of the big toe occurred
4. Once big toe response was confirmed, the intensity was lowered to 10–25 mA
5. Stimulation is applied for 20 min

Patients underwent daily 20-min sessions for 6 months. In the patients who had urinary leakage, 83% were continent at the 6-month period, as measured by the Schurch score for urine. In the patients with fecal leakage, 63% no longer leaked, 25% improved, and 13% did not respond, as measured by Jorge-Wexner score for defecation. This retrospective study suggested that transcutaneous PTNS is potentially an effective treatment option in patients with refractory fecal and urinary incontinence due to various organic pathologies.

PTNS and the Future

With recent studies showing that PTNS shows promise in managing children with voiding issues, there has been increased interest in making this treatment option more tolerable and convenient for these patients. The transcutaneous approach, as discussed above, eliminates the aspect of a needle, which has been shown to deter some of these patients from treatments. With regard to convenience, because classic PTNS requires weekly or semiweekly visits for application of treatments, some researchers have developed devices that can be used by patients in their homes. Lecompte and colleagues specifically focused on patients with complex pathology that require daily treatments, which made the home-device very useful and almost necessary for these patients. Ferroni and colleagues recently described a novel at-home, transcutaneous technique for managing nocturnal enuresis in children [17]. Their approach focused on stimulating peripheral branches of the tibial nerve at the plantar surface of the foot. The equipment used included a commercially available transcutaneous electrical nerve stimulation (TENS) device and two electrode pads. The treatment sessions consisted of the following steps:

1. Place one electrode across the plantar bridge (negative) and the other more proximal over the medial edge of the foot inferior to the medial malleolus (positive)
2. Set TENS device settings to the following: 5 Hz frequency, 0.02 ms pulse width
3. Increase current amplitude (0–100 mA) to the maximal intensity comfortable to the child and when observable involuntary great toe contraction
4. Continue treatment for 60 min

This was a 6-week study, where baseline voiding information was collecting in the first 2 weeks, treatment sessions conducted in the second 2 weeks, and follow-up in the final 2 weeks. In the 22 pediatric patients who were studied, there was a significant reduction in mean total wet nights per week during the stimulation period and a sustained reduction during the follow-up sessions. This study shows promise with this novel technique; however, randomized-controlled studies and long-term data are lacking to support its efficacy.

In summary, PTNS is an exciting technique that should be considered in pediatric patients who are refractory to conventional treatments. There are various approaches to providing PTNS treatments and these options should be included in a discussion between the patient, their family, and their urologist.

References

1. Snodgrass W. Relationship of voiding dysfunction to urinary tract infection and vesicoureteral reflux in children. Urology. 1991;38(4):341–4.
2. Homsy YL. Dysfunctional voiding syndromes and vesicoureteral reflux. Pediatr Nephrol. 1994;8(1):116–21.
3. Nevéus T, von Gontard A, Hoebeke P, et al. The standardization of terminology of lower urinary tract function in children and adolescents: report from the Standardisation Committee of the International Children's Continence Society. J Urol. 2006;176:314–24.
4. von Gontard A, Lettgen B, Olbing H, et al. Behavioural problems in children with urge incontinence and voiding postponement: a comparison of a paediatric and child psychiatric sample. Br J Urol. 1998;81:100–6.

5. Nevéus T, Sillén U. Lower urinary tract function in childhood; normal development and common functional disturbances. Acta Physiol. 2013;207(1):85–92.
6. Nijman RJ. Diagnosis and management of urinary incontinence and functional fecal incontinence (encopresis) in children. Gastroenterol Clin N Am. 2008;37(3):731–48.
7. Bani-Hani AH, Vandersteen DR, Reinberg YE. Neuromodulation in pediatrics. Urol Clin North Am. 2005;32(1):101–7.
8. Tanagho EA. Neuromodulation in the management of voiding dysfunction in children. J Urol. 1992;148(2):655–7.
9. McGuire EJ, Zhang SC, Horwinski ER, et al. Treatment of motor and sensory detrusor instability by electrical stimulation. J Urol. 1983;129(1):78–9.
10. Yu K-W, Lin C-L, Hung C-C, et al. Effects of electroacupuncture on recent stroke in patients with incomplete bladder emptying: a preliminary study. Clin Interv Aging. 2012;7:469–74.
11. Vandonick V, Van Balken MR, Finazzi Agro E, et al. Posterior tibial nerve stimulation in the treatment of voiding dysfunction: urodynamic data. Neurourol Urodyn. 2004;23(3):246–51.
12. Hoebeke P, Renson C, Petillon L, et al. Percutaneous electrical nerve stimulation in children with therapy resistant nonneuropathic bladder sphincter dysfunction: a pilot study. J Urol. 2002;168(6):2605–8.
13. De Gennaro M, Capitanucci ML, Silveri MM, et al. Percutaneous tibial nerve neuromodulation is well tolerated in children and effective for treating refractory vesical dysfunction. J Urol. 2004;171(5):1911–3.
14. Boudaoud N, Binet A, Line A, et al. Management of refractory overactive bladder in children by transcutaneous posterior tibial nerve stimulation: a controlled study. J Pediatr Urol. 2015;11(3):138.
15. Patidar N, Mittal V, Kumar M, et al. Transcutaneous posterior tibial nerve stimulation in pediatric overactive bladder: a preliminary report. J Pediatr Urol. 2015;11(6):351.
16. Lecompte JF, Hery G, Guys JM, et al. Evaluation of transcutaneous electrical posterior tibial nerve stimulation for the treatment of fecal and urinary leaks in children: preliminary results. J Pediatr Surg. 2015;50(4):630–3.
17. Ferroni MC, Chaudhry R, Shen B, et al. Transcutaneous electrical nerve stimulation of the foot: results of a novel at-home, noninvasive treatment for nocturnal enuresis in children. Urology. 2017;101:80–4.

15 Parasacral Transcutaneous Electrical Nerve Stimulation (TENS) in Pediatric Bladder Dysfunction

Paul J. Guidos and Douglas W. Storm

Abbreviations

BBD	Bladder and bowel dysfunction
DSD	Detrusor sphincter dyssynergia
DV	Dysfunctional voiding
EMG	Electromyogram
ENS	Electrical nerve stimulation
NMNE	Non-monosymptomatic nocturnal enuresis
OAB	Overactive bladder
PMNE	Primary monosymptomatic nocturnal enuresis
PTENS	Parasacral transcutaneous electrical nerve stimulation

Introduction

The use of electroneurostimulation (ENS) for bladder dysfunction has been well established within the adult population, with indications for treatment of urinary retention and the symptoms of overactive bladder, including urinary urge incontinence and significant symptoms of urgency-frequency. It has also been trialed in children with lower urinary tract symptoms (LUTS), with promising results [1–3]. There is a suggested advantage to ENS use in children versus adults, in that there may be increased neuroplasticity, which could allow for improved long-term outcomes [1]. However, this has not been established within the literature and remains purely theoretical.

Childhood LUTS may be secondary to bladder and bowel dysfunction (BBD) which can lead to recurrent urinary tract infections (UTIs), vesicoureteral reflux, kidney damage, and incontinence, all of which have a serious impact on the health and quality of life of affected children and their families [4–6]. Pediatric BBD is commonly believed to be secondary to learned misbehaviors, where the child may prolong having a bowel movement or voiding. This holding behavior may lead to pain when the child does defecate or urinate, which may make it less likely for them to use the restroom when necessary, perpetuating these issues. In fact, BBD has been described as the second most common chronic condition of childhood [1]. Pediatric BBD may lead to an overactive bladder (OAB) and dysfunctional voiding (DV). OAB in children is thought to be secondary to detrusor overactivity during the bladder storage phase, whereas DV is due to a failure of normal relaxation of the external urethral sphincter during the voiding phase [4, 7]. Children with OAB commonly present with urinary urgency, frequency, and incontinence.

P. J. Guidos · D. W. Storm (✉)
Department of Urology, University of Iowa Hospitals and Clinics, Iowa City, IA, USA
e-mail: paul-guidos@uiowa.edu; douglas-storm@uiowa.edu

J. P. Gilleran, S. A. Alpert (eds.), *Adult and Pediatric Neuromodulation*,
https://doi.org/10.1007/978-3-319-73266-4_15

Dysfunctional voiding may be manifested by a staccato voiding pattern, urinary straining, and incomplete bladder emptying, which may result in recurrent urinary tract infections and urinary incontinence. In children with DV, an uroflow with electromyogram (EMG) or a videourodynamic study may demonstrate an intermittent uroflow pattern along with excessive EMG activity due to contraction of the sphincter during voiding. DV is similar to detrusor sphincter dyssynergia (DSD), except that DSD, by definition, only occurs in patients with a concurrent neurological disorder; as such DV is also known as non-neurogenic neurogenic voiding or Hinman's syndrome [4].

Management of pediatric OAB and DV is varied and targeted at the individual patient, but traditional therapies include timed voiding, management of any concurrent constipation through the use of medications or dietary changes, anticholinergics, biofeedback, and pelvic floor physical therapy. In rare cases, clean intermittent catheterization and surgery may be necessary. Despite management, it is estimated that 20–40% of pediatric OAB and DV cases are resistant to conservative traditional treatment [1]. ENS can thus be a useful adjunct. A wide variety of ENS methods have been utilized and reported to be effective, including intravesical electrical stimulation, anal and vaginal stimulation, and transcutaneous electrical nerve stimulation (TENS) of the suprapubic region, posterior tibial nerve, and parasacral nerve roots [1–3, 8]. Of these locations, transcutaneous parasacral TENS, which involves electrical nerve stimulation of the second and third sacral dermatomes through the use of surface electrodes, has been the most widely utilized and studied in the treatment of pediatric bladder and bowel dysfunction [1].

This chapter discusses utilization of parasacral transcutaneous electrical nerve stimulation in the pediatric population. A review of normal bladder neuroanatomy and physiology, PTENS technique and its theorized mechanism of action, as well as the indications, treatment outcomes, and side effects of PTENS therapy is presented.

Normal Bladder Neuroanatomy and Physiology

A full understanding of normal bladder filling and emptying is imperative for distinction of bladder dysfunction and related symptoms. During normal bladder filling, stimulation of the sympathetic hypogastric plexus at the spinal level of T10–T12 results in detrusor muscle relaxation as well as contraction of the intrinsic sphincter, inhibiting micturition. Once the bladder is full, stimulation of the pelvic parasympathetic plexus at the spinal level of S2–S4 causes detrusor muscle contraction and relaxation of the intrinsic sphincter, facilitating micturition [9]. Somatic innervation of the pelvic floor and external urethral sphincter at the spinal level of S2–S4 through the pudendal nerve is more complex, but allows for both afferent and efferent pathways between the bladder and the central nervous system. There are two types of bladder afferent, A-δ fibers from mechanoreceptors in the bladder wall which detect fullness and C-fibers which relay discomfort or pain [1]. Normal bladder storage and micturition cycles depend on intact neural pathways in the central nervous system at the cortical and pontine micturition centers which allow for smooth coordination between the two states.

Normal bladder filling and emptying and the related neuroanatomy are depicted in Fig. 15.1 and can be divided into (1) urinary storage and (2) voiding. During the storage of urine, distention of the bladder produces low-level vesical afferent firing. This in turn stimulates the sympathetic outflow in the hypogastric nerve to the bladder outlet (the bladder base and the urethra) and the pudendal outflow to the external urethral sphincter. These responses occur by spinal reflex pathways and represent guarding reflexes, which promote continence. Sympathetic firing also inhibits contraction of the detrusor muscle and modulates neurotransmission in bladder ganglia. A region in the rostral pons (the pontine storage center) might increase striated urethral sphincter activity.

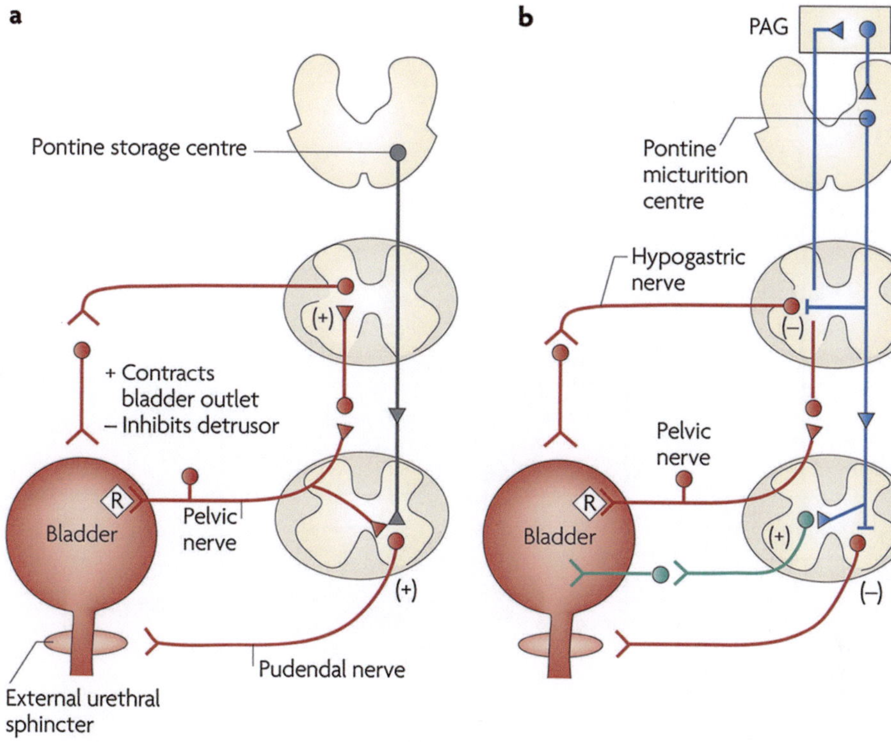

Fig. 15.1 Neuroanatomy and innervation of the bladder, pelvic floor, and urethral sphincter that control continence and micturition. (**a**) Urine storage reflexes. (**b**) Voiding reflexes. From Fowler et al., The neural control of micturition. Nat Rev. Neurosci 2008;9:453–66. Reprinted with permission from Nature Publishing Group

During the elimination of urine, intense bladder-afferent firing in the pelvic nerve activates spinobulbospinal reflex pathways that pass through the pontine micturition center. This stimulates the parasympathetic outflow to the bladder and to the urethral smooth muscle and inhibits the sympathetic and pudendal outflow to the urethral outlet. Ascending afferent input from the spinal cord might pass through relay neurons in the periaqueductal grey (PAG) before reaching the pontine micturition center.

Proposed Mechanism of Action of ENS on the Lower Urinary Tract

The exact mechanism of action of ENS on the lower urinary tract is unclear, but there are several theories (Fig. 15.2) [10]:

1. Affecting the neuroaxis at various levels and restoring the balance between excitatory and inhibitory regulation within the peripheral and central nervous systems
2. Activation of afferent bladder somatosensors with input to micturition center in the brain and/or activation of hypogastric sympathetic nerves
3. Downregulation of bladder response with recurrent, repetitive electrical stimulation and subsequent reduction in detrusor muscle activity
4. Afferent sacral nerve stimulation which increases inhibitory stimuli to efferent pelvic nerve and reduction in detrusor contractility
5. Hypogastric nerve stimulation through activation of sympathetic fibers and low bladder volumes, with stimulation of pudendal nerve nuclei in spinal cord at maximal bladder volume

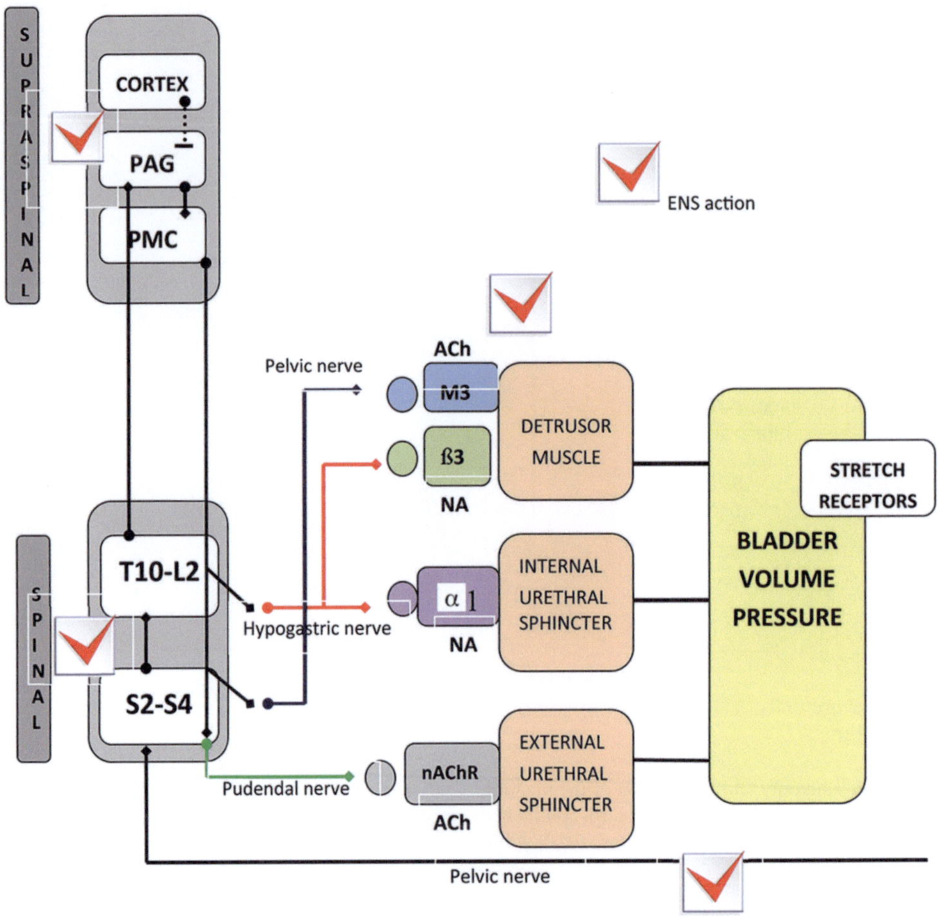

Fig. 15.2 Neurophysiology of the lower urinary tract and the proposed sites of action of ENS action. The proposed sites of ENS action are depicted with the red check marks and include (1) affecting the neuroaxis at various levels, (2) activation of afferent bladder somatosensors, (3) downregulation of bladder response, (4) afferent sacral nerve stimulation, and (5) hypogastric nerve stimulation. From Wright et al. [1]. Reprinted with permission from Elsevier, Ltd

Pediatric PTENS Technique

Parasacral transcutaneous electrical nerve stimulation machines utilize electrical energy at various frequencies and disposable adhesive surface electrodes, which are placed at the sacral region (Fig. 15.3). The typical placement of electrodes is over the second and third sacral dermatomes (lateral border of each electrode over the posterior superior iliac crest, inside border 1 finger-width from the midline). This therapy can be done in-office but is often done at home, with children placing the surface electrodes and wearing them for a specified length of time. The electrodes can be attached using either inexpensive carbon rubber electrodes (requiring adhesive tape along with an electrolyte gel) or self-adhesive electrodes. The current frequency most commonly utilized is 10 Hz, which has been established within the adult literature as the frequency that causes inhibition of detrusor activity [11]. The pulse duration allows for optimal depolarization of the motor and sensory fibers at a minimum charge per pulse and in the adult population has been reported as between 100 and 300 μs for sensory fibers and 200 μs for motor fibers [12]. Most studies on the use of

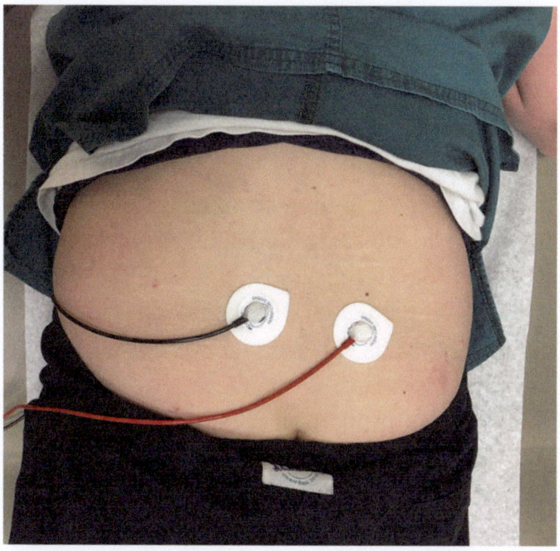

Fig. 15.3 PTENS surface electrode placement. The lateral border of each electrode typically is over the posterior superior iliac crest and the inside border should be one finger width from the midline

PTENS in children have utilized a pulse duration ranging from 150 to 700 μs. Stimulus intensity has been reported as a range from 0 to 60 mA, but is adjustable based on the child's tolerance level. The electrodes are placed and each session typically lasts 20 min, performed twice daily three times a week, for a total of 20 sessions, but can vary depending on patient improvement and tolerance to therapy [2, 3, 13–18]. Complete resolution of symptoms has been reported in as few as three sessions in some cases, with 55–60% resolution after 20 sessions [19].

Indications for Pediatric PTENS

PTENS over the S2–S3 sacral foramina has been utilized for all forms of childhood lower urinary tract dysfunction. The most common pediatric indication for therapy is overactive bladder, which is defined as urinary urgency, which may be accompanied by urinary frequency with or without urinary incontinence [4]. PTENS has also been utilized in the treatment of pediatric nocturnal enuresis, dysfunctional voiding, and constipation. In this section, we will discuss the various pediatric bladder and bowel conditions in which PTENS has been utilized and the results of studies regarding the usage of PTENS in the treatment of these abnormalities.

Overactive Bladder

Classically, pediatric OAB has been managed with urotherapy and anticholinergics [4]. Urotherapy is considered by most practitioners to be a first-line therapy for OAB in children and typically involves education of the child and family, routine hydration and regular optimal, timed voiding regimens and bowel programs. Routine treatment may also include anticholinergics and physical therapy and biofeedback training. While these treatments can be effective, there is a significant percentage of patients who fail conservative therapy. In addition, while the reported rate of response to anticholinergics is high (70–80%) [20], the rate of complete symptom resolution is much lower, ranging from 14 to 35% [20, 21]. Treatment with anticholinergics also has several drawbacks, including the necessity of long-term administration, poor long-term compliance, and undesirable side effects, which lead to discontinuation in up to 10% of children [22].

The first reported use of PTENS for the treatment of pediatric overactive bladder was by Bower et al. in 2001, with treatment performed twice daily at home for 1 h, over a period of 1–6 months (average 2 months) [3]. Complete resolution of symptoms was found in 68% of children, with 39% of parents reporting improvement in urgency and 73% with reduced number of incontinence episodes. Hoebeke et al. also reported similar findings with children treated with PTENS in combination with anticholinergics, with a 51% overall cure rate at 1 year, 23% decrease in urgency symptoms, and 66% improvement in weekly incontinence episodes [2]. Malm-Buatsi et al. also retrospectively examined the use of PTENS in a treatment-resistant group of children with OAB, with a reported 13% cure and 66–73% improvement rate in urgency and incontinence symptoms, respectively [13].

Several prospective trials have since been performed, with promising results. Barroso et al. used PTENS in a predominately treatment-naive group of children with OAB for a mean of 4.4 weeks, with a 63% cure and 32% improvement rate [14]. Wright et al. examined 84 treatment-resistant (failed standard urotherapy and at least one anticholinergic) children treated with home-based PTENS for 1 h daily for 12 weeks and reported a 16.6% cure rate, with improvement in 43% of patients, with no serious adverse effects [1]. In another study of treatment-resistant patients, a complete response to therapy was seen in 70%, with an 82% improvement in urgency and 81% improvement in incontinence symptoms [15].

Randomized prospective trials are limited, but there are two reported which compare PTENS with sham treatment. Lordêlo et al. examined a treatment-naive group of children who underwent 20 PTENS sessions of 20 min each (10 Hz), performed three times weekly [16]. When compared to a scapular electrical stimulation group, 62% of parents reported complete improvement of symptoms, with no cases of complete resolution in the sham group ($p < 0.001$). Significant improvement of symptoms was found in 38.1% of patients in the test group and 31.3% of those in the sham group. Similar findings were found by Hagstroem et al. in a treatment-resistant group of children with refractory daytime urinary urge incontinence and demonstrable detrusor overactivity on urodynamics [18]. In this group of children, a 61% partial response rate (improvement 50–90%) was seen, with a significant decrease in incontinence scores, wet days, number of daily urge incontinence episodes, and improved response to urgency.

Long-term results of pediatric PTENS are not yet well established in the literature. However, Lordêlo et al. reported a response rate of 84% of children with a history of OAB, a 74% response rate for children suffering from daytime incontinence and a 78% response rate for all children suffering from LUTS at 2 years after treatment initiation [17]. They identified a 10% recurrence rate of LUTS in their study population.

PTENS has been compared in several trials to conventional therapy, with mixed results. Sillén et al. compared children with symptoms of OAB and incontinence treated with standard urotherapy (behavioral therapy and lifestyle changes, including timed voiding and management of constipation) to those treated with urotherapy and PTENS [23]. In this study, children treated with PTENS did not achieve a significant reduction in number of voids or incontinence episodes compared to standard urotherapy. However, there were a higher proportion (67%) of children in the PTENS group who were completely dry after treatment, compared to 46% in the urotherapy-only group, but this result was not statistically significant. Quintiliano et al. also compared pediatric PTENS to oxybutynin in a randomized, prospective trial of 28 children with OAB symptoms and found complete symptom resolution in 46% of patients treated with PTENS versus 20% with oxybutynin alone [24]. This was also not statistically significant, likely due to small sample size.

One published comparison study between pediatric PTENS and posterior tibial nerve stimulation (PTNS) found a 70% parent-reported symptom response rate in the PTENS group compared to 9% in the PTNS group [8]. However, there was no statistically significant difference between the groups using a standardized pre- and post-treatment symptom questionnaire, suggesting that the difference may have been due to different electrical parameters used or placebo effect, as PTENS treatment required more frequent office visits.

The effect of pediatric PTENS is less clear with regard to pre- and post-treatment urodynamics. Borch et al. examined the effect of PTENS on natural-fill urodynamics in a double-blind, placebo-controlled study of 24 children with severe OAB and daytime urinary incontinence [25]. After 24 h of baseline investigation, the children were randomized to either active continuous PTENS or placebo PTENS. In this study, PTENS had no immediate objective effect on bladder capacity or number of bladder contractions. Barroso et al. performed urodynamic evaluation in children with idiopathic isolated OAB immediately before and after the first session of parasacral TENS, as well as immediately after the last session (7 weeks later) [26]. There was no change in the urodynamic parameters immediately after the first session of stimulation, and after the last session, bladder capacity was the only urodynamic finding that showed improvement, although this was not statistically significant. Table 15.1 provides a summary of studies focusing on the use of PTENS in children with OAB.

Dysfunctional Voiding

As described in the introduction, pediatric dysfunctional voiding is defined as a fluctuating flow rate due to intermittent contractions of the periurethral striated or levator ani muscles during voiding in neurologically normal children, resulting in staccato-type voiding. Dysfunctional voiding can be diagnosed by the presence of sphincter activity on electromyography during voiding [4]. The first-line therapy for DV is biofeedback, and success rates are typically high, around 90–100% [7]. However, there are some children who fail conventional therapy, and in this population PTENS has been utilized with some benefit.

There are limited studies evaluating the use of PTENS in children with DV. Tugtepe et al. examined the effect of PTENS in a mixed cohort of treatment-resistant children with OAB and DV [15]. The majority of patients (60%) fell into the DV category and had previously failed 6 months of treatment with either biofeedback or alpha-adrenergic blockers. After 3 months of treatment with daily PTENS, there was a 64% improvement in fractionated voiding as well as a statistically significant increase in bladder capacity and Qmax on uroflow-electromyogram. There was an overall cure rate of 70% among all children treated with PTENS. Barroso et al. also examined the effect of PTENS in children with DV who did not have complete resolution of symptoms after biofeedback. In this small subset of patients, four had complete improvement of symptoms, with the other two patients reporting 90 and 40% improvement [14]. Table 15.2 provides a summary of studies focusing on the use of PTENS in children with DV.

Nocturnal Enuresis

The etiology of nocturnal enuresis (NE) is multifactorial. It is observed in 15–20% of children at the age of 5, which decreases to 1–2% by the age of 17 years [27]. This condition can be subdivided into primary monosymptomatic nocturnal enuresis (PMNE), where the only symptom is loss of urine during sleep, and non-monosymptomatic nocturnal enuresis (NMNE), where nocturnal enuresis is associated with any other daytime lower urinary tract symptom, such as urinary urgency, urge incontinence, or frequency [4]. Standard first-line therapy for patients with PMNE includes limiting fluids prior to bedtime, as well as the use of bedwetting alarms and medications, including desmopressin and imipramine. In children with NMNE, treatments may include those utilized for PMNE, but should also include treatment of the daytime issues as well. This may include the use of timed toileting, anticholinergics, and the treatment of constipation. The treatment of the daytime symptoms in children with NMNE is important as studies have demonstrated a treatment failure rate of 50% for anticholinergics and 53% for bedwetting alarm therapy use alone [28].

In some children, PTENS has been considered to be a promising alternative option in the treatment of pediatric NE, although there are limited studies evaluating this utilization. There has been one randomized prospective trial of children with PMNE who underwent treatment with behavioral therapy as well as PTENS, which showed a 62% improvement in number of dry nights after ten sessions, compared to 37% in the control group [29]. Neither gender nor age influenced the effects of PTENS on improving percentage of wet nights. A small non-randomized controlled trial of children with NMNE showed a 42% rate of complete resolution of NE, with 21% of patients reporting a reduction in enuresis to less than once per week [28]. In a subgroup analysis of patients with OAB who also had NE, Barroso et al. found a cure rate of 38%, with decreased severity of symptoms in 53% after treatment with PTENS [14]. Further studies have found a 14% rate of complete resolution [13] and 41% improvement in NMNE with patients treated

Table 15.1 PTENS studies in children with overactive bladder

	Study design	No. of patients	Pre-treatment conventional urodynamics	TENS location	Current intensity	Pulse width	Pulse frequency	Periodicity	Prior/concomitant urotherapy	Concomitant anticholinergic use	Treatment-refractory	Length of treatment	Complete resolution/cure rate	OAB/DV symptom improvement	Incontinence symptom improvement	Mean voided volume	Relapse rate
Bower et al. 2001	Pilot study, no control group	17	No	S2/S3, supra-pubic	Maximum tolerated	Not stated	10 Hz, 150 Hz	1 h BID	No	Some patients	Some patients	1–5 months	68.0%	39.0%	73.0%	Increased	Not reported
Hoebeke et al. 2001	Pilot study, no control group	41	Yes, docu-mented DO	S3	Not reported	150 µs	2 Hz	2 h/day	Prior	Yes	All patients	1–6 months	51.2%	22.8%	66.0%	Increased	25%
Mal-Buatsi et al. 2007	Retrospective chart review	18	No	S2/S3	Until 60 mA, maximum tolerated	Not stated	100 Hz	20 min BID	Prior	Some patients	All patients	8 ± 7 months	13.0%	66.0%	73.0%	No change	Not reported
Barroso et al. 2006	Prospective	17	No	S3	Mean (range) of 22.2 mA (6–42), maximum tolerated	Not stated	10 Hz	20 min 3×/week	Prior	No	All patients	Mean 4.3 weeks (1–6.6)	63.0%	15.7%	15.7%	Not reported	Not reported
Lordelo et al. 2009	Prospective	49	No	S3	Mean of 22.2 mA (6–42), maximum tolerated	700 µs	10 Hz	20 min 3×/week	Prior	No	Not stated	Not stated (max of 6.6 weeks)	76.0%	Not reported	Not reported	Not reported	10%
Barroso et al. 2013	Prospective	37	No	S2/S3	Not stated, maximum tolerated	700 µs	10 Hz	20 min 3×/week	Con-comitant	No	No	Not stated (max of 6.6 weeks)	70.0%	78.0%	80.0%		
Wright et al. 2014	Prospective	84	Not reported	S3	Not stated, maximum tolerated	Not stated	10 Hz	1 h daily	Prior	Not reported	All patients	12 weeks	16.6%	43.0%	Not reported	Not reported	2%
Tugtepe et al. 2015	Prospective	27	No	S3	Not reported	350 µs	10 Hz	20 min daily	Prior	Yes	All patients	12 weeks	70.4%	82.4%	81.3%	Increased	Not reported

Veiga et al. 2016	Prospective	51	No	S2-S4	Not stated, maximum tolerated	700 μs	10 Hz	20 min 3×/week	Con-comitant	No	None	6.6 weeks	49.0%	Not reported	Not reported	Not reported	Not reported
Lordelo et al. 2010	Randomized, controlled, single-blind	37	No	S2/S3 or scapu-lar	Median 37.5 mA, max of 40 mA	700 μs	10 Hz	20 min 3×/week	Con-comitant	No	Not stated	Not stated, max of 6.6 weeks	62.0%	Not reported	Not reported	Increased	11%
Hagstroem et al. 2009	Randomized, controlled, double-blind	25	Yes, docu-mented DO	S2/S3	Not stated, maximum tolerated	200 μs	10 Hz	2 h/day	Prior	No	All patients	Median 3.8 weeks, max of 4 weeks	0.0%	Not reported	61.0%	No change	Not reported
Sillen et al. 2014	Randomized, controlled	62	No	S2/S3	Maximum 40 mA	Not stated	10 Hz	20 min BID	Con-comitant	No	Some patients	12 weeks	67.0%	63.0%	80.0%	No change	Not reported
Quintiliano et al. 2015	Randomized, controlled, single-blind	28	No	S2/S3	Not reported, maximum tolerated	700 μs	10 Hz	20 min 3×/week	Prior	Crossover	No	Not stated, max of 6.6 weeks	46.0%	Not reported	Not reported	Improved	Not reported

Table 15.2 PTENS studies in children with dysfunctional voiding

	Study design	No. of patients	Pre-treatment conventional urodynamics	TENS location	Current intensity	Pulse width	Pulse frequency	Periodicity	Prior/concomitant urotherapy	Concomitant anticholinergic use	Treatment-refractory	Length of treatment	Complete resolution/cure rate	OAB/DV symptom improvement	Incontinence symptom improvement	Mean voided volume	Relapse rate
Tugtepe et al. 2015	Prospective	27	No	S3	Not reported	350 μs	10 Hz	20 min daily	Prior	Yes	All patients	12 weeks	70.0%	64.0%	–	Increased	Not reported
Barroso et al. 2006	Prospective	6	No	S3	Mean (range) of 22.2 mA (6–42), maximum tolerated	Not stated	10 Hz	20 min 3×/week	Prior	No	All patients	Mean 4.3 weeks (1–6.6)	66.0%	Not reported	–	Not reported	Not reported

Table 15.3 PTENS studies in children with nocturnal enuresis

	Study design	No. of patients	Pre-treatment conventional urodynamics	TENS location	Current intensity	Pulse width	Pulse frequency	Periodicity	Prior/concomitant urotherapy	Concomitant anticholinergic use	Treatment-refractory	Length of treatment	Complete resolution/cure rate	OAB/DV symptom improvement	Incontinence symptom improvement	Mean voided volume	Relapse rate
NE																	
Fajardo et al. 2015	Randomized, controlled, single-blind	45	No	S2/S3	Not reported, maximum tolerated	700 μs	10 Hz	20 min 3×/week	Con-comitant	No	None	3.3 weeks	15.0%	–	62%	Not reported	Not reported
Lordelo et al. 2010	Randomized, controlled, single-blind	37	No	S2/S3 or scapular	Median 37.5 mA, max of 40 mA	700 μs	10 Hz	20 min 3×/week	Con-comitant	No	Not stated	Not stated, max of 6.6 weeks	42.0%	–	21.0%	Increased	11%

with PTENS [14]. Table 15.3 provides a summary of studies focusing on the use of PTENS in children with NE.

Constipation

There is a strong association between bowel and bladder dysfunction, and it has been well established that improvement in bowel habits can significantly improve bladder dysfunction. Traditional treatment of constipation in children includes increasing dietary fiber, the use of polyethylene glycol, avoiding postponement of defecation, and laxatives [30].

PTENS has been studied and utilized in children who have failed these standard therapies. Transcutaneous nerve stimulation has been shown to significantly improve colonic transit time, with subsequent resolution or improvement in constipation [31]. In a double-blind placebo-controlled study of children with OAB, PTENS was found to result in a significant increase in the number of rectal contractions as measured by rectal manometry during 48-h urodynamic monitoring [30]. Other studies have supported the role for TENS in constipation, although they have utilized interferential stimulation, with lead placement over the anterior abdominal wall as well as along the paraspinal region between T9 and L2 [31, 32]. Literature supporting the use of parasacral TENS is limited, although Veiga et al. found an 85.7% improvement in constipation symptoms based on Rome III criteria after PTENS therapy [19]. Quintiliano also examined children with OAB and constipation and found that use of PTENS improved constipation in 100% of those treated, although this was not statistically significant [24]. A recent prospective study in children with OAB and constipation found that treatment with PTENS resulted in a 49% cure rate for OAB symptoms and 60% cure rate for constipation. The cure rate for OAB was not associated with either the presence or absence of constipation before treatment, and PTENS resolved OAB irrespective of its positive effect on constipation [32]. Table 15.4 provides a summary of studies focusing on the use of PTENS in children with OAB.

Adverse Effects, Dropout, and Recurrence Rates

PTENS is typically well tolerated. The most common side effects are skin sensitivity from electrode pads, discomfort or pain related to the intensity of the TENS machine, and sensation of decreased need to void [2, 11, 13, 19]. Given that the child or provider can easily titrate the TENS intensity up or down, any discomfort is usually transient and an intensity level can be chosen that is comfortable. The dropout rate in one study was found to be 22% [2]. Early discontinuation of therapy (less than 2 weeks) has been reported at 11%, with compliance of therapy beyond 2 weeks reported at 78%. The most common reason for discontinuing therapy is typically due to lack of motivation and/or inconvenience of the treatment [13]. The recurrence rate for parasacral TENS ranges from 2 to 17%, depending on the follow-up interval [1, 2, 16, 17].

Discussion

The use of parasacral TENS is best established in the pediatric OAB population, although there is evidence to support its use in patients with dysfunctional voiding, nocturnal enuresis, and constipation. The majority of patients with OAB report at least some improvement in symptoms with PTENS. The overall cure rate is highly variable, ranging from 13 to 76% (average 50%), which may be due to lack of consistency in TENS technical parameters, severity of pre-treatment symptoms, as well as number and duration of stimulation sessions completed by patients among available studies [1–3, 8, 13–18, 23, 24]. However, PTENS has clear improvement over the reported rate of spontaneous resolution of pediatric OAB [2]. PTENS therapy also has the advantage of being well tolerated with minimal, if any, reported side effects. There is an added benefit to PTENS, in that it acts on the same sacral nerve roots involved in bowel function, and has high success in improving constipation along with OAB symptoms [19, 24, 32]. This is important, as constipation is a common issue in

Table 15.4 PTENS studies in children with constipation

	Study design	No. of patients	Pre-treatment conventional urodynamics	TENS location	Current intensity	Pulse width	Pulse frequency	Periodicity	Prior/concomitant urotherapy	Concomitant anticholinergic use	Treatment-refractory	Length of treatment	Complete resolution/cure rate	OAB/DV symptom improvement	Incontinence symptom improvement	Mean voided volume	Relapse rate
Quintiliano et al. 2015	Randomized, controlled, single-blind	28	No	S2/S3	Not reported, maximum tolerated	700 μs	10 Hz	20 min 3×/week	Prior	Crossover	No	Not stated, max of 6.6 weeks	100.0%	–	–	–	–
Veiga et al. 2016	Prospective	51	No	S2-S4	Not stated, maximum tolerated	700 μs	10 Hz	20 min 3×/week	Concomitant	No	None	6.6 weeks	60.0%	–	–	–	–

children with lower urinary tract symptoms and dysfunction.

The long-term results of PTENS appear to be promising, although there is only one published study with over 2 years of follow-up. This study reported that 78% of children experienced a durable response to therapy [17]. Given that pediatric lower urinary tract dysfunction is common and often does not respond adequately to traditional treatments such as anticholinergics and standard urotherapy, PTENS is a unique noninvasive mode of treatment that can be offered as second-line therapy to parents and children who have persistent symptoms. In addition, PTENS may be an attractive option for parents and children who are considering posterior tibial nerve stimulation, given that it appears to have similar efficacy and does not require the use of needles [8].

Unfortunately, there is a lack of high-quality evidence that can substantiate the reported efficacy and response rates to therapy in PTENS use in children with OAB. Most of the available studies are not comparable due to differences in study design and definitions of "cure" and "improvement in symptoms." There is inconsistent use of International Children's Continence Society standardization of terminology for diagnosis of OAB and dysfunctional voiding, which creates difficulty in interpreting actual success rates of treatment. Specific details regarding presence, severity, and frequency of incontinence are often not reported. Electrical parameters such as the pulse duration, stimulation frequency, intensity, and number and duration of stimulation sessions are highly variable among studies, which reinforces that there is not a universally established regimen for treatment. The use of concurrent anticholinergic medication in many studies acts as a confounding variable that may influence the reported success rates of treatment. ENS studies in general are challenging to perform with a credible sham treatment, which allows for a significant placebo effect, especially given that many studies evaluate outcomes based on subjective symptom scores, rather than objective measures such as voiding diaries, uroflowmetry, or urodynamic studies. While the recurrence rate ranges from 2 to 25%, this is from a small subset of studies with short-term follow-up.

The evidence supporting the use of PTENS for other conditions, including dysfunctional voiding and nocturnal enuresis, is also not robust. DV has high success rates with biofeedback therapy, roughly 90–100% [7]. However, in a treatment-resistant population of patients, PTENS may have some benefit, with limited evidence reporting approximately 66% improvement in symptoms. The success of NE depends on whether concomitant symptoms of OAB are present. In patients with primary monosymptomatic nocturnal enuresis, PTENS has a 25% improvement in number of dry nights, but has not been associated with complete resolution of symptoms [29]. Success rates for patients with non-monosymptomatic NE are slightly better, with >60% of patients reporting improvement in number of dry nights. However, nearly 50% of children showed persistence of NE despite resolution of their daytime OAB symptoms [28]. Thus, PTENS may be offered as a second-line therapy option for patients with NE, with the understanding that there will likely be improvement but not complete cure.

Conclusion

The use of PTENS in children with lower urinary tract symptoms is best established and studied within the OAB population, and has success rates of approximately 50% among all available studies. It may also serve as a treatment modality in children with dysfunctional voiding, nocturnal enuresis, and constipation. Comparisons between available studies are difficult due to the heterogeneity of treatment populations, lack of consistent electrical parameters, duration and total number of sessions, and risk of placebo effect and confounding variables. Nevertheless, PTENS remains an attractive noninvasive option for patients suffering from bladder and bowel dysfunction.

References

1. Wright AJ, Haddad M. Electroneurostimulation for the management of bladder bowel dysfunction in childhood. Eur J Paediatr Neurol. 2017;21(1):67–74.
2. Hoebeke P, Van Laecke E, Everaert K, Renson C, De Paepe H, Raes A, et al. Transcutaneous neuromodulation for the urge syndrome in children: a pilot study. J Urol. 2001;166:2416–9.
3. Bower WF, Moore KH, Adams RD. A pilot study of the home application of transcutaneous neuromodulation in children with urgency or urge incontinence. J Urol. 2001;166:2420–2.
4. Austin PF, Bauer SB, Bower W, Chase J, Franco I, Hoebeke P, et al. The standardization of terminology of lower urinary tract function in children and adolescents: update report from the standardization committee of the International Children's Continence Society. J Urol. 2014;191:1863–5.
5. Koff SA, Wagner TT, Jayanthi VR. The relationship among dysfunctional elimination syndromes, primary vesicoureteral reflux and urinary tract infections in children. J Urol. 1998;160:1019–22.
6. Naseer SR, Stenhardt GF. New renal scars in children with urinary tract infections, vesicoureteral reflux and voiding dysfunction: a prospective evaluation. J Urol. 1997;158:566–8.
7. Chase J, Austin P, Hoebeke P, McKenna P. The management of dysfunctional voiding in children: a report from the standardisation committee of the International Children's Continence Society. J Urol. 2010;183(4):1296–302.
8. Barroso U Jr, Viterbo W, Bittencourt J, Farias T, Lordelo P. Posterior tibial nerve stimulation vs parasacral transcutaneous neuromodulation for overactive bladder in children. J Urol. 2013;190(2):673–7.
9. Clemens JQ. Basic bladder neurophysiology. Urol Clin North Am. 2010;37(4):487–94.
10. Kumsar S, Keskin U, Akay A, Bilgilisoy UT, Erdem SR, Peskircioglu CL, et al. Effects of sacral neuromodulation on isolated urinary bladder function in a rat model of spinal cord injury. Neuromodulation. 2015;18(1):67e74.
11. Bower WF, Moore KH, Adams RD, Shepherd R. A urodynamic study of surface neuromodulation versus sham in detrusor instability and sensory urgency. J Urol. 1998;160:2133–6.
12. Plevnik S, Vodušek DB, Vrtačnik P, Janež J. Optimization of pulse duration for electrical stimulation in treatment of urinary incontinence. World J Urol. 1986;4:22–3.
13. Malm-Buatsi E, Nepple KG, Boyt MA, Austin JC, Cooper CS. Efficacy of transcutaneous electrical nerve stimulation in children with overactive bladder refractory to pharmacotherapy. Urology. 2007;70(5):980–3.
14. Barroso U Jr, Lordêlo P, Lopes AA, Andrade J, Macedo A Jr, Ortiz V. Nonpharmacological treatment of lower urinary tract dysfunction using biofeedback and transcutaneous electrical stimulation: a pilot study. BJU Int. 2006;98(1):166–71.
15. Tugtepe H, Thomas DT, Ergun R, Kalyoncu A, Kaynak A, Kastarli C, et al. The effectiveness of transcutaneous electrical neural stimulation therapy in patients with urinary incontinence resistant to initial medical treatment or biofeedback. J Pediatr Urol. 2015;11(3):137.e1–5.
16. Lordêlo P, Teles A, Veiga ML, et al. Transcutaneous electrical nerve stimulation in children with overactive bladders: a randomized clinical trial. J Urol. 2010;184:683–9.
17. Lordêlo P, Soares PVL, Maciel I, Macedo A, Barroso U. Prospective study of transcutaneous parasacral electrical stimulation for overactive bladder in children: long-term results. J Urol. 2009;182(6):2900–4.
18. Hagstroem S, Mahler B, Madsen B, Djurhuus JC, Rittig S. Transcutaneous electrical nerve stimulation for refractory daytime urinary urge incontinence. J Urol. 2009;182(4 Suppl):2072–8.
19. Veiga ML, Queiroz AP, Carvalho MC, Braga AANM, Sousa AS, Barroso U Jr. Parasacral transcutaneous electrical stimulation for overactive bladder in children: an assessment per session. J Pediatr Urol. 2016;12(5):293.e1–5.
20. Kilic N, Balkan E, Akgoz S, Sen N, Dogruyol H. Comparison of the effectiveness and side-effects of tolterodine and oxybutynin in children with detrusor instability. Int J Urol. 2006;13(2):105–8. https://doi.org/10.1111/j.1442-2042.2006.01240.x.
21. Reinberg Y, Crocker J, Wolpert J, Vandersteen D. Therapeutic efficacy of extended release oxybutynin chloride, and immediate release and long acting tolterodine tartrate in children with diurnal urinary incontinence. J Urol. 2003;169(1):317–9.
22. Chapple CR, Yamanishi T, Chess-Williams R. Muscarinic receptor subtypes and management of the overactive bladder. Urology. 2002;60:82–9.
23. Sillén U, Arwidsson C, Doroszkiewicz M, Antonsson H, Jansson I, Stålklint M, et al. Effects of transcutaneous neuromodulation (TENS) on overactive bladder symptoms in children: a randomized controlled trial. J Pediatr Urol. 2014;10(6):1100–5.
24. Quintiliano F, Veiga ML, Moraes M, Cunha C, de Oliveira LF, Lordelo P, et al. Transcutaneous parasacral electrical stimulation vs oxybutynin for the treatment of overactive bladder in children: a randomized clinical trial. J Urol. 2015;193(5 Suppl):1749–53.
25. Borch L, Rittig S, Kamperis K, Mahler B, Djurhuus JC, Hagstroem S. No immediate effect on urodynamic parameters during transcutaneous electrical nerve stimulation (TENS) in children with overactive bladder and daytime incontinence—a randomized, double-blind, placebo-controlled study. Neurourol Urodyn. 2017;36(7):1788–95. https://doi.org/10.1002/nau.23179.
26. Barroso U Jr, Carvalho MT, Veiga ML, Moraes MM, Cunha CC, Lordêlo P, et al. Urodynamic outcome of parasacral transcutaneous electrical neural stimu-

lation for overactive bladder in children. Int Braz J Urol. 2015;41(4):739–43. https://doi.org/10.1590/S1677-5538.IBJU.2014.0303.

27. Houts AC, Berman JS, Abramson H. Effectiveness of psychological and pharmacological treatments for nocturnal enuresis. J Consult Clin Psychol. 1994;62(4):737–45. http://dx.doi.org.proxy.lib.uiowa.edu/10.1037/0022-006X.62.4.737.
28. Lordêlo P, Benevides I, Kerner EG, Teles A, Lordêlo M, Barroso Jr U. Treatment of non-monosymptomatic nocturnal enuresis by transcutaneous parasacral electrical nerve stimulation. J Pediatr Urol. 2010;6(5):486–9.
29. Fajardo L, Oliveria D, Iliada L, de Figueiredo AA, de Bessa Junior J, Netto JMB, et al. Transcutaneous parasacral electrical neural stimulation in children with primary monosymptomatic enuresis: a prospective randomized clinical trial. J Urol. 2013;190(4):1359–63.
30. Moeller Joensson I, Hagstroem S, Siggaard C, Bower W, Djurhuus JC, Krogh K. Transcutaneous electrical nerve stimulation increases rectal activity in children. J Pediatr Gastroenterol Nutr. 2015;61(1):80–4.
31. Chase J, Robertson VJ, Southwell B, Hutson J, Gibb S. Pilot study using transcutaneous electrical stimulation (interferential current) to treat chronic treatment-resistant constipation and soiling in children. J Gastroenterol Hepatol. 2005;20(7):1054–61.
32. Clarke MCC, Chase JW, Gibb S, Robertson VJ, Catto-Smith A, Hutson J, et al. Decreased colonic transit time after transcutaneous interferential electrical stimulation in children with slow transit constipation. J Pediatr Surg. 2009;44(2):408–12.

Neuromodulation for Treatment of Pediatric Defecatory Disorders

16

Peter L. Lu and Desale Yacob

Abbreviations

PTNS Posterior tibial nerve stimulation
SNM Sacral neuromodulation
TES Transcutaneous electrical stimulation

Introduction

Defecatory disorders, namely constipation and fecal incontinence, are common among children. Constipation and fecal incontinence can occur secondary to a variety of disease processes, but the majority of children with these symptoms have functional constipation [1]. Population-based studies estimate the prevalence of pediatric functional constipation to be 12% [2]. In children, fecal incontinence is most commonly seen as a result of poorly controlled constipation that leads to overflow incontinence, with the involuntary passage of soft stools around a fecal impaction [3]. Constipation accounts for up to 10% of visits to the general pediatrician and up to 25% of referrals to pediatric gastroenterologists [4]. A study of data from 2003 to 2004 found that the cost of care for pediatric constipation resulted in an additional healthcare cost of $3.9 billion per year in the United States, and with recent evidence of rising costs of hospital care for constipation, this figure is likely now much higher [5, 6].

Conventional treatment of pediatric constipation and fecal incontinence generally consists of education, toilet training, and oral laxatives. Although the majority of children with constipation and fecal incontinence respond to conventional medical and behavioral treatment, a sizable proportion of children will have symptoms that remain refractory to conventional treatment [7]. Unfortunately, treatment options for these children are fairly limited. Traditionally, treatment for these more challenging cases consists of surgical creation of a cecostomy or appendicostomy for antegrade continence enema administration, partial or total colonic resection, or creation of an ileostomy or colostomy. However, these procedures are generally invasive and can be associated with complications [8, 9].

P. L. Lu (✉) · D. Yacob
Division of Gastroenterology, Hepatology and Nutrition, Department of Pediatrics, Nationwide Children's Hospital, Columbus, OH, USA
e-mail: peter.lu@nationwidechildrens.org; desalegn.yacob@nationwidechildrens.org

J. P. Gilleran, S. A. Alpert (eds.), *Adult and Pediatric Neuromodulation*,
https://doi.org/10.1007/978-3-319-73266-4_16

There clearly remains a need for less invasive treatment options that are effective and safe for children with refractory defecatory dysfunction. Over the past decade, there has been growing interest in the use of neuromodulation for the treatment of this population, particularly as its use in adults with refractory constipation and fecal incontinence has grown. Although experience with neuromodulation in children with refractory defecatory disorders remains relatively limited, several treatment modalities have shown promise. In this chapter, we will review current applications of neuromodulation for the treatment of pediatric defecatory disorders and discuss its potential future applications.

Sacral Neuromodulation

Sacral neuromodulation (SNM) is the most established of the neuromodulation-based treatments that have been used for children with refractory defecatory disorders. SNM involves the application of low-amplitude electrical stimulation to the sacral nerve root through an electrode placed in the sacral foramen. This electrode is connected to a pulse generator and battery that is implanted into a subcutaneous pocket in the buttock. Permanent implantation can occur after demonstration of clinical response during a temporary percutaneous nerve evaluation period, during which the pulse generator and battery remain external to the patient [10]. SNM has been used for adults with urinary or defecatory symptoms for nearly three decades, but experience in children is limited to the last decade.

Sacral Neuromodulation for Pediatric Bowel and Bladder Dysfunction

In the years following its approval by the United States Food and Drug Administration for the treatment of adults with urinary incontinence in 1997, SNM was initially used for children with refractory urinary dysfunction. However, even the early studies of children primarily treated with SNM for urinary symptoms suggested benefit for defecatory symptoms as well. In 2004, Guys and colleagues published a randomized controlled trial of 42 children with neurogenic bladder, many of whom had underlying spina bifida. Participants were randomized to either SNM treatment or conventional treatment with anticholinergic medications, antibiotic treatment for urinary tract infections, and bulking agents for urinary continence. Nine of the 21 patients (43%) treated with SNM reported subjective improvement in intestinal transit based on symptom diaries, while none of the control patients reported corresponding improvement [11]. While encouraging, it was unclear whether these patients truly had constipation at baseline and whether decreasing anticholinergic use was associated with reported improvements.

In 2006, Humphreys and colleagues described a multicenter series of 23 children with bowel and bladder dysfunction who were treated with SNM between 2001 and 2003. Twenty-one of 23 children progressed to permanent SNM implantation. After an average of 13.3 months of follow-up, 12 of 15 patients reported improvement in constipation and 4 of 10 patients reported improvement in fecal incontinence, although the reported improvement was not quantified [12]. In 2008, Roth and colleagues described a series of 20 children with bowel and bladder dysfunction who were treated with SNM between 2002 and 2005. Eighteen of 20 children progressed to permanent SNM implantation. After a median of 27 months of follow-up, 7 of 17 patients reported resolution of constipation and 5 of 17 reported improvement. Fecal incontinence was not assessed. Interestingly, 2 of 18 patients were able to undergo stimulator removal after a prolonged period of symptom resolution and they remained improved at follow-up [13].

In 2010, Haddad and colleagues published the results of a multicenter, randomized, crossover study of 33 children with urinary incontinence and/or fecal incontinence. Five of 33 participants had fecal incontinence alone and 19 of 33 had both fecal and urinary incontinence. After SNM implantation, participants were randomized to having the stimulator turned on or kept off for 6 months, after which the stimulator was then switched to the opposite setting for another

6 months. The authors found that significantly more participants reported a decrease in fecal incontinence frequency of >50% when SNM was turned on compared to when it was turned off (78% vs. 17%), and concluded that SNM was more effective than conservative management for both fecal and urinary incontinence [14].

In 2014, Dwyer and colleagues published a follow-up study to the earlier studies by Humphreys and Roth. The authors included 105 children with bowel and bladder dysfunction who had been treated with SNM for a median of 2.7 years. The majority (88%) of their cohort had concurrent constipation, and 79% of these children reported improvement in constipation at follow-up, which was defined as any increase in bowel movement frequency or decrease in the frequency of painful defecation. Forty percent of these children reported resolution of constipation. Fecal incontinence was not assessed [15].

Sacral Neuromodulation for Constipation and Fecal Incontinence

Experience with the use of SNM to treat children with severe constipation refractory to conventional treatment has been growing over the past few years. In 2012, van Wunnik and colleagues described the use of SNM to treat 12 adolescent females with functional constipation refractory to conventional treatment. After a median of 7 months of SNM treatment, patients reported significant clinical improvement, including improvement in defecation frequency, abdominal pain, and overall constipation severity as measured by the Cleveland Clinic Constipation Score [16]. In 2015, Sulkowski and colleagues published the short-term outcomes of the first 29 patients treated with SNM at our institution. This cohort included 22 children with constipation, 9 children with fecal incontinence, and 4 children with both symptoms, and 8 of these children had a history of anorectal malformation. The authors reported significant improvement in gastrointestinal symptoms and quality of life after a median of 5 months of SNM treatment [17].

Both of these institutions have recently begun to describe the long-term outcomes of SNM treatment for children with refractory constipation. In the Netherlands, van der Wilt and colleagues published a follow-up to van Wunnik's earlier study and reported the outcomes of 27 females, ages 10–20 years, who underwent SNM treatment for refractory functional constipation. At a median of 22 months of treatment, the authors reported continued clinical improvement, including improvement in defecation frequency, abdominal pain, and overall constipation severity as measured by a validated questionnaire. However, 15 of 27 were considered not to have had a successful response to SNM, which was defined as having >2 bowel movements per week, and 6 of 15 underwent subsequent colectomy and SNM removal [18].

Our institution recently described the long-term outcomes of 25 children and adolescents, ages 6–19 years, who had been treated with SNM for constipation for at least 2 years. This was a heterogeneous cohort and included 16 patients with functional constipation, 6 patients with a history of anorectal malformation, 2 patients with a history of tethered spinal cord, and 1 patient with Hirschsprung's disease. At a median of 27 months of treatment, patients reported continued improvement in clinical symptoms, including significant decreases in concurrent fecal and urinary incontinence, and quality of life. Patients were able to decrease the use of laxatives and antegrade continence enemas. Seventeen of 25 patients were considered to have successfully responded to SNM, which was defined as having >2 bowel movements per week and <1 episode of fecal incontinence per week. Six of these 17 patients met our criteria for successful response without concurrent use of laxatives or antegrade continence enemas. Families were contacted after a median of 27 months of SNM treatment to assess perceived health-related patient benefit and parent satisfaction. Fifteen of 16 responders reported positive patient benefit and all parents reported that they would recommend SNM to other children with similar symptoms [19].

While it is generally accepted that SNM treatment should only be considered for children with refractory constipation after symptoms have persisted despite optimal conventional treatment, the role of SNM in relation to other surgical treatment options, like appendicostomy or cecostomy for antegrade continence enema treatment or colonic resection, remains unclear. Both studies by van der Wilt and Lu included patients receiving antegrade continence enemas [18, 19]. A recent study examined the outcomes of 22 children who underwent SNM treatment for continued constipation despite antegrade continence enema treatment. SNM treatment allowed a steady decrease in antegrade continence enema use over the first year of treatment, from a median of 7 antegrade continence enemas per week prior to device implantation to 1 antegrade continence enema per week at 12 months after SNM initiation. After a median of 18 months of follow-up, 10 of 22 patients were not only able to discontinue antegrade continence enema treatment, but had undergone elective closure of their appendicostomy or cecostomy. While there was no comparison group included in this study, the proportion of patients able to discontinue antegrade continence enema treatment during this time period was dramatically higher than what has been previously reported among children treated with antegrade continence enemas. It therefore appears that SNM may be a promising treatment option for children with severe constipation who are dependent on antegrade continence enemas or inadequately treated with antegrade continence enemas [20].

The existing literature on the use of SNM for children with defecatory disorders has primarily focused on children with severe constipation, with or without concurrent fecal incontinence. However, it is important to recognize that in adults, SNM is primarily used for the treatment of fecal incontinence and a number of recent studies have raised doubts regarding its efficacy for constipation. Two recent randomized crossover studies of adults with severe constipation did not find SNM treatment to be more effective than sham stimulation [21, 22]. Unlike in adults, fecal incontinence in children is most commonly the result of poorly controlled constipation leading to overflow incontinence, and there have not been any studies of SNM treatment specifically for children with non-retentive fecal incontinence [3]. In our recent study on long-term outcomes of SNM for children with constipation, comparisons were made between children with constipation alone and children with constipation and concurrent fecal incontinence. Although our analysis was limited by sample size, there were no differences in the ability to discontinue laxative or antegrade continence enema use, health-related patient benefit, or parent satisfaction between these two groups. Therefore, our results suggested that SNM could be beneficial for children with constipation regardless of the presence or absence of fecal incontinence [19].

Complications

Unfortunately, SNM treatment for children with defecatory disorders is associated with a fairly high rate of complications requiring further surgery. In the two long-term studies of SNM treatment for children with constipation, 24–44% of the cohort experienced complications requiring at least one further surgical procedure. These procedures included lead revision, device removal, and device replacement and were performed as a result of lead displacement or malfunction, local pain or numbness, or local infection [18, 19]. This complication rate is consistent with that reported in studies of SNM treatment for children with bowel and bladder dysfunction. In the large series published by Dwyer and colleagues, 49% of the cohort experienced complications requiring further surgery after a median of 2.7 years of treatment. In their series, the majority of subsequent surgeries resulted from device malfunction [15].

Mechanism and Predicting Response

The mechanism by which SNM leads to improvement in constipation and fecal incontinence remains unclear and our understanding of the physiological effects of SNM is limited.

A review of adult studies evaluating various potential mechanisms of SNM treatment concluded that SNM likely modulates anorectal function at the afferent or central level. However, adult studies have not identified consistent effects on specific measurements of anorectal function or colonic motility [23]. In their randomized crossover study of children with urinary and fecal incontinence, Haddad and colleagues did not find any differences in anorectal parameters or colonic transit between when the stimulator was on or off, although the methods by which these variables were assessed were not clearly described [14]. There have not yet been any further studies comparing measurements of anorectal function or colonic motility before and after SNM treatment in children.

There has been interest in identifying prognostic factors predictive of response to SNM, particularly given the sizable risk of complications following stimulator implantation. Unfortunately, identifying prognostic factors has been challenging, in part because of our limited understanding of the mechanism by which SNM acts and the limited sample sizes available. In addition, patients treated with SNM tend to be a heterogeneous group with varying degrees of bladder and/or bowel dysfunction. In a recent study evaluating the prognostic value of selected patient characteristics and manometry testing in predicting response to SNM for children with constipation, we did not find associations between response and concurrent fecal incontinence, concurrent urinary symptoms, or anorectal malformation. In 20 children who underwent anorectal manometry testing prior to SNM and in 7 children who underwent colonic manometry testing prior to SNM, we did not find an association between response and any of the manometry parameters we studied. Response was defined as having >2 bowel movements per week and <1 episode of fecal incontinence per week at follow-up. We concluded that abnormal anorectal manometry or colonic manometry should not preclude children with refractory constipation from consideration of SNM treatment [24].

Abdominal Transcutaneous Electrical Stimulation

A number of therapies involving transcutaneous electrical stimulation (TES) have been used for the treatment of children with defecatory disorders. Abdominal TES is perhaps the best studied of these therapies, with growing experience with its use for the treatment of children with constipation over the past decade. Abdominal TES was first applied to children with constipation after gastrointestinal effects were noted during its use for children with urinary symptoms [25]. Abdominal TES involves the placement of two surface electrodes on the anterior abdomen at the level of the umbilicus and another two on the lower back at the level of the lower thoracic/upper lumbar spine. These electrodes are then used to generate two sinusoidal currents that cross within the abdomen, thereby applying interferential electrical current to the abdomen. This current is applied at an intensity that is below the motor threshold [25–27].

Abdominal Transcutaneous Electrical Stimulation for Constipation and Fecal Incontinence

In 2005, Chase and colleagues published a pilot study using abdominal TES to treat eight children with constipation and fecal incontinence refractory to laxatives and behavioral treatment. Abdominal TES was applied in 20–30 min sessions, three times per week, for 9–12 sessions. Treatment was well tolerated without any adverse effects. The authors found improvements in bowel movement frequency and fecal incontinence in the majority of their cohort, with three children reporting continued improvement even at 3 months [25]. In 2009, Clarke and colleagues followed the pilot study with a randomized controlled trial evaluating the impact of abdominal TES on quality of life in 33 children with slow-transit constipation. The authors described a significant improvement in self-reported quality of life after TES when compared to sham stimulation [28]. However, clinical improvement after abdominal TES has been less consistent in subsequent studies. A recent Cochrane review summarized the results of a randomized controlled trial performed by the same group that evaluated the efficacy of abdominal TES in the treatment of 42 children with slow-transit constipation. Children were randomized to receiving either abdominal TES, consisting of 20-minute treatments performed three times weekly for 4 week, or sham stimulation. The authors reported that there were no significant differences in the number of patients with normal bowel movement frequency or improvement in fecal incontinence, colonic transit, or quality of life between children who received abdominal TES and sham stimulation. The authors concluded that abdominal TES, at least as administered in the manner studied, does not clearly benefit children with slow-transit constipation [27].

In 2009, Ismail and colleagues demonstrated the feasibility of home-based abdominal TES in a group of 11 children with slow-transit constipation who had relapsed or did not respond to an initial trial of clinic-based abdominal TES [29]. This was followed by a 2012 report by Yik and colleagues on outcomes of home-based abdominal TES in 32 children with slow-transit constipation. TES was administered for an hour each day for 3–6 months and, in a proportion of patients, led to increased bowel movement frequency, decreased fecal incontinence, and decreased abdominal pain. The authors concluded that approximately 50% of their cohort benefitted from treatment [30]. Yik and colleagues recently applied abdominal TES to a cohort of ten children with constipation secondary to anorectal retention rather than slow colonic transit. The authors found significant improvements in bowel movement frequency and fecal incontinence in 9 of 10 children after 3 months of treatment [31].

Experience with the use of abdominal TES in treating children with constipation has generally been limited to children with functional constipation thus far. However, Ladi-Seyedian and colleagues recently described the use of abdominal TES to treat 30 children with Hirschsprung's disease who had constipation postoperatively. The authors randomized children to receiving either behavioral therapy alone or behavioral therapy with abdominal TES, and found significant improvements in bowel movement frequency, fecal incontinence, and abdominal pain in the group treated with both behavioral therapy and abdominal TES. The authors concluded that abdominal TES is an effective adjunctive treatment for constipation and fecal incontinence in postoperative Hirschsprung's disease patients [32].

Mechanism

The mechanism by which abdominal TES leads to improvement in constipation and fecal incontinence remains unclear. There is some evidence that abdominal TES can improve colonic transit in children with slow-transit constipation [27]. A study of 8 children with slow-transit constipation who underwent colonic manometry testing before and after abdominal TES showed an increase in the frequency of colonic propagating contractions even 2–7 months after treatment [26]. In the study by Ladi-Seyedian and colleagues of children with Hirschsprung's disease, anorectal manometry testing before and 6 months after abdominal TES initiation showed decreases in anal sphincter resting pressure and balloon volume required for recto-anal inhibitory reflex in children treated with abdominal TES [32].

Posterior Tibial Nerve Stimulation

The use of posterior tibial nerve stimulation (PTNS) for the treatment of adults with defecatory disorders has been growing over the past 15 years, but experience in children remains very limited. PTNS involves electrical stimulation of the posterior tibial nerve at the level of the ankle delivered either in a percutaneous manner through a needle electrode or in a transcutaneous manner through an electrode pad. PTNS is thought to modulate urinary and defecatory function by stimulating the sacral nerve roots, and therefore may exert an effect similar to that of

SNM [33, 34]. Much like SNM and abdominal TES, PTNS was initially used for urologic indications before application to defecatory disorders.

In 2003, Shafik and colleagues reported the first application of PTNS to adults with fecal incontinence [35]. A number of subsequent studies have since supported the efficacy of PTNS for the treatment of fecal incontinence in adult patients [34]. Evidence for the use of PTNS for the treatment of constipation is more limited. In 2012, Collins and colleagues reported the successful treatment of 18 women with slow-transit constipation with percutaneous PTNS, with significant improvements in constipation severity and quality of life after treatment [33]. In 2015, Iqbal and colleagues reported more measured improvement after transcutaneous PTNS in a study of 15 adults with constipation. The authors concluded that PTNS led to improvement in approximately a quarter of their cohort [36].

Lecompte and colleagues recently published the only report of PTNS treatment for children with defecatory disorders. The authors described the use of PTNS in a series of 8 children with fecal incontinence secondary to anorectal malformation, neurological anomaly, or Hirschsprung's disease. Patients were instructed to perform home-based transcutaneous PTNS for 20 min a day for a total duration of 6 months. Five of 8 patients experienced resolution of fecal incontinence and 2 of 8 reported improvement. Treatment was well tolerated without any adverse events [37].

Conclusion

Defecatory disorders are relatively common in children and can have a significant detrimental impact on a child's quality of life. Treatment options for constipation and fecal incontinence refractory to conventional treatment are limited and often require more invasive and permanent procedures such as cecostomy or appendicostomy. Neuromodulation is a promising minimally invasive, non-destructive treatment modality for this population, but the body of evidence thus far for its use remains fairly limited. Further studies of the use of SNM to treat children with refractory constipation and fecal incontinence have been growing over the past decade, and there are reports of improved clinical response in children with a variety of underlying disorders, including functional constipation, anorectal malformation, and spinal cord abnormalities. However, sacral neuromodulation is associated with a sizable risk of complication requiring further surgery, which emphasizes the need for high-quality evidence evaluating the efficacy of SNM in comparison to more established treatment options for refractory constipation. Further studies are also needed to identify prognostic factors predictive of response and development of complications. Less invasive forms of neuromodulation which do not require surgery or an implantable device, like abdominal TES and PTNS, have been used for children with defecatory disorders to a limited extent and with mixed results. However, because of the significant safety and potential cost advantages of abdominal TES and PTNS when compared to SNM and other more invasive treatment options, these treatment modalities warrant further investigation if the durability of treatment response remains high.

References

1. Tabbers MM, DiLorenzo C, Berger MY, Faure C, Langendam MW, Nurko S, et al. Evaluation and treatment of functional constipation in infants and children: evidence-based recommendations from ESPGHAN and NASPGHAN. J Pediatr Gastroenterol Nutr. 2014;58(2):258–74. Epub 2013/12/19.
2. Mugie SM, Benninga MA, Di Lorenzo C. Epidemiology of constipation in children and adults: a systematic review. Best Pract Res Clin Gastroenterol. 2011;25(1):3–18. Epub 2011/03/09.
3. Koppen IJ, von Gontard A, Chase J, Cooper CS, Rittig CS, Bauer SB, et al. Management of functional nonretentive fecal incontinence in children: recommendations from the International Children's Continence Society. J Pediatr Urol. 2016;12(1):56–64. Epub 2015/12/15.
4. Mugie SM, Di Lorenzo C, Benninga MA. Constipation in childhood. Nat Rev Gastroenterol Hepatol. 2011;8(9):502–11. Epub 2011/08/03.
5. Liem O, Harman J, Benninga M, Kelleher K, Mousa H, Di Lorenzo C. Health utilization and cost impact of

childhood constipation in the United States. J Pediatr. 2009;154(2):258–62. Epub 2008/09/30.
6. Park R, Mikami S, LeClair J, Bollom A, Lembo C, Sethi S, et al. Inpatient burden of childhood functional GI disorders in the USA: an analysis of national trends in the USA from 1997 to 2009. Neurogastroenterol Motil. 2015;27(5):684–92. Epub 2015/03/27.
7. van Ginkel R, Reitsma JB, Buller HA, van Wijk MP, Taminiau JA, Benninga MA. Childhood constipation: longitudinal follow-up beyond puberty. Gastroenterology. 2003;125(2):357–63. Epub 2003/08/02.
8. Kuizenga-Wessel S, Koppen IJ, Zwager LW, Di Lorenzo C, de Jong JR, Benninga MA. Surgical management of children with intractable functional constipation; experience of a single tertiary children's hospital. Neurogastroenterol Motil. 2017;29(5). Epub 2016/12/14.
9. Koppen IJ, Kuizenga-Wessel S, Lu PL, Benninga MA, Di Lorenzo C, Lane VA, et al. Surgical decision-making in the management of children with intractable functional constipation: what are we doing and are we doing it right? J Pediatr Surg. 2016;51(10):1607–12. Epub 2016/06/23.
10. Thaha MA, Abukar AA, Thin NN, Ramsanahie A, Knowles CH. Sacral nerve stimulation for faecal incontinence and constipation in adults. Cochrane Database Syst Rev. 2015;8:CD004464. Epub 2015/08/25.
11. Guys JM, Haddad M, Planche D, Torre M, Louis-Borrione C, Breaud J. Sacral neuromodulation for neurogenic bladder dysfunction in children. J Urol. 2004;172(4 Pt 2):1673–6. Epub 2004/09/17.
12. Humphreys MR, Vandersteen DR, Slezak JM, Hollatz P, Smith CA, Smith JE, et al. Preliminary results of sacral neuromodulation in 23 children. J Urol. 2006;176(5):2227–31. Epub 2006/10/31.
13. Roth TJ, Vandersteen DR, Hollatz P, Inman BA, Reinberg YE. Sacral neuromodulation for the dysfunctional elimination syndrome: a single center experience with 20 children. J Urol. 2008;180(1):306–11; discussion 11. Epub 2008/05/24.
14. Haddad M, Besson R, Aubert D, Ravasse P, Lemelle J, El Ghoneimi A, et al. Sacral neuromodulation in children with urinary and fecal incontinence: a multicenter, open label, randomized, crossover study. J Urol. 2010;184(2):696–701. Epub 2010/06/22.
15. Dwyer ME, Vandersteen DR, Hollatz P, Reinberg YE. Sacral neuromodulation for the dysfunctional elimination syndrome: a 10-year single-center experience with 105 consecutive children. Urology. 2014;84(4):911–7. Epub 2014/08/07.
16. van Wunnik BP, Peeters B, Govaert B, Nieman FH, Benninga MA, Baeten CG. Sacral neuromodulation therapy: a promising treatment for adolescents with refractory functional constipation. Dis Colon Rectum. 2012;55(3):278–85. Epub 2012/04/04.
17. Sulkowski JP, Nacion KM, Deans KJ, Minneci PC, Levitt MA, Mousa HM, et al. Sacral nerve stimulation: a promising therapy for fecal and urinary incontinence and constipation in children. J Pediatr Surg. 2015;50(10):1644–7. Epub 2015/04/11.
18. van der Wilt AA, van Wunnik BP, Sturkenboom R, Han-Geurts IJ, Melenhorst J, Benninga MA, et al. Sacral neuromodulation in children and adolescents with chronic constipation refractory to conservative treatment. Int J Colorectal Dis. 2016;31:1459–66. Epub 2016/06/14.
19. Lu PL, Koppen IJ, Orsagh-Yentis DK, Leonhart K, Ambeba EJ, Deans KJ, et al. Sacral nerve stimulation for treatment of constipation in children: long-term outcomes, patient benefit, and parent satisfaction. Gastroenterology. 2016;150(4):S227–S8.
20. Lu PL, Asti L, Lodwick DL, Nacion KM, Deans KJ, Minneci PC, et al. Sacral nerve stimulation allows for decreased antegrade continence enema use in children with severe constipation. J Pediatr Surg. 2017;52(4):558–62. Epub 2016/11/27
21. Dinning PG, Hunt L, Patton V, Zhang T, Szczesniak M, Gebski V, et al. Treatment efficacy of sacral nerve stimulation in slow transit constipation: a two-phase, double-blind randomized controlled crossover study. Am J Gastroenterol. 2015;110(5):733–40. Epub 2015/04/22.
22. Zerbib F, Siproudhis L, Lehur PA, Germain C, Mion F, Leroi AM, et al. Randomized clinical trial of sacral nerve stimulation for refractory constipation. Br J Surg. 2017;104(3):205–21. Epub 2016/10/26.
23. Carrington EV, Evers J, Grossi U, Dinning PG, Scott SM, O'Connell PR, et al. A systematic review of sacral nerve stimulation mechanisms in the treatment of fecal incontinence and constipation. Neurogastroenterol Motil. 2014;26(9):1222–37. Epub 2014/08/30.
24. Lu PL, Koppen IJ, Yacob D, Deans KJ, Minneci PC, Diefenbach KA, et al. The prognostic value of manometry testing in children with constipation treated with sacral nerve stimulation. J Pediatr Gastroenterol Nutr. 2016;63(Suppl 2):S97–S8.
25. Chase J, Robertson VJ, Southwell B, Hutson J, Gibb S. Pilot study using transcutaneous electrical stimulation (interferential current) to treat chronic treatment-resistant constipation and soiling in children. J Gastroenterol Hepatol. 2005;20(7):1054–61. Epub 2005/06/16.
26. Clarke MC, Catto-Smith AG, King SK, Dinning PG, Cook IJ, Chase JW, et al. Transabdominal electrical stimulation increases colonic propagating pressure waves in paediatric slow transit constipation. J Pediatr Surg. 2012;47(12):2279–84. Epub 2012/12/12.
27. Ng RT, Lee WS, Ang HL, Teo KM, Yik YI, Lai NM. Transcutaneous electrical stimulation (TES) for treatment of constipation in children. Cochrane Database Syst Rev. 2016;7:CD010873. Epub 2016/07/06.
28. Clarke MC, Chase JW, Gibb S, Hutson JM, Southwell BR. Improvement of quality of life in children with slow transit constipation after treatment with trans-

cutaneous electrical stimulation. J Pediatr Surg. 2009;44(6):1268–72; discussion 72. Epub 2009/06/16.
29. Ismail KA, Chase J, Gibb S, Clarke M, Catto-Smith AG, Robertson VJ, et al. Daily transabdominal electrical stimulation at home increased defecation in children with slow-transit constipation: a pilot study. J Pediatr Surg. 2009;44(12):2388–92. Epub 2009/12/17.
30. Yik YI, Ismail KA, Hutson JM, Southwell BR. Home transcutaneous electrical stimulation to treat children with slow-transit constipation. J Pediatr Surg. 2012;47(6):1285–90. Epub 2012/06/19.
31. Yik YI, Stathopoulos L, Hutson JM, Southwell BR. Home transcutaneous electrical stimulation therapy to treat children with anorectal retention: a pilot study. Neuromodulation. 2016;19(5):515–21. Epub 2016/06/14.
32. Ladi-Seyedian SS, Sharifi-Rad L, Manouchehri N, Ashjaei B. A comparative study of transcutaneous interferential electrical stimulation plus behavioral therapy and behavioral therapy alone on constipation in postoperative Hirschsprung disease children. J Pediatr Surg. 2017;52(1):177–83. Epub 2016/08/16.
33. Collins B, Norton C, Maeda Y. Percutaneous tibial nerve stimulation for slow transit constipation: a pilot study. Colorectal Dis. 2012;14(4):e165–70. Epub 2011/09/14.
34. Edenfield AL, Amundsen CL, Wu JM, Levin PJ, Siddiqui NY. Posterior tibial nerve stimulation for the treatment of fecal incontinence: a systematic evidence review. Obstet Gynecol Surv. 2015;70(5):329–41. Epub 2015/05/15.
35. Shafik A, Ahmed I, El-Sibai O, Mostafa RM. Percutaneous peripheral neuromodulation in the treatment of fecal incontinence. Eur Surg Res. 2003;35(2):103–7. Epub 2003/04/08.
36. Iqbal F, Collins B, Thomas GP, Askari A, Tan E, Nicholls RJ, et al. Bilateral transcutaneous tibial nerve stimulation for chronic constipation. Colorectal Dis. 2016;18(2):173–8. Epub 2015/09/04.
37. Lecompte JF, Hery G, Guys JM, Louis-Borrione C. Evaluation of transcutaneous electrical posterior tibial nerve stimulation for the treatment of fecal and urinary leaks in children: preliminary results. J Pediatr Surg. 2015;50(4):630–3. Epub 2015/04/04.

Pediatric Sacral Neuromodulation for Voiding Dysfunction

17

Spencer C. Hiller and Megan S. Schober

Introduction

Voiding dysfunction accounts for approximately 30% of outpatient visits to the pediatric urologist's office [1]. Children typically present with any combination of fecal and urinary complaints including incontinence, enuresis, urinary tract infections, incomplete bladder emptying, constipation, fecal incontinence, urinary frequency or urgency, posturing, and/or bladder pain [2]. Previously termed "Dysfunctional Elimination Syndrome" (DES), this complex of symptoms is now known as "Bowel Bladder Dysfunction" (BBD). It is well established that functional gastrointestinal problems, particularly constipation, play a prominent role in the spectrum of BBD. First-line therapy remains behavioral therapy, including timed voiding and management of constipation.

Pharmacologic agents for urinary symptoms are reserved for second-line therapy. It is important to always address and treat any constipation issues prior to considering any anti-cholinergic medication as these are significantly constipating and may paradoxically exacerbate voiding symptoms if utilized in a very constipated child.

While SNM is well recognized as a third-line treatment option for adult patients with overactive bladder (OAB), urinary urgency and frequency, non-obstructive urinary retention, and fecal incontinence, this technique is not currently approved by the United States Food and Drug Administration (FDA) for children less than 16 years of age. Despite this, neuromodulation via sacral nerve stimulation has been performed successfully in the pediatric population for more than a decade. Unique concerns of SNM in a pediatric population include somatic growth with subsequent lead migration, multiple surgeries for battery replacement over the lifetime of the patient, possibility of child requiring future magnetic resonance imaging, and the general paucity of long-term follow-up data in this patient population.

Sacral Neuromodulation in the Pediatric Population

BBD without a discernable neurologic etiology remains a frequent complaint within the pediatric urology office. First-line treatment includes behavioral modifications, particularly timed and double voiding, avoidance of dietary bladder irritants, and aggressive treatment for constipation.

S. C. Hiller
Department of Urology, William Beaumont Hospital, Royal Oak, MI, USA
e-mail: spencer.hiller@beaumont.org

M. S. Schober (✉)
Division of Pediatric Urology, William Beaumont Hospital, Royal Oak, MI, USA
e-mail: mschober@urologist.org

J. P. Gilleran, S. A. Alpert (eds.), *Adult and Pediatric Neuromodulation*,
https://doi.org/10.1007/978-3-319-73266-4_17

Pediatric voiding dysfunction is typically categorized as neurogenic or non-neurogenic; both of which can be responsive to neuromodulation under the appropriate circumstances.

Neurogenic bladder dysfunction in children can be due to underlying congenital defects such as spina bifida, sacral agenesis, tethered cord, or cord lipoma as well as the result of tumor or trauma [3]. Neurogenic bladder dysfunction often leads to progressive bladder and upper urinary tract deterioration secondary to high pressures generated in the bladder.

Traditionally, therapies have been aimed at decreasing the intravesical pressures and includes clean intermittent catheterization, anticholinergics, and in severe cases, enterocystoplasty [3]. There is an abundance of literature in the adult patient population demonstrating the ability of SNM to improve voiding function to those with refractory urge incontinence/OAB. In general, SNM has been utilized effectively in pediatric populations with both storage and non-obstructive voiding disorders. It should be reserved to motivated, select patients and families with refractory symptoms who have failed medical and behavioral therapies. Literature to date has been unsuccessful in identifying a universally accepted urodynamic study finding that would be predictive of response to SNM [4, 5].

Pediatric Sacral Neuromodulation

The use of neuromodulation in the pediatric population is relatively novel. In 2001, Hoebeke and colleagues demonstrated transcutaneous electrical nerve stimulation with surface electrodes placed over the level of the S3 nerve root can improve symptoms of detrusor over activity as well as improve bladder capacity in children [6]. Symptom improvement was also maintained for up to a year in some of these patients. In this study, 51% of patients were deemed "definitively cured" after 1 year. After demonstrating promising results from transcutaneous neuromodulation in children, the next step was permanent device placement. One of the first published studies by Humphreys et al. investigated a cohort of 23 patients with significant BBD refractory to behavioral and medical therapy. The study excluded any patient with known underlying neurological pathology (i.e., cerebral palsy, spina bifida, or spinal cord injury). A total of 21 patients (91%) underwent permanent device placement with mean follow-up greater than 13 months. Patients reported a statistically significant reduction in urinary incontinence, enuresis, incomplete emptying, urinary urgency/frequency complaints, UTI episodes, and constipation postoperatively. Additionally, there was also a significant reduction on the number of medications required per patient after device placement [2].

In the adult population, data has been mixed regarding the pre-operative predictive value of urodynamic findings in patient response to SNM. In regards to post-op urodynamic assessment, data is also conflicting regarding correlation of SNM success and urodynamic parameters. The clinical improvement associated with SNM is not always associated with a demonstrable improvement in urodynamic parameters. Schober et al. sought to determine if there is a measurable effect on urodynamic parameters after SNM by performing pre- and postoperative urodynamic studies (UDS) in pediatric patients [4]. Complete UDS data was available in 22 patients with OAB/incontinence. They found a significant decrease in the number of uninhibited contractions and maximum detrusor pressure during filling cystometry after SNM. Additionally, they found a significant improvement in post void residual in a small group of pediatric patients with urinary retention/incomplete emptying.

In 2014, Dwyer and colleagues reported data on their single institution 10-year experience with pediatric SNM [7]. In the largest study to date, a total of 105 patients were followed prospectively for a median of 2.72 years. Ninety-four percent of their patients experienced an improvement in at least one of their symptoms. Urinary incontinence was the most commonly improved symptom, with 88% of patients reporting an improvement and 41% reporting complete resolution of symptoms. Similarly, patients with constipation, frequency and/or urgency and enuresis demonstrated a statistically significant improvement in symptoms. The above studies were conducted in patients without any identified bladder neuropathy. Guys et al. however, utilized SNM in a neurogenic bladder population of 42 patients, aged 5–21 years who were refractory to medical therapy or sacral neuromodulation [3]. The neuromodulation group observed a significant increase in leak point pressure up to 1 year after implantation, theorized by the authors to allow for potentially higher continence rates with the continuation of clean intermittent catheterization (CIC). Patients also demonstrated a significant subjective improvement in symptoms. Nine patients also had an improvement in fecal transit.

Haddad and colleagues reported a multicenter, open label, randomized, cross-over study investigating the use of SNM in 33 pediatric patients with urinary and/or fecal incontinence [8]. Response was defined as resolution of urinary leakage and/or fecal soiling, or a decrease of more than 50% in the number of leaks and/or soiling with minimum protection. At the termination of the study, 81% reported a statistically significant reduction in urinary incontinence and 78% reported a statistically significant reduction in fecal incontinence. All patients undergoing CIC preoperatively continued to require catheterization postoperatively, however, despite response to SNM.

Further evidence of efficacy of pediatric SNM was demonstrated in a 2008 study, in which a total of 20 children with BBD underwent first stage SNM implant, with 90% proceeding to stage two generator implant. Median follow-up was 25 months and in a subset of primary urinary retention patients 82% reported a subjective reduction or resolution of incontinence episodes. There was also a significant improvement in patient-reported enuresis, urinary urgency, urinary frequency, and constipation [9].

Stephany and colleagues reported on a total of 14 patients with non-neurogenic lower urinary tract dysfunction who underwent sacral nerve modulator placement. They focused on clinical responses to validated questionnaires because their results seemed to correlate more to patient satisfaction than objective measures. All patients completed the Vancouver NLUTD/DES questionnaire and the PedsQ 4.0 General Core Scales. Median follow-up was relatively short at 6 months, however, 14 patients demonstrated decreased voiding symptom scores from 23 preoperatively to 10.5 postoperatively following lead placement ($p < 0.001$). As demonstrated by the aforementioned studies, there is a near-uniform improvement in symptomology reported by patients [10].

Complication rates quoted in pediatric studies are comparable to those in adults. In the largest study to date, Dwyer and colleagues did report a reoperation rate of 56%, of which 35% were for device malfunction such as lead breakage and 10% for wound infection [7]. Haddad et al. reported an 18.8% complication rate in their population of 33 patients. Their most common complication was infection followed by electrode migration [8].

Specific Issues Related to the Pediatric Population

As with all surgical procedures, but with pediatric patients in particular, attempts are typically made to minimize invasiveness, morbidity, pain, cost, hospitalization, and maintain good cosmesis. Radiation exposure is also of particular concern in the pediatric population due to possible consequences later in life from accumulated exposure. Traditionally, the implantation of the SNM device is performed in a two-stage procedure. McGee and colleagues describe an incisionless first and second stage without fluoroscopy. The procedure was performed on 27 patients, median age of 10.1 years. During the first stage procedure, the extender leads of the device are tunneled laterally along the line of the gluteal cleft to the axillary line of the patient using a 14-french ureteral access sheath. After placing the quadripolar tined lead and temporary external lead through the subcutaneous tract, the eventual site of the pulse generator was marked with a methylene blue temporary tattoo, obviating the need for fluoroscopy during the second stage procedure [11]. The described procedure was similar to the standard in terms of operative time, postoperative pain, hospital stay, and interval between first and second stage, but fluoroscopy time and number of incisions was reduced.

Voiding function improves gradually after SNM placement, particularly in congenital neurogenic patients. Thus, it has been proposed to forgo the temporary test stimulation period in pediatric patients [3]. The test simulation period used in adults is considered too short to induce a response in children with neurologic conditions [8]. Roth and colleagues reserved a second stage procedure for patients who exhibited a 50% or greater improvement in voiding dysfunction during the trial period, which ranged from 14 to 34 days [9]. Alternatively, Stephany and colleagues patients underwent a 1-week trial period and performed a second stage if they reported any improvement in symptoms with no significant side effects [10]. Schober et al. also utilized a 2–3 week test period and proceeded to second stage if patients demonstrated a significant subjective improvement in symptoms [4]. By eliminating a "test period" and utilizing a single-stage approach, patients undergo only a single anesthetic and surgical morbidity may be decreased. However, restrictions on single-stage procedure eligibility for pediatric patients placed by insurance companies may not allow widespread use of this option in practical terms.

Developmentally, the child must have sufficient communication skills to respond and interact to allow for modification during the testing phase. Careful consideration must be given to proper patient selection. Another consideration unique to the pediatric population is the expected somatic growth that may lead to recurrent lead migration and repeated procedures. Clark and colleagues reported on a small group of 4 pediatric patients, average age of 12.1 years. In this study, 3 patients (75%) required a total of 5 revisions due to lead malfunction with an average of 1.5 years between surgeries. They found patients averaged 8.1 cm of growth between revisions. This revision rate is striking compared to their reported 5% revision rate in an adult population. All of their revisions were performed safely and with return of prior device efficacy [12].

Overall, safety and efficacy of SNM in the pediatric population have been repeatedly demonstrated in multiple studies despite the current status of not having FDA approval for this procedure in patients less than 16 years old. As the pediatric SNM patient population ages and further longitudinal studies are possible, long-term success and complication rates will be key in determining the utility of and ideal candidacy for neuromodulation in young patients.

References

1. Rushton HG. Wetting and functional voiding disorders. Urol Clin North Am. 1995;22:75.
2. Humphreys MR, Vandersteen DR, Slezak JM, Hollatz P, Smith CA, Smith JE, et al. Preliminary results of sacral neuromodulation in 23 children. J Urol. 2006;176(5):2227–31.
3. Guys JM, Hadid M, Planche D, Torre M, Louis-Borrione C, Breaud J. Sacral neuromodulation for neurogenic bladder dysfunction in children. J Urol. 2004;172:1673.
4. Schober MS, Sulkowski JP, Lu PL, Minneci PC, Deans KJ, Teich S, et al. Sacral nerve stimulation for pediatric lower urinary tract dysfunction: development of a standardized pathway with objective urodynamic outcomes. J Urol. 2015;194(6):1721–7.
5. Groenendijk P, Lycklama ANA, Ouwerkerk T, van den Hombergh U. Five-year follow-up after sacral neuromodulation: single center experience. Neuromodulation. 2007;10(4):363–8.
6. Hoebeke P, Van Laecke E, Everaert K, Renson C, De Paepe H, Raes A, et al. Transcutaneous neuromodulation for the urge syndrome in children: a pilot study. J Urol. 2001;166(6):2416–9.
7. Dwyer ME, Vandersteen DR, Hollatz P, Reinberg Y. Sacral neuromodulation for the dysfunctional elimination syndrome: a 10-year single-center experience with 105 consecutive children. Urology. 2014;84:911–8.
8. Haddad M, Besson R, Aubert D, Ravasse P, Lemelle J, El Ghoneimi A, et al. Sacral neuromodulation in children with urinary and fecal incontinence: a multicenter, open label, randomized, crossover study. J Urol. 2010;184(2):696–701.
9. Roth TJ, Vandersteen DR, Hollatz P, Inman BA, Reinberg YE. Sacral neuromodulation for the dysfunctional elimination syndrome: a single center experience with 20 children. J Urol. 2008;180(1):306–11.
10. Stephany HA, Juliano TM, Clayton DB, Tanaka ST, Thomas JC, Adams MC, et al. Prospective evaluation of sacral nerve modulation in children with validated questionnaires. J Urol. 2013;190(4 Suppl):1516–22.
11. McGee SM, Routh JC, Granberg CF, Roth TJ, Hollatz P, Vandersteen DR, et al. Sacral neuromodulation in children with dysfunctional elimination syndrome: description of incisionless first stage and second stage without fluoroscopy. Urology. 2009;73:641–4.
12. Clark C, Ngo T, Comiter CV, Anderson R, Kennedy W. Sacral nerve stimulator revision due to somatic growth. J Urol. 2011;186:1576–80.

Index

J. P. Gilleran, S. A. Alpert (eds.), *Adult and Pediatric Neuromodulation*,
https://doi.org/10.1007/978-3-319-73266-4

Q

R

S

MIX
Papier aus verantwortungsvollen Quellen
Paper from responsible sources
FSC® C105338

If you have any concerns about our products,
you can contact us on
ProductSafety@springernature.com

In case Publisher is established outside the EU,
the EU authorized representative is:
Springer Nature Customer Service Center GmbH
Europaplatz 3, 69115 Heidelberg, Germany

Printed by Libri Plureos GmbH
in Hamburg, Germany